1996

The Problem That Won't Go Away

The Problem That Won't Go Away

Reforming U.S. Health Care Financing

Henry J. Aaron
Editor

THE BROOKINGS INSTITUTION
Washington, D.C.

Copyright © 1996 by
THE BROOKINGS INSTITUTION
1775 Massachusetts Avenue, N.W., Washington, D.C. 20036

Library of Congress Cataloging-in-Publication data

The problem that won't go away : reforming U.S. health care financing
/ Henry J. Aaron, ed.
   p.   cm.
Includes bibliographical references and index.
ISBN 0-8157-0010-5 (cl : alk. paper). — ISBN 0-8157-0009-1 (pa :
alk. paper)
   1. Health care reform—United States. 2. Medical care—United
States—Finance. 3. National health insurance—United States.
I. Aaron, Henry J.
RA395.A3P756   1995
338.4'33621'0973—dc20   95-37621
                                              CIP

9 8 7 6 5 4 3 2 1

The paper used in this publication meets the minimum
requirements of the American National Standard for
Information Sciences—Permanence of Paper for Printed
Library Materials, ANSI Z39.48-1984

Typeset in Sabon

Composition by Harlowe Typography, Inc.
Cottage City, Maryland

Printed by R. R. Donnelley and Sons, Co.
Harrisonburg, Virginia

B THE BROOKINGS INSTITUTION

The Brookings Institution is an independent organization devoted to nonpartisan research, education, and publication in economics, government, foreign policy, and the social sciences generally. Its principal purposes are to aid in the development of sound public policies and to promote public understanding of issues of national importance.

The Institution was founded on December 8, 1927, to merge the activities of the Institute for Government Research, founded in 1916, the Institute of Economics, founded in 1922, and the Robert Brookings Graduate School of Economics and Government, founded in 1924.

The Board of Trustees is responsible for the general administration of the Institution, while the immediate direction of the policies, program, and staff is vested in the President, assisted by an advisory committee of the officers and staff. The by-laws of the Institution state: "It is the function of the Trustees to make possible the conduct of scientific research, and publication, under the most favorable conditions, and to safeguard the independence of the research staff in the pursuit of their studies and in the publication of the results of such studies. It is not a part of their function to determine, control, or influence the conduct of particular investigations or the conclusions reached."

The President bears final responsibility for the decision to publish a manuscript as a Brookings book. In reaching his judgment on the competence, accuracy, and objectivity of each study, the President is advised by the director of the appropriate research program and weighs the views of a panel of expert outside readers who report to him in confidence on the quality of the work. Publication of a work signifies that it is deemed a competent treatment worthy of public consideration but does not imply endorsement of conclusions or recommendations.

The Institution maintains its position of neutrality on issues of public policy in order to safeguard the intellectual freedom of the staff. Hence interpretations or conclusions in Brookings publications should be understood to be solely those of the authors and should not be attributed to the Institution, to its trustees, officers, or other staff members, or to the organizations that support its research.

Foreword

THREE YEARS AGO, President Clinton made reform of health care financing and the achievement of universal coverage his top domestic policy objective. Two years later that effort collapsed. Shortly thereafter the Republican opposition wrested control of Congress from the Democrats. In their drive for a balanced budget, they too made changes in one part of health care financing a priority: the federal programs of medicare and medicaid. Meanwhile, revolutionary changes in private financing and organization of health care have led to turmoil in the management of hospitals and the organization of physicians.

Although President Clinton's efforts were unsuccessful, they revealed much about the American people's attitudes toward large-scale change in a fundamental institution. Furthermore, the specifics of the president's proposals—emphasis on managed care and cutbacks in medicare and medicaid—have remained on the public agenda. The initiative was a watershed for at least three reasons: it promoted the idea of managed care, which others have taken up and used for different purposes; it showed that changes in private health insurance, were they to occur, would not be led from Washington; and it became a central symbol in the political debate preceding the elections of 1994.

In collaboration with the journal *Health Affairs*, the Brookings Institution organized a conference held on January 23 and 24, 1995, to try to draw lessons from the health care reform debate of 1993 and 1994. Why did President Clinton's initiative fail so totally? Did it ever stand much chance of passage?

Although understanding the past is challenging and educational, the conference also sought to draw lessons for the future. Did the misfortunes of the Clinton plan remove health reform from the national agenda? Or would it reappear, in new or familiar guise, after a few years? Meanwhile, what changes in health care financing deserve immediate consideration because they could move the financing system incrementally in a desirable direction over the long term?

The health policy experts in this book, representing a wide range of political perspectives, address these questions. Although their analyses and recommendations differ, they support the judgment embodied in the title of this book. Reform of health care financing and organization remain on the national agenda for the foreseeable future. This problem, most assuredly, will not go away.

This conference was supported by the Kaiser Foundation Health Plan, the Commonwealth Fund, FHP International Corporation, Health Net, the Prudential Foundation, U.S. Healthcare, the Henry J. Kaiser Family Foundation, and the California Wellness Foundation. The chapters included in this volume (other than the introduction) first appeared in slightly different form in a special issue of *Health Affairs*.

At Brookings, Theresa Walker edited the manuscript, Cynthia Iglesias and Stephanianna Lozito verified it, and Victoria Agee prepared the index. Kathleen M. Bucholz, Michelle A. Johnson, Paige Oeffinger, Anita G. Whitlock, and Kathleen Elliott Yinug prepared the manuscript for publication.

The views expressed here are those of the authors and should not be ascribed to the institutions that supported this work, or to the trustees, officers, or staff members of the Brookings Institution.

MICHAEL H. ARMACOST
President

October 1995
Washington, D.C.

Contents

1. The Problem That Won't Go Away   1
   Henry J. Aaron

Part One: Why Did the Clinton Plan Fail?

2. Clinton's Health Reform in Historical Perspective   15
   Hugh Heclo

3. The Rise and Resounding Demise of the Clinton Health   34
   Security Plan
   Theda Skocpol
   Comments: Margaret Weir   54
             James J. Mongan   58

4. The Debate That Wasn't: The Public and the Clinton Health   70
   Care Plan
   Daniel Yankelovich
   Comments: Drew E. Altman   91
             Karlyn H. Bowman   95
             Uwe Reinhardt   100

5. Interest Groups in the Health Care Debate   110
   Graham K. Wilson
   Comments: Julie Kosterlitz   130
             Fred Grandy   135

Part Two: How Can Information Be Improved?

6. Estimating the Effects of Reform 147
   Linda Bilheimer and Robert Reischauer
   Comments: John F. Shiels 165
        Len M. Nichols 169
        Kenneth Thorpe 174

Part Three: What Does the Future Hold?

7. Market-Based Reform: What to Regulate and by Whom? 185
   Alain C. Enthoven and Sara J. Singer

8. How Does Antitrust Enforcement Fit In? 207
   Steven C. Sunshine
   Comments: William L. Roper 213
        Helen Darling 217

Part Four: Incremental Reform

9. Steps toward Universal Coverage 225
   Judith Feder and Larry Levitt

10. The Conservative Agenda 236
    Stuart M. Butler

11. Cutting Costs and Improving Health 250
    David M. Cutler

12. Bite-Sized Chunks of Health Care Reform: 266
    Where Medicare Fits In
    Gail R. Wilensky

13. Using Tax Credits for Health Insurance and Medical Savings 274
    Accounts
    Mark V. Pauly and John C. Goodman

Contributors   291

Index   293

Tables

11-1.   Characteristics of Health Insurance, by Firm Size, 1991   254
13-1.   Detailed Calculations of Cost Implications of Medical
        Savings Accounts   281
13-2.   Examples of Maximum Deductible and Out-of-Pocket
        Limits under a Medical Savings Account Proposal   283

Figures

3-1.   Slippery Slope from Universality to Diminished Coverage   60
6-1.   Existing Data on Health Care Delivery and Financing   172
10-1.   Lewin-VHI, The Individual Tax Credit Program:
        Estimated Cost and Impacts   241
11-1.   Growth of Health Costs per Enrollee   256

CHAPTER ONE

The Problem That Won't Go Away

Henry J. Aaron

THE WORDS "pivotal" and "watershed" are much overused but hard to avoid in describing the glorious birth and inglorious death of President Clinton's bid to reform the U.S. health care system. The events of the debate invite grand interpretations. Bill Clinton wins a hard-fought election victory promising a new form of Democratic leadership. He commits himself to winning congressional approval of a plan to assure health insurance to all Americans and to control costs. He releases the agonizingly detailed plan to initial plaudits that quickly give way to doubt, then confusion, and finally, scorn. The plan never even comes to a floor vote in either house of Congress and serves as exhibit 1 in an extravagantly successful Republican campaign against the Democrats as the party of bloated bureaucracy, which ends in devastating Democratic electoral defeat.

Lessons from the Past

Generals revisit great battles to improve strategy and tactics. For similar reasons, practical politicians and scholars of public policy will revisit the debate over the Clinton health plan. What did planners do right? How can the mistakes of that experience be avoided in the future? In addition to creating a superlative teaching tool for future study, the Clinton plan and the failed effort to enact it did something far more—they definitively ended the health care financing debate as we know it.

This debate began six decades ago and has flared up sporadically since. The prospect that the federal government should orchestrate some com-

I wish to thank Joseph Milano for research assistance, Gary Burtless and Theda Skocpol for comments, and Joseph P. Newhouse for the citation to Machiavelli.

bination of public and private actions to bring about universal coverage has been part of the "unfinished agenda" of the political left at least since enactment of the Social Security Act in 1935. The Committee for Economic Security, which designed the Social Security Act, had believed in national health insurance but did not recommend it. They feared that doing so would have doomed its principal recommendations for a new old age retirement system and for unemployment insurance. President Harry S Truman advanced a proposal for national health insurance, but he was narrowly elected and confronted a Congress that had no interest in acting on his proposal. Many saw the enactment of medicare and medicaid in 1965 as the first step in resuming the unfinished journey to national health insurance. Presidents Nixon and Carter also advanced proposals to extend universal coverage to the nonaged and, in addition, to control growth of medical costs. For various reasons, these efforts failed and nothing happened for the next thirty years after enactment of medicare beyond marginal expansions in medicaid coverage and the introduction of new methods of paying hospitals and physicians under medicare. The passage of nearly thirty years without further major action might have been read as a bad omen for ultimate success, but many advocates of national health insurance saw it as evidence that ultimate success, which they never doubted, was that much closer. President Clinton's proposal to provide all Americans with health insurance "that is always there" and to slow the growth of health care spending was thus part of a historical mission Democrats had been striving to complete for more than half a century.

That mission, it is now apparent, will not be completed in a form recognizable by traditional advocates of national health insurance. For reasons that in prospect seemed evident to some and in retrospect seem clear to most, President Clinton had no real chance to win congressional acceptance of a single bill transforming the financing of American health care. To begin with, he was politically weak. Elected by barely two-fifths of voters and having run behind most congressional Democrats in contested elections, he had little leverage with members even of his own party. Second, changes in congressional rules and in methods of financing and managing congressional campaigns that weakened party discipline had diminished the capacity of a president to force through costly and complex legislation important to most members of Congress. Third, and most important, no legislation remotely approximating the size and complexity of the Clinton health reform plan had ever been enacted in the United States except during war or major depression. Unlike earlier legislation that created land grant colleges or retirement pensions, the proposed legislation to reform health care financing was not filling a vacuum—after all, about 85 percent of nonaged Americans already had insurance and one-seventh of the U.S. economy was devoted to producing health care services.[1] Thus, health reform required the reconstruction of whole industries, putting jobs and investments at risk, and confronting most Americans with the prospect of seeing familiar and comfortable arrangements for gaining access to a life-or-death service radically transformed. As Charles Schultze observed, it was as if the president had proposed to remake an entity as large as all of France in a single piece of legislation. The legislation affected the vital interests of hospitals, physicians, other health providers, medical device manufacturers, pharmaceutical companies, small businesses and large corporations, and organized labor. And since one goal of reform was to slow the growth of spending, the proposal had to reduce the expected incomes of these groups.

Four centuries ago, Machiavelli captured the risks associated with large-scale reforms with a clarity scarce in Washington in 1993:

> It should be borne in mind that there is nothing more difficult to arrange, more doubtful of success, and more dangerous to carry through than initiating changes in a state's constitution. The innovator makes enemies of all those who prospered under the old order, and only lukewarm support is forthcoming from those who would prosper under the new. Their support is lukewarm partly from fear of their adversaries, who have the existing laws on their side, and partly because men are generally incredulous, never really trusting new things unless they have tested them by experience. In consequence, whenever those who oppose the changes can do so, they attack vigorously, and the defense made by the others is only lukewarm. So both the innovator and his friends are endangered together. But to discuss this subject thoroughly we must distinguish between innovators who stand alone and those who depend on others, that is between those who to achieve their purposes can force the issue and those who must use persuasion. In the second case, they always come to grief.[2]

The collapse of the effort to reform health care financing and the subsequent Republican electoral victory in November 1994 have erased government-led reform of private health insurance from the national agenda for the foreseeable future. It now seems unlikely that any administration or Congress will take up this issue again in the way that President Clinton—or, earlier, Presidents Carter, Nixon, and Truman—did. They all saw the national government as the agent for enforcing universal national health insurance. The mechanisms varied, but all agreed on four key points: that universality was important; that the only way to reach that goal was a legal mandate requiring everyone to be insured; that only the federal government could enforce such a mandate; and that such a mandate was an acceptable instrument of social policy.

In the aftermath of the Clinton health plan and the Republican electoral victory, it is hard to find any major political figure who will advance these views. In the course of the political debate in 1994, the concept of universal insurance underwent an Orwellian transformation from its traditional meaning of essentially 100 percent coverage to 97 percent or 95 percent coverage, although such redefined "universality" would have left many of the prereform uninsured population still uncovered. The view that universal health insurance coverage is desirable but not vital has gained new respectability. The reason for the abandonment of universality as a goal was the realization, born of the complexity of the Clinton proposal, that the means necessary to achieve it were more than the country would tolerate. As James Mongan recounts in this volume, the stages of erosion of the commitment to universal coverage stand as milestones in the demise of the Clinton plan.

Several of the chapters of this book recount the history of the Clinton health plan and its collapse. Theda Skocpol considers several alternative strategies the administration might have pursued and concludes that none was a good bet to have achieved the administration's goals of universal coverage and cost containment. The chapters by Hugh Heclo, Graham Wilson, Daniel Yankelovich, and Linda Bilheimer and Robert Reischauer, and comments on those papers, support the view that the administration, Congress, and the nation lacked the political consensus and the information to credibly describe the effects of any single bill to reform the U.S. health care system.

If they are correct, the only option available to the administration was to reach for goals far more modest than those it sought—the initiation of a *process* of change that would begin with modest, incremental steps, entering wedges to eventually achieve universal coverage and general reform. This approach would not have promised immediate cuts in federal health care spending, but in the end estimates of the Congressional Budget Office confirmed that the president's own proposal failed that test, at least for the first decade after enactment. Covering the costs of extended coverage would take all the feasible savings from reduced growth of spending and more besides. To contribute to deficit reduction, planners discovered, would take sizable tax increases, a step that in 1993 and 1994 seemed the political equivalent of public indecency. A strategy of small steps couched in a vision of longer-term reform would not have made the giant strides toward reestablishing the conviction among the American people that limited government can achieve major social objectives. But the administration lacked the political resources to do more and, reaching for vastly more, it squandered its limited capacity even to advance a bit its most cherished programmatic and political objectives.

Looking Forward

The events of 1993 and 1994 may have put proposals for government-guaranteed universal coverage and cost control in the deep freeze, but they assuredly did not cool political interest in health care policy. The federal role in financing health care will remain a hot political issue for at least three reasons. First, the pressure to cut public spending to balance the budget means that medicare and medicaid will be in the legislative spotlight. These two programs represent 22 percent of projected federal government spending in the year 1996 (apart from interest on the debt), and the increase in spending on these two programs as a share of gross domestic product accounts for all of the projected increase in the federal deficit between 1996 and 2002.[3] Second, the retirement of the baby-boom generation over the quarter century from 2010 to 2035 promises large additional increases in the cost of medicare, which pays for acute care for the elderly and disabled, and of medicaid, which pays about half of the national cost of long-term care. Third, a seemingly inexhaustible flood of new and costly medical technologies will continue to put financial pressure on everyone responsible for paying for health insurance, including not only federal and state governments, but also the private sector. Real health care spending has grown about 5 percent annually for more than four decades. Despite anecdotal information suggesting that growth is slowing, overall spending continues to rise at about that rate.[4]

For all of these reasons, health care financing as a national political issue will not go away. But the nature of the debate in the years after the demise of the Clinton plan will be altogether different from that of the past several decades. Public and private policy in the United States are combining to transform the health care financing system in ways that were not widely foreseen when the Clinton administration made health care reform its number one domestic priority. To understand the changes that are under way, it is necessary to recognize some key features of the current system.

A Brief Sketch of U.S. Health Care Financing

Most Americans continue to enjoy rather good health insurance coverage. Some earn coverage at work. Others receive coverage through public programs, principally medicare and medicaid. Some of the uninsured pay for their own health care, but many receive "uncompensated" care. Indeed, uncompensated care is the balm that has made socially tolerable the abrasive fact that one nonaged person in six is without insurance at any given time. The term "uncompensated" is really a misnomer. In fact, providers are generally compensated by "cross subsidies" from those who pay for insurance for the covered population—companies that finance care for their employees and government programs that cover the aged and disabled—who have paid more than the full cost of the care for the patients they were covering.

The Demise of Uncompensated Care

That system has come under increasing pressure from two directions. First, the flow of cross subsidies is drying up. Medicare, like private insurers, once paid more than full cost for hospital services. After a decade of slow increases in fees, medicare now pays less than full cost, as does medicaid. Private companies, appalled at the rapid and unpredictable increase in the cost of insuring their employees, have begun to negotiate aggressively for discounted prices from hospitals, physicians, and other providers. One of the most important services provided by many managed care organizations is just such aggressive bargaining. In the simplest terms, each payer is trying to make sure that it pays just for the services used by the people for whom it is responsible. Buying services from preferred-provider organizations can be characterized, with some lack of charity but little inaccuracy, as a way to make sure that one does not pay cross subsidies. But if no payer provides cross subsidies, providers can render uncompensated care only to the extent that they are prepared to render charity.[5]

Second, the number of uninsured has increased, stretching ever thinner any given capacity to finance uncompensated care. The population of uninsured was 24 million in 1980 and has risen since, to 31.3 million in 1985 and 41 million in 1994. This increase has occurred although medicare covers almost all of the elderly, and medicaid coverage has increased from 21.8 million in 1985 to 33.4 million in 1993. The proportion of Americans with private insurance coverage has fallen from 83 percent in 1980 to 70 percent in 1991.[6] In 1984 medicare moved from paying hospitals based on estimated costs to prepayment based on diagnosis at admission. Increases in these payments have been below increases in actual costs and in 1993 covered about 89 percent of cost. Medicaid reimbursements, as low as 76 percent of cost in 1989, now cover an estimated 93 percent of cost. Medicaid and medicare payments to physicians average 60 percent and 73 percent of private payments, respectively.[7]

All of these forces are likely to continue and intensify. Both short-term deficit reduction goals and long-term cost projections make likely sizable cuts in medicare and medicaid. Some savings may be achieved through increased efficiency. Some savings will be achieved through further restraint on the growth of payments to providers; but this source of savings will reduce the capacity of providers to provide uncompensated care. Cost pressures on private payers will increase as well. The avalanche of new and costly medical technologies shows no signs of diminishing and may be increasing.[8] In addition, the average age of the active labor force is increasing, adding further to medical costs. For all of these reasons, private companies will have every reason to bargain for discounts with unflagging zeal. And companies that provide health insurance coverage and other fringe benefits to their workers will have a continuing incentive to contract with other companies that do not provide such fringe benefits for goods and services that parent companies once produced themselves. If the new suppliers do not have to return in increased cash wages all of the savings from the omitted fringe benefits, the contracting company can reduce costs.

Private Market Developments

Under the pressure of rising costs, private companies are transforming the organization of the delivery of health care in the United States. These changes, summarized under the vague term "managed care," encompass a variety of techniques that share one characteristic—someone other than the patient or the health care provider reviews the provision of health care to determine whether the right services are being provided and whether cost of provision is minimized. This agent has the power to influence patterns of care, staffing of hospitals, access to physicians, salaries and fees of providers, and other aspects of the delivery of health care.

One might think that insurers would always have performed at least some of these functions. Once they have enrolled clients, however, insurers have customarily paid bills and done little more. Furthermore, as employers increasingly have "self-insured," by paying all costs of health care for their employees, they intentionally used insurance companies or some other organization only to pay bills. The rapid growth of health care costs under such arrangements has led private companies to hire organizations to manage care. These intermediary organizations take many forms. Some are traditional health maintenance organizations (HMOs) that hire physicians or contract with physicians to provide services. HMOs exercise direct control over staffing, equipment and other facilities, and practice patterns of affiliated physicians. HMOs may allow enrolled members to secure service from physicians or other providers outside the HMO for an additional charge under so-called point-of-service plans. Independent practice associations are networks of physicians that agree to provide stipulated services to enrolled customers at a fixed periodic charge, but, unlike HMOs, typically pay physicians on a fee-for-service basis. In other cases, hospitals are affiliating with physician groups and offering services for preset fees. Profit-making companies have gotten into the business and have enrolled millions of patients.

These new organizations are forming with impressive speed. Most insured working-age Americans now receive care through an organization that uses at least some practices associated with managed care, and within a few years nearly everyone is expected to be under such arrangements. These developments are well advanced in selected areas. In Minneapolis and St. Paul, for example, three managed care plans enroll 75 percent of the area population. Similar trends are emerging in Boston. In fact, managed care companies are regulating patients' choice of physicians and access to treatment and medication with an aggressiveness that would surely evoke outrage and uproar if attempted by government.

As the number of surviving managed care plans falls, an old issue in economic policy will emerge—whether government should regulate an industry in which only one or a small number of companies controls the market. In such situations, the public has reacted in various ways. When so-called natural monopolies exist, which means that one company can supply, at lower cost than two or more companies can, all of a product that a market will buy, the customary reaction has been economic regulation to prevent the companies from charging excessive prices. Leading examples have been public utilities of various kinds. Even when natural monopoly does not exist, one or a small number of companies may come to control the market. In such cases, the traditional intervention has been antitrust enforcement.

Some health services are natural monopolies in most markets. Such services include many hospital-based diagnostic and therapeutic procedures. For hospital services in general, one hospital can satisfy all of the demands in many smaller communities, and the number of such communities is rising as modern technology lowers admissions and lengths of stay. In the case of health care plans, additional issues likely to provoke regulatory intervention arise. Is the general quality of care adequate? Is the plan providing adequate treatment for particular conditions? Are facilities located in areas that are convenient to residents of all parts of a community? Does the plan provide enough charity care? Are the inevitable errors of medical judgment adequately investigated and is corrective action sufficient? Will the community accept judgments of plan managers when the managers conclude that benefits from costly diagnostic or therapeutic procedures are so small for patients with particular conditions that these patients should be denied access to those technologies? As the number of health plans in a given community falls, issues such as these are likely to cause demands for government involvement in regulating the delivery of health care to reemerge.

These trends are playing themselves out in an era when the demand for curtailing the reach of government is in flood tide. The combination of trends in insurance coverage, of the curtailment of public programs to insure the poor, the elderly, and the disabled, and of the emergence and consolidation of powerful managed care organizations imply a period of great turmoil in health care financing. They will result, I believe, in pressures for a revived and heightened role of government. Three stages are likely.

Stage 1. In the first stage, the number of uninsured will rise and their access to care will decline because of continued private and public cost cutting. At the same time, the mass of the U.S. population will come increasingly to secure care through managed care organizations of one kind or another. These organizations will compete aggressively to hold down costs and to increase enrollments, thereby giving themselves added leverage with providers. To keep down costs, these organizations will try to curtail services that produce small benefits relative to costs or that patients undervalue. In plain English, these organizations will ration care, husbanding savings so that their members can enjoy the fruits of new medical technologies and the growth of medical costs can be kept to a socially acceptable rate. People with high incomes or unusually strong tastes for medical care will retain the option of buying care through more costly organizations that do not ration care, but even this group will find that hospitals, whose staffing and equipment depend on the general availability of resources, will be more Spartan than in the past.

Stage 2. Popular discontent will grow as the numbers of uninsured increase and their choice of providers and access to care diminishes. The traditional method of dealing with problems of inequality and poverty in the United States has been one form or another of government assistance. This assistance could take the form of publicly supported clinics and hospitals. Or it could take the form once again of public support for measures to increase insurance coverage. At the same time, concern about the behavior of the few large managed care plans that will dominate most communities will cause government intervention to regulate health plans.

Step 3. Health care delivery organizations will come to be seen as a kind of public utility and treated as such by governments. Governments will take steps to assure the delivery of health care to those who are uninsured or who, but for government policy, would be uninsured. Through this circuitous route, all Americans will achieve access to health care. Government will play a principal part in setting the policies of health care providers, although that role will differ from that envisaged by advocates of government-sponsored national health insurance and be far more extensive than that desired by its opponents. The course to this outcome will be much longer and more indirect than advocates of government-sponsored health insurance to ensure universal coverage ever imagined. In fact, the result may well be a collection of ad hoc prohibitions, mandates, standards, and subsidies quite different from the government role envisaged in past plans for national health insurance. This process will result in a system that is uniquely American but confirms that health care is too important for any modern society to permit many of its citizens to lack.

Postscript

Many readers may not find the vision of how health care financing arrangements will evolve that I have just outlined to be as probable as I do. They may doubt that insurance coverage will narrow, that access to care for the insured will waste away, or that health plans will ever achieve as much market power as I envisage. They may see other scenarios as more likely than the one I have sketched. Some may fear that a loss of access to health care by the poor may not cause the majority to intervene, because the poor have little political power. Others may hold, perhaps sensibly, that the current situation is so chaotic that any course is possible and none particularly likely. What is certain, however, is that the very events that make health care financing so dynamic will prevent it from leaving the center of the political stage for years, if not decades. For that reason more than any other, it behooves anyone interested in health care or American political life to examine the effort to reform health care financing that began so energetically in 1993 and ended so ignominiously in 1994.

Notes

1. Employee Benefit Research Institute, "Sources of Health Insurance and Characteristics of the Uninsured: Analysis of the March 1993 Current Population Survey," Washington, January 1994; author's calculations using data from *Survey of Current Business*, vol. 75 (June 1995), p. 5; and Prospective Payment Assessment Commission, *Medicare and the American Health Care System, Report to the Congress* (Washington, June 1995), p. 16.

2. Niccolo Machiavelli, *The Prince* (Penguin, 1961), sect. 6, pp. 51–52.

3. Authors' calculations based on Congressional Budget Office, *The Economic and Budget Outlook: Fiscal Years 1996–2000* (Washington, January 1995), p. 58.

4. Between the first quarter of 1994 and the first quarter of 1995, real personal health care spending rose 5.1 percent. For further discussion of these issues, see Henry J. Aaron, "Thinking Straight about Medical Costs," *Health Affairs*, vol. 13 (Winter 1994), pp. 8–13; and Haiden A. Huskamp and Joseph P. Newhouse, "Is Health Spending Slowing Down?" *Health Affairs*, vol. 13 (Winter 1994), pp. 32–38.

5. The issue is complicated by the distinction between average and marginal costs. Where overhead is significant, the additional cost for serving one more patient may be below the average cost of serving all patients. A hospital with half its beds empty, for example, can typically serve an additional patient at lower

than average cost because the overhead costs are paid by those already using the facility. Underused facilities are therefore particularly vulnerable to demands for discounts by powerful buyers. As more and more buyers form groups to increase their leverage, the pressure on hospitals and other high-overhead operations becomes increasingly severe.

6. Author's calculations based on data from Alan L. Sorkin, *Health Economics: An Introduction*, (Lexington books, 1992), pp. 172, 199; Prospective Payment Assessment Commission, *Medicare and the American Health Care System*, p. 5; and Department of Health and Human Services, *Health United States* (Washington, 1994), p. 246. See also Jack A. Meyer and Sharon Silow-Carroll, eds., *Building Blocks for Change: How Health Care Reform Affects Our Future* (Washington: Economic and Social Research Institute, 1993), p. 44.

7. Prospective Payment Assessment Commission, *Medicare and the American Health Care System*, p. 21.

8. William B. Schwartz, "In the Pipeline: A Wave of Valuable Medical Technology," *Health Affairs*, vol. 13 (Summer 1994), pp. 70–79.

PART ONE

Why Did the Clinton Plan Fail?

social reform efforts of this century. For better or worse, there were constellations of political forces that made the reform happen.

What constitutes the population of "big and bold" reforms versus smaller incremental changes is of course a matter of judgment. As used here, the term "major reform effort" refers to social policy claims that were, and were seen to be, fundamental transformations in national policy commitments as against the inherited course of the status quo. Despite the many gray areas, one can reasonably claim that major reforms were at hand in trying to create a federal inspection system for food and drugs, national prohibitions on the sale of alcohol or use of child labor, old age retirement insurance, comprehensive civil rights laws, or federal standards for water and air pollution.[2] In these and other instances there were precedents at the margins of public policy, but advocates and opponents were under no illusion that a policy transformation of major proportions was at stake if the reform effort succeeded. Thus the historical focus in this chapter will be on those rare instances when reformers succeeded in enacting comprehensive national changes in the structure and presumptions of American social policy broadly understood.

For convenience, I group characteristics associated with successful major reform efforts in three general categories: the nature of reform objectives, the resources of the political environment, and what I am calling gestation periods.

The Nature of Reform Objectives

The success of major reform efforts should have something to do with the character of the ends being sought.

For example, any major proposal is likely to contain an immensely complex series of explicit, implicit, and often crosscutting purposes. But it often seems to help when these can be encapsulated in a concrete, easily understandable action to express the objective. "Prohibit the sale of alcohol," "guarantee minority voting rights," "prohibit environmental pollution"—such simple messages can provide a rallying point around which to mobilize reform efforts, even if they do vastly oversimplify the work at hand. By contrast more ambiguous statements of purpose, such as "cleaning up the welfare mess," may have trouble distilling reform into a simple action message (though "stop welfare for teenage mothers" comes close). The 1964 Equal Opportunity Act's "War on Poverty" is perhaps a leading example of a successful major reform effort that did not enjoy the advantage of such a T-shirt accessible statement of immediate purpose.

At the same time it can be argued that clear-cut action objectives have also had the effect of mobilizing opposition and that vague reform goals allow appeals to larger, if less single-minded, coalitions. In the end one should probably make only modest claims for the helpfulness of simple, concrete action objectives.

A much stronger case can be made regarding what has been called the "breakthrough" versus the "consolidating" character of reform objectives.[3] Some major reform initiatives deal largely with new subject matter in the sense that federal public policy is being asked to move into a heretofore relatively unoccupied field for the first time. Establishing the first national standards for water and air pollution would be an example.[4] Major consolidating reforms, however, are efforts to reformulate in some comprehensive way a policy area in which a great many program commitments and interests are already in place. The fundamental 1990 revisions to the Clean Air Act, for example, would fall into this category.[5]

Anyone who has both designed a new house from scratch and thoroughly remodeled an old house will appreciate the different challenges posed by these two policy categories. Major reform efforts to break new ground in a relatively open policy field face the formidable initial task of justifying such unprecedented action. However, if the principle of federal policy action can win acceptance as needed and legitimate, reformers enjoy considerable latitude in designing the substance of that initiative. Their task is then more technical than political because there is little by way of a preexisting infrastructure of political interests that have to be accommodated. Major reform, however, in a policy field already well populated by public or private arrangements is bound to encounter resistance from powerful stakeholders already organized around prevailing approaches. Hence modest, incremental initiatives are often the order of the day, and big and successful reform efforts with consolidating objectives seem especially rare.

Something like this balance of advantages helps explain why the major social policy reform of the 1930s consisted of federal old age insurance rather than federal health insurance. The meager union pensions and company retirement schemes that existed in the 1920s (mainly in the railway, public utility, and metal products industries) had been devastated by the Great Depression. The handful of state old age pension plans effectively on the statute books provided little more than charity grants to fewer than 200,000 persons and offered no competition to federal social insurance planners.[6] In short, the field of contributory old age insurance was uncongested with well-organized interests, offering reformers major policymaking opportunities if they could gain constitutional legitimacy for breaking into that field. It is true that at the same time there was no public policy presence in health insurance either,[7] and commercial and nonprofit groups offering sickness insurance were few and far between. But even at this early time, policy reformers' mere intimation of federal health insurance ran headlong into a dense thicket of established interests, namely, the going concern represented by millions of remuneration arrangements between doctors and their patients. National health insurance portended a consolidation of these arrangements under comprehensive federal standards that would include "reasonably adequate remuneration to medical practitioners and institutions."[8] Vehement protests from physicians and their organizations led President Roosevelt to back off a minimal promise merely to study health insurance in the proposed social security board, lest the rest of the social security plan be jeopardized.

After 1935 subsequent developments only served to complicate and thicken this infrastructure of health insurance interests. As a defensive measure, doctors and hospitals turned to promote private health insurance for their own services (Blue Shield and Blue Cross, respectively); wartime wage restraint and federal tax policy encouraged the growth of a massive employer-based health insurance system, and reformers eventually circumvented the opponents of comprehensive reform by erecting a categorical health security structure for the elderly and poor (medicare and medicaid in 1965). By the time comprehensive health insurance reform was revisited in the Carter years, a vast complex of powerful inertial forces were in place to resist any major consolidating reform.

Finally in the category of objectives is another obvious but important point. Successful efforts at major social reform have generally sought policy ends that claim to benefit self-conscious and at least moderately powerful constituencies. There was a time in the nineteenth century when religiously driven moral claims were a vibrant part of social reform movements.[9] In our more secular century, appeals to social solidarity, altruism, and other noble ends have made little headway unless linked to concrete interests and politically weighty beneficiary groups. Thus for many decades resolution of the moral dilemma between the American creed and American racism only inched its way through the courts with the help of NAACP lawyers. It was the discovery of their political *and* moral power as a mass civil rights movement that brought blacks the sweeping legal reforms of the 1964 and 1965 civil rights statutes.[10] Likewise, vast numbers of Americans have been potential beneficiaries of environmental protection, but federal clean air and clean water initiatives depended more directly on pressures from a mobilizing if nascent environmental movement, from mayors and governors eager for federal grants, and from businesses fearing the growth of diverse state standards. Again, an exception to this generalization was the antipoverty initiative enacted in the mid-1960s, when no powerful constituency pushing the issue was in sight.[11] On the other side of the ledger to this exception could be put the failed efforts at comprehensive welfare reform in the Nixon and Carter administrations.

All of these considerations about objectives overlap with what might be said about the nature of resources in the political environment, resources that major reform efforts need to draw upon in order to survive.

Environmental Resources

Successful efforts to enact major social reforms may or may not build political credit for the future, but they inevitably make heavy demands on political assets that have been accumulated up to the present. Thus such efforts are often characterized by a movement-based brand of politics, in the sense that the concrete objective in question has put significant numbers of people in many places "on the move" from neutrality or passive support to active and sustained advocacy. For such people, elections are merely part of a larger policy campaign to win on "their" issue. Although reform movements are sometimes confined largely to elites (as seems to be the case with social insurance before 1935), those that are successful most often appear to combine elite and mass levels. The drawn-out campaigns for child labor, civil rights, and pure food and drug legislation are only a few prominent examples.[12]

Additional advantages seem to accrue to those reform movements that have their assets in the form of what might be called "federated" support for their cause. By this I mean a reform movement organized in parallel with the formal state and local structure of the federal system.[13] Not only has this arrangement allowed piecemeal victories at state level to build momentum for national action; it has also permitted a close articulation between the reform movement activists and the geographical bases of congressional power. The temperance movement is a dramatic example. So well articulated was the Prohibitionists' federated power that the supporters of repeal wisely prescribed ratification of the Twenty-First

Amendment through special state conventions rather than state legislatures, the only time this constitutional provision has been used.

Observers have frequently noted a pendulum swing in the political environment's resources for reform.[14] At some times but not others, social reform is said to be "in the air." In such periods public sentiments are thought to favor a tempo of faster change, more energetic innovation, and greater activism in dealing with the public's problems.

However, such assessments of the public psyche need to be tempered with an appreciation of *realpolitik*. The historic record suggests that major social reform efforts have not prospered simply because a mood of change and reform has been prevalent. The rare periods of fundamental policy reform have typically been associated with the appearance of powerfully unified party majorities in Congress and the White House. More than mere numerical majorities, these have been party formations unified on the heels of an election repudiating what has been portrayed as a regime of the status quo.[15] The Democrats' capture of the progressive reform banner in 1912 and 1932 are familiar examples that ushered in a series of successful social reform efforts.

The contrast with Democratic victories in 1948 and 1960 is informative. On both of these latter occasions, reform and activism were said to be in the air, and Harry S Truman and John F. Kennedy enjoyed numerical majorities in Congress. But these were far from pro-reform, activist, philosophical majorities. Truman's promised comprehensive national health insurance reform ran afoul of a Democratic congressional party that was deeply divided over Truman's liberal civil rights position, among other things. Kennedy faced a comparable problem with the conservative wing of the Democratic party in Congress. Having run as an "activist," Kennedy proposed and bargained for major social reforms that had grown to be part of the Democratic party agenda. But he was willing to see most of those reform proposals blocked (medicare, federal aid for education, Youth Conservation Corps, and others) or deferred (civil rights enforcement, fair employment practices, and so on) rather than risk defeat in major public battles with Congress. As Kennedy explained, "There is no sense in raising hell . . . in putting the office of the Presidency on the line on an issue, and then being defeated." He allegedly went on to quote Thomas Jefferson that "great innovations should not be forced on slender majorities."[16]

The breakthrough to successful major reform enactments awaited the remarkable events of 1963–64. A presidential assassination, the uniquely (for Americans) ideological challenge from a disunited Republican party and overwhelming Democratic majorities in 1964 all combined to produce a rare political environment. Forthcoming were ground-breaking reforms in civil rights, federal education funding, health care, environmental and antipoverty programs. The peculiarity of that situation was already becoming clear by the end of 1966, as the single-minded Democratic majority unraveled under the impact of racial tensions and Vietnam.

More typical was the experience with major social reform efforts in the Nixon and Carter years. With weak or nonexistent majorities in Congress, both administrations unsuccessfully sought major changes in the welfare system and health care policy. For Carter the problems were exacerbated by a more fragmented "reformed" Congress and its ability to frustrate efforts to assemble political resources behind any given reform plan.

Then too, the 1970s marked the closing of a period when the costs of major social reform efforts seemed irrelevant or easily manageable. Heretofore, successful reform proposals had often carried meager spending implications, depending as they did on new legal and regulatory stipulations (for example, temperance, compulsory social security contributions without general revenue funds, environmental protection standards, civil rights). But by the 1970s the residue of past reform successes was itself becoming a dense regulatory thicket of competing purposes. Moreover, those postwar reforms with major budgetary implications (for example, medicare, federal aid to elementary and secondary education) had enjoyed a favorable political environment of easy financing through rapid economic growth, declining relative defense spending, and unindexed tax brackets. By the late 1970s concerns about pressures from spending and inflation on the budget were mounting, economic growth and tax revenues were lagging, and signs of taxpayer resistance were appearing on the political landscape. Social reform efforts were entering a political environment that brought, not good news about painless possibilities of engineering social progress, but bad news about zero-sum conflicts. Not surprisingly, Carter health reform strategists sensed the need to enact new cost control reforms before expanding health insurance coverage as promised in the 1976 campaign. And no less surprisingly, such reform proved a political orphan, given the diffuse, latent constituency that would benefit from cost controls, the well-organized medical interests that would bear the costs of restraint, and the president's philosophically unfocused majority in Congress.

Gestation Periods

At risk of straining the language, one might say that successful major reform efforts have been characterized by a sustained, multicentered gestation process. I do not mean by this simply that reforms typically have a long history or that in our complicated political system reformers will not at first succeed and must try, try, and try again. All that is true, but gestation suggests something more. It means a gradual working through and ripening of arguments surrounding an issue. Because they are so important, major reform efforts profit from the extensive, if messy, deliberative process through which the complex political system achieves not so much a consensus but a clarification of the lines of dissent. Through this process factual claims are tested and countered, the "problem" defined and redefined, alternatives advanced and attacked. Thus, for example, the warrant for major federal reforms in the 1960s was gradually built in the 1950s through the ongoing interactions and arguments of congressional, interest group, and executive branch policy activists. There, and in the press, major new reform proposals were politically tested and reworked on issues having to do with the environment, civil rights, education, and health care for the elderly, among other things.[17] As a seasoned political observer put it, Kennedy "was 'getting the country moving' by sending back to Congress legislation that had been debated many times, in some cases for decades."[18]

Desultory as all the hearings, debates, and other exchanges may seem over the years prior to a successful reform effort, such a gestation process plays an important role in preparing the political ground. The very ability to sustain the policy argument over time helps persuade people to the view that there is a real problem that will not go away until something is done. Almost unnoticed, a presumption for policy action can grow. In time, opportunities can present themselves for reformers to split the opposition between those who deny a major need for reform and those who acknowledge the problem but reject the reformers' specific proposals. The ongoing deliberations among so many participants also help create the raw materials for potential working partnerships. Particular circumstances will decide whether some of these participants coalesce into a larger reform coalition, but the gestation process draws out the political opportunities for that to happen. Thus years of apparent frustration with proposals for federal aid to elementary and secondary education eventuated in a policy formula and coalition that was able to sidestep the historic roadblock posed by church/state and racial issues.[19] By the same token, as health care reformers endured year after year of delay, "progress" toward the major 1965 medicare reform was occurring indirectly as congressional opponents inched forward with ineffective half-measures (for example, the 1956 Old Age Assistance program and 1960 Kerr-Mills package).[20]

The notion of a long-term gestation process across and within the political branches seems in tension with the conventional view of the modern presidency as leader of the national agenda and font of major policy reform proposals. Yet we would do well to moderate that textbook vision. If Franklin Roosevelt is the exemplar for that view, then the image does not fit well at the outset of the modern presidency in the New Deal. Major reforms that may have become known as New Deal-presidential measures were often policy initiatives that were already in progress (for example, Agricultural Adjustment Act, Reconstruction Finance Corporation, Wagner Act), or that FDR initially opposed but could be persuaded to take credit for (for example, Federal Deposit Insurance) or that he held at arm's length in the planning process (for example, 1934 Committee on Economic Security, 1943 Wagner-Murray-Dingell health insurance bill). Arguably the most profound reform of social security occurred in 1939, largely outside the public view of any presidential involvement.

Of course, none of this denies that presidential advocacy and leadership have been crucial in focusing the national policy debate. However, it does raise doubts about associating successful reform efforts with a strictly president-centric view of the process. From that perspective the track record does not look particularly good. For example, as opposed to FDR's position on the issue, national health insurance did seem to become personally identified with President Truman in 1948, mainly to the proposal's disadvantage when the president's standing sank under pressure from other forces. In more recent decades presidents have in fact tried to shoulder more of the reform burden by mobilizing academic experts, task forces, and special working groups to design presidential policy initiatives. The expectations appear to have been exaggerated and the results generally disappointing.[21] One prominent example of a successful major reform effort that was ungestated and assembled on short order within the presidency is the Kennedy/Johnson "War on Poverty" enactments in the mid-1960s. But again, this helped make reform commitments a hostage to the fortune of Johnson's personal popularity.

These then seem to be some of the background conditions associated with successful major efforts to reform national social policy commitments. How does the Clinton experience compare?

The Clinton Reform Effort

Participants in the 1993–94 health care debate have offered a variety of reasons for the failure of President Clinton's reform proposal.[22] Some claim that the plan was too complex and bureaucratic, that the planning process was too secret, too partisan in thrust, and too long delayed. Reform backers have contended that the Clinton initiative succumbed to massive spending by the health insurance industry, relentless Republican obstructionism in Congress, and a public campaign of misinformation.

Surely these and many other factors are relevant to what happened. However, from a broader historical perspective the interesting question is not which particular nail in the horseshoe was faulty, thereby losing the horse, the rider, and the kingdom. The issue is why, in the first place, the kingdom should be in a position to be vulnerable to any one or more of these factors. Making retrospective predictions would be a cheap shot. The purpose here is simply to assess the background conditions that pushed the probabilities for success in one direction or another.

Nature of the Objective

Since complexity is inherent in virtually any major social reform, it makes little sense to fault the Clinton plan for its complicated design. However, it does seem fair to say that the president's reform effort did not enjoy the advantage of a single, easily understood objective. Far from encapsulating a simple message, the reform action to be taken pointed variously toward controlling runaway health costs, and to covering the 36–37 million uninsured, and to securing uninterrupted and adequate coverage to persons already insured. Over the course of time, between 1992 and 1994, the Clinton reform effort cycled among these appeals, ending in the summer of 1994 on the theme of security: "Health Care That's Always There."

On substantive grounds a good case could be made that these were mutually supportive objectives. Without cost controls, universal coverage would be too expensive, and without universal coverage in a single system the control of overall costs would be very difficult. However, the fact of life in the public arena was that these overlapping objectives did not translate into an easily understandable call to action. By the 1990s "health care reform," like "welfare reform," inevitably represented an ambiguous rallying cry. Still, since the Carter experience showed that decoupling major cost control reform from coverage expansion was also no royal road to success, one may not wish to make too much of this point.

The second consideration concerning reform objectives deserves greater weight. When reformers revisited national health insurance in the 1990s, there could be no question that the ends in view were what we have referred to above as consolidating rather than breakthrough in nature. Reference to the Clinton plan as affecting "one-seventh of the economy" was really a shorthand way of saying that an enormous array of existing arrangements now crowded the policy landscape, an array of economic and political stakeholders far beyond anything imagined sixty years earlier when FDR demurred from taking on the powers of the status quo in health financing.

On the one hand, this meant that Clinton had the advantage of not having to make and win a "breakthrough" policy argument with the general public (or courts). By 1992 a major federal government role in the health care system was widely accepted on all sides as legitimate. On the other hand, it also meant that the president had embarked on a campaign for sweeping reform in a field full of powerful groups with an immense stake in the status quo. Here was a pre-existing condition in health care with profound political implications.

To be sure, all of the components of the Clinton plan (employer mandates, community rating, managed competition) were familiar from past policy debates. What was new—and what enters the Clinton initiative in that rarest category of "big and bold" consolidating reforms— was the aim of incorporating everyone and all health industry interests into a single, federally designed structure of regulation. The implication is clear: the fundamental work of health reform would be a thorough-going struggle of political power, not the technical design of good policy or negotiation about incremental changes.

At the same time, such comprehensive reform aimed to benefit most directly a quite diffuse constituency: the uninsured, workers fearful of losing coverage, and those hard-pressed to pay escalating private insurance premiums. Without doubt this represented a large number of Americans, but they were Americans who posed the classic problem of collective action by a poorly organized, nonaffluent body of people. Reformers could hope for collateral support by adding sweeteners in the plan for the elderly and others. And too, the financial interests of businesses already insuring their workers could offer some additional, though low-intensity, support to the reform cause. The fact remained, however, that at its core the reform effort was directed to a politically weak constituency, who would gain, and a well-organized and financed set of interests centered in the insurance industry, who would lose.

Thus, as far as the objectives of the Clinton health reform effort are concerned, the structure of the situation firmly nudged the probabilities of success in an unfavorable direction.

Environmental Resources

The election of 1992 appears as one of those times when the pendulum of public sentiments had swung toward a pro-activist approach to social and economic problems. Business as usual was widely perceived to have fallen before the demand for change. To this extent the political setting seemed generally favorable for the president's reform effort.

At the same time, from a comparative historical perspective, the Clinton reform was born into an extraordinarily resource-poor environment. In the first place, there is little evidence that health care reform enjoyed anything like what was termed earlier to be a movement-based politics, much less federated ligaments into the mass body politic. On the contrary, the November 1991 Senate victory of Harris Wofford in Pennsylvania appeared as a surprising and overinterpreted event precisely because there had heretofore been so little sign of grass-roots public interest in health care issues. At best, public opinion polls showed a vague, simple-minded disposition toward cost-free health reform. Clearly, there was nothing resembling a serious reform movement except perhaps within the policy-wonk elite. Instead, as is typical in the modern era of political consultants, the appearance of grass-roots mobilization was orchestrated from above after the partisan policy lines had been drawn in Washington. In the fall of 1993, tens of thousands of "personal" solicitation letters from the president were mailed through the Democratic National Committee. What was envisioned, beyond donations, was a network of citizen groups in all 435 congressional districts (the Democratic Action Network) that would organize speakers' bureaus, rallies, petition and ad campaigns on behalf of the Clinton plan. The actual political results appear to have been negligible. Indeed, the major forms of grass-roots power in home districts were small business interests and conservative talk-radio programs opposed to the Clinton plan.

Second, Clinton's major reform effort was launched from what appears historically as an extremely narrow base of presidential political capital. For Clinton, health reform represented the hope of building a new Democratic majority rather than the consequence of already having a proreform majority behind him. In part this was reflected in the president's meager 43 percent of the popular vote and continued public doubts about him personally. But in part too, the Democrats' continued numerical majority in Congress concealed rather than expressed any credible claims for a mandate of transformative reform from the White House. For all his criticisms of Reaganomics in 1992, candidate Clinton could not launch a thorough, repudiating attack on the prevailing political order commensurate with the public's distaste for that order. This was because the Democratic establishment in Washington was a major part of that received order. It was old Democrats, not Clintonesque "new Democrats," who returned to Congress in 1992. Thus the wind of reform that blew into town with the new president was not of a strength likely to intimidate opponents of major change, in health care or anything else. While Clinton publicly likened his health plan to the great reforms of social security and medicare in earlier Democratic generations, his political situation resembled that of Kennedy and Carter much more than that of FDR in 1934 or Johnson in 1964.

In fact, President Clinton's command over political resources was actually diminished from the time of either Kennedy or Carter. This was due to long-run trends in public trust and public finances that predated anything Clinton might do. Although it went unrecognized at the time, Kennedy enjoyed the luxury of a large stock of public confidence in the capabilities of government and institutional leadership more generally. His and Johnson's era of reform was also a time of relatively painless choices in taxing and spending, as economic growth drove up revenues and budget deficits had yet to accumulate. Both of these political assets had diminished significantly by the Carter presidency, but Carter's situation was positively rosy compared with the budgetary problems and public distrust of government in place by 1992.[23]

On these counts, the resources in the political environment did not bode well for President Clinton's effort at comprehensive health reform.

Gestation Periods

No one could claim that national health insurance has gone undebated in the United States. Since Theodore Roosevelt raised the issue in his

1912 presidential campaign, federally supported health insurance has been a recurring, if intermittent, item on the national policy agenda. The question here, however, is not how long the subject has been around but how well worked through were the important substantive and political issues prior to risking political capital on a major reform effort at a given time.

Judgments will no doubt differ on the matter, but the position advanced here is that, compared with other major social reform enactments, the Clinton project falls into the unfortunate category of poorly gestated initiatives envisioned by the textbook presidency. This is not to say that the presidential task force was inadequate in its work, only that for the longer term prior to that work the larger political system had not been particularly involved in thrashing out the political arguments and policy realities underlying such an effort.

The political debate on national health insurance largely disintegrated in 1979 at the end of the Carter administration. By then, for a variety of reasons that need not concern us here, the president's health reform initiatives had stalled in Congress. Senator Edward Kennedy, who was labor's champion on health insurance reform, had launched an internal party challenge to the president's leadership, and mounting concerns about the federal budget only increased the frustration and exhaustion on all sides. Republican control of the White House and mounting deficits in the 1980s added to the sense that major reforms in health insurance were probably unattainable. Reformers in Congress settled for cheaper incremental changes such as mandated expansions in state medicaid coverage.

For all practical purposes, the immediate gestation period for the current round of major health reform battles began in the hothouse political atmosphere surrounding the 1992 election. Harris Wofford's surprising 1991 Senate victory and subsequent media attention to health issues prompted the Bush White House to hastily frame a proposal for tax credits and deductions that claimed to make health insurance affordable for all Americans. Unveiled in the president's January 1992 State of the Union Address, these initiatives were never seriously taken up by Congress. Meanwhile, campaign speeches by Democrats in Congress and on the presidential primary trail advanced a variety of health reform schemes. Some would impose government requirements on employers to provide basic health insurance to all employees or contribute to a public plan providing the insurance entitlement (play or pay). Some proposed a nationalized program making the federal government the single payer of health insurance benefits. Still others advocated reorganization of the health system to strengthen the ability of market forces to control spending. None of these ideas and their costs could be seriously deliberated upon in a political system now absorbed with the momentum and staged media events of the presidential campaign.[24]

For example, early permutations of the Clinton health reform effort evolved largely in response to immediate campaign needs, especially the felt need to avoid any discussion of costs and new taxes to pay for health reform.[25] In the New Hampshire primary Democratic challengers were countered with a modified pay or play proposal. With no new taxes, government coverage of all uninsured Americans would be paid for with savings from cost controls and management efficiencies. The June 1992 manifesto for launching the general election campaign (*Putting People First*) deliberately avoided any mention of whether health reform would cost or save money. By the fall, Bush attacks on Clinton as another big government, tax-and-spend liberal elicited a more detailed plan from the Clinton campaign, again with minimal analysis of financial realities. Universal coverage would be achieved by requiring employers to pay for workers' insurance, by providing government coverage of the unemployed, and subsidized insurance premiums for small businesses. Health costs would be held down by managed competition among providers and national limits on overall health spending.

Thus by the time 1992 drew to an end, comprehensive health reform had come to be defined, and explicitly promised, as a purely presidential initiative that would be fully worked out, presented to Congress in the first one hundred days, and passed in the first year of the new administration. And it would all apparently happen with little if any cost to the taxpayer. The danger was that lacking a more extensive and genuine gestation process—that is, a sustained and fully engaged debate in the political system on the difficult issues of financing and other contentious trade-offs implied by comprehensive change—the real politics of such a reform (both in Washington and the public's limits of acceptability) remained unknown territory. More even than in the heady 1960s, when Kennedy and Johnson reform efforts had profited from gestational scars of the 1950s and from the advantage of far more abundant political resources, reform in 1993 became a White House deduction about what would work technically and politically.

Heading the health care task force with the first lady and managing it through Clinton's personal friend and policy adviser Ira Magaziner only made obvious in January 1993 what had been implicit in White House operations since the election: the health reform effort was to be a continuation of the political campaign to sell a Clinton presidency to the public and rebuild a Democratic majority. As with Johnson's War on Poverty, but without Johnson's political resources, serious reform was now becoming hostage to a president's personal popularity.

Although the White House task force consulted widely, its arguments and decisions were made in secret so as to produce a coherent, integrated Clinton plan. The plan itself would anticipate and embody the compromises needed to circumvent public fears of big government and higher taxes. Not only did this further dim prospects for educating Washington and the public to the difficult trade-offs at stake. It also all but prohibited prenegotiated arrangements with those in and around Congress who could be potential allies. From this perspective, any alternatives from congressional Republicans who backed universal coverage or Democrats who advocated a different approach to cost controls could be—and were—seen as a presumptive threat to the political and technical integrity of the Clinton plan. Health reform was to be a triumph of synoptic policy design and a personal political victory for the president, pointing toward 1996. A number of Republican strategists needed no encouragement to try to turn that partisan challenge into a personal defeat. Eventually, negotiators in 1994 would try to produce a single Democratic compromise, but by then it was too late. The great confusion known in the public mind as "health reform" was in full flower.

In sum, conditions were in place firmly to nudge probabilities for a major reform effort toward failure. The enormous challenge of enacting a comprehensive social policy transformation in America's complex political system had been telescoped into an in-house presidential thought experiment and a frenzied White House campaign to sell the resulting brainchild to the public. In the modern history of major social reform efforts, never had a president with so few political resources tried to do so much.

Notes

1. Paul A. Colinvaux, *Why Big Fierce Animals Are Rare: An Ecologist's Perspective* (Princeton University Press, 1978).

2. A sampling of such "big, bold" transformative reforms would include the following: first national intervention in favor of consumer protection in the mass commercial market (American Pure Food and Drug and Meat Inspection Act of 1906); national prohibition of manufacture, sale, or transportation of alcoholic

beverages (congressional passage of the Eighteenth Amendment, December 1919, and enabling Volstead Act of January 1920); national social insurance system for old age pensions (Social Security Act of 1935) federal commitment of a responsibility for educational quality throughout the United States (National Defense Education Act of 1958); national standards for general environmental protection (Clean Air and Clean Water Acts, 1963–65); federal system of social insurance for health care (Medicare Act of 1965); first modern civil and voting rights guarantees for minorities (Voting Rights Act of 1965 and Civil Rights Act of 1964); first federal funding for general precollege schooling (Elementary and Secondary Education Act of 1965). For an attempt to classify proposals in terms of their innovativeness and scale, and evidence on the inability of postwar presidents to dominate congressional responses to such "big bold" domestic reforms, see Mark A. Peterson, *Legislating Together: The White House and Capitol Hill from Eisenhower to Reagan* (Harvard University Press, 1990), pp. 152–54.

3. Lawrence D. Brown, *New Policies, New Politics: Government's Response to Government's Growth* (Brookings, 1983).

4. Clean Air Act of 1963, Clean Air and Solid Waste Disposal Act of 1965, Water Quality Act of 1965.

5. Clean Air Amendments Act of 1990.

6. Only 150,000 Americans were in receipt of industrial and trade union pensions according to *The Report of the Committee on Economic Security of 1935 and Other Basic Documents Relating to the Development of the Social Security Act* (Washington: National Conference on Social Welfare, 1985), p. 44, with 6.5 million Americans then over the age of 65.

7. This is apart from industrial accident and occupation disease provisions of various workmen's compensation laws.

8. *Report of the Committee on Economic Security*, p. 62.

9. Timothy L. Smith, *Revivalism and Social Reform in Mid-Nineteenth Century America* (Johns Hopkins University Press, 1980).

10. This observation should not be interpreted to downplay the immensely powerful moral claims mobilized by the religious institutions associated with the civil rights movement in midtwentieth century America. Black and white churches, revivalist, and other groups were crucial to the mass mobilization movement for equal rights.

11. If agreeing on nothing else, this seems to be the consensus view of contemporary policy historians. Cf. James T. Patterson, *America's Struggle against Poverty 1900–1980* (Harvard University Press, 1981); Henry J. Aaron, *Politics and the Professors: The Great Society in Perspective* (Brookings, 1978); and Nicholas Lemann, *The Promised Land: The Great Black Migration and How It Changed America* (Alfred A. Knopf, 1991).

12. Morton Keller, *Regulating a New Society: Public Policy and Social Change in America, 1900–1933* (Harvard University Press, 1994).

13. Theda Skocpol, *Protecting Soldiers and Mothers: The Political Origins of Social Policy in the United States* (Cambridge: Belknap Press, 1992), pp. 530, 537–38.

14. James L. Sundquist, *Politics and Policy: The Eisenhower, Kennedy, and Johnson Years* (Brookings, 1968), p. 500; John W. Kingdon, *Agendas, Alternatives*

and Public Policies (Little Brown and Co., 1984), p. 198; and Albert O. Hirschman, *Shifting Involvements: Private Interest and Public Action* (Princeton University Press, 1982).

15. Stephen Skowronek, *The Politics Presidents Make: Leadership from John Adams to George Bush* (Cambridge: Belknap Press, 1993).

16. Arthur M. Schlesinger, Jr., *A Thousand Days: John F. Kennedy in the White House* (Houghton Mifflin, 1965), quotation on page 709.

17. Sundquist, *Politics and Policy*.

18. Harry McPherson, *A Political Education* (Little Brown, 1972), p. 189.

19. Sundquist, *Politics and Policy*, pp. 206–15.

20. Theodore R. Marmor, *The Politics of Medicare* (Aldine, 1973).

21. Robert C. Wood, *Whatever Possessed the President?: Academic Experts and Presidential Policy, 1960–1988* (University of Massachusetts Press, 1993).

22. Robin Toner, "The Health Care Debate: News Analysis—Autopsy on Health Care," *New York Times*, September 27, 1994, p. A1. See also James Fallows, "A Triumph of Misinformation," *Atlantic Monthly*, January 1995, pp. 26–37.

23. C. Eugene Steuerle, "Financing the American State at the Turn of the Century," in Elliott Brownlee, ed., *Funding the Modern American State* (Washington: Woodrow Wilson International Center for Scholars, forthcoming); and Times-Mirror Center for the People and the Press, *The People, the Press, and Politics: The New Political Landscape*, Los Angeles, mimeo, 1994.

24. For a realistic account of how policy ideas are used and abused in such a situation, see David Blumenthal, "Health Policy on the High Wire: Thirteen Days with a Presidential Campaign," *Journal of Health Politics, Policy, and Law*, vol. 17 (Summer 1992), pp. 353–73.

25. Summary press accounts can be found in Robert Pear, "The 1992 Campaign: Issues—Health Care; Health Care Policy," *New York Times*, August 12, 1992, p. A1; Susan B. Garland and Mike McNamee, "Health Reform Hits the Campaign Trail," *Business Week*, August 30, 1993, pp. 34–35; Michael Duffy and Dick Thompson, "Behind Closed Doors," *Time*, September 20, 1993, pp. 60–63; Burt Solomon, "Clinton's Inscrutable Health Plan," *National Journal*, September 18, 1993, pp. 2260–61; Adam Clymer, Robert Pear, and Robin Toner, "The Health Care Debate: What Went Wrong?" *New York Times*, August 29, 1994, p. A1; and Toner, "The Health Care Debate: News Analysis."

CHAPTER THREE

The Rise and Resounding Demise of the Clinton Health Security Plan

Theda Skocpol

O N SEPTEMBER 22, 1993, President Bill Clinton stirred Congress and the nation with a speech calling for "America to fix a health care system that is badly broken . . . giving every American health security—health care that is always there, health care that can never be taken away."[1] Millions listened to the president, and polls taken soon after the speech registered strong support.[2] "The Clinton Plan Is Alive On Arrival," trumpeted the *New York Times*, as moderate Republicans and leaders of groups with a stake in the health care system promised to cooperate in working out reforms.[3]

Historic themes resonated in the Clinton plan. Its very title "Health Security" harkened back to the Social Security Act of 1935; and the "health security card" that the president said every American would receive was obviously meant to encourage a sense of safe and honorable entitlement such as Americans feel they have in social security. How ironic, then, that just a bit over one year later both the Clinton Health Security plan and the Democratic party—the legatee of the very New Deal whose achievements President Clinton had hoped to imitate and extend—lay in a shambles. Voters went to the polls on November 8, 1994, and provided widespread victories to Republicans, not only those running for statehouses, governorships, and the U.S. Senate, but also those running for the House of Representatives, which changed partisan hands for the first time in four decades. Many of the Republicans who won in 1994 are ideologically hostile to governmental social provision, and their Contract with America called for dismantling social programs and hobbling the federal government.[4] The New Deal tradition is dead, postelection commentators declared.

The collapse of the 1993–94 campaign for health care reform lurked like a brooding ghost in the electoral upheavals of November. Polls showed that many voters were punishing Democrats for having been in charge during a time when Washington was "a mess" and not delivering desired results. A crucial minority of voters—particularly "swing" independents and former Ross Perot voters—were disappointed in President Clinton in part because they believed he had proposed a "big government solution" to health care reform.[5] An election-night survey of voters sponsored by the Kaiser Family Foundation found that a substantial majority (and especially those who voted Republican) believed that the Democrats' reform plans entailed too much "government bureaucracy" and could have reduced the quality of their own health care.[6]

The demise of President Clinton's Health Security plan was not just a proposal that fizzled out, leaving the same terrain clear for a revised attempt to solve the same problems from a similar starting point. The presentation and decisive defeat of the Clinton plan was a pivotal moment in U.S. politics. To understand why the 1993–94 attempt at comprehensive health reform failed, and to speak intelligently about what should and could have been done differently, one must begin by asking why President Clinton devised a plan that not only failed in Congress but also helped to fuel a massive political upheaval. Only against the backdrop of the upheaval, moreover, can we make sense of possibilities for the future.

A Way Through the Middle? The Fashioning of Clinton's Plan

Looking back over the two years before the September 1993 Health Security speech, the president and his advisers had every reason to believe that they were acting with the tide of U.S. politics. By 1990 public opinion polls indicated that public support for national health reform was at a forty-year high and that Americans overwhelmingly believed insurance coverage should be available to everyone.[7] In the fall of 1991, Harris Wofford's improbable triumph in a special senatorial election in Pennsylvania suddenly brought the issue of health care reform to the front burner in Washington, D.C.[8] The financing of health care had become a middle-class issue as well as a problem for the working near-poor, whose jobs often do not carry health benefits. Middle-class concerns focused on "dramatic increases in health care costs," as more and more employers shifted expenses toward covered employees, and on "fear of losing all or part of their health care benefits in our employment-based system of health insurance," particularly during a period of extensive corporate down-sizing. As opinion analysts Robert Blendon and Karen Donelan summed up, "60 percent [of Americans] worry that they will not be adequately insured . . . in the future.[9]

Bold proposals for reforms of health care financing proliferated inside and outside of government. Two dozen reform bills were introduced during the 102d Congress.[10] Reform proposals, many of them sweeping, also came from business groups, trade unions, insurance companies, and assorted health policy experts.[11] Even the American Medical Association, historically the bitterest of all enemies of governmental-sponsored health reforms, came up with its own plan for universally guaranteed health insurance.[12]

Committed presidential leadership was lacking while George Bush remained in office, yet the American people wanted it to be forthcoming. In early 1992, as the presidential campaign was getting under way, the public told pollsters that health care reform ranked right after the economy and foreign affairs as a policy topic it wanted addressed by presidential candidates.[13] Most Americans looked to the federal government for action and believed that Democrats were more likely than Republicans to promote desired health care reforms.[14] Not surprisingly, the leading Democratic presidential candidates, including Bill Clinton of Arkansas, committed themselves to pursue national heath care reform if elected.[15] Health care reform, after all, looked like an excellent issue for 1990s Democrats. The party needed to overcome racial divisions on issues such as welfare reform and affirmative action; it had to highlight issues that could unite more and less privileged Americans. Successful sponsorship of national health care reform could revive the electoral fortunes of the Democratic party, provided that ways could be found simultaneously to extend insurance to low-wage working families and to make coverage for the middle class more secure and less costly.

The Clinton administration has been accused of championing a "liberal," "government-takeover" approach to health reform. On the contrary, during the 1992 presidential campaign, Bill Clinton gravitated toward competition with a budget, an approach to national health care reform distinct from previously defined liberal as well as conservative alternatives. Once he found this middle way, Clinton never wavered from it.

Back in 1991 and 1992, the major visible alternatives in the simmering national debate over health care reform were three, and it was clear that Bill Clinton would not accept two that appeared to be on the right and left. Incremental "market-oriented" reforms not aiming for universal coverage or cost controls were identified with the Republicans, and they had very little appeal for Democrats (and little backing from health policy experts, for that matter).[16] Apparently at the other end of the partisan spectrum a few health policy experts, various advocacy groups, a sizable group of congressional Democrats, and Democratic presidential hopeful Senator Robert Kerrey favored various sorts of Canadian-style "single-payer" schemes, calling for taxes to displace private health insurance.[17] An excellent technical case could be made that a single-payer approach could save more than enough on simplified administrative costs to cover all of the uninsured, and the Canadian experience after the 1970s suggested that it could also significantly slow the increase of national health care expenditures, while sustaining the day-to-day autonomy of patients and health providers.[18] Nevertheless, most U.S. politicians feared to endorse a single-payer scheme, because it would necessitate switching from employer-provided insurance and private insurance premiums toward explicit general or payroll taxation. Frank talk about raising taxes was considered the kiss of death. Walter Mondale had apparently shot himself in the foot with such talk in 1984; and George Bush was in trouble during the 1992 presidential campaign for having broken his "read my lips" pledge never to raise taxes. Not surprisingly, Bill Clinton rejected the single-payer approach.[19] Determined to win middle-class votes for the Democratic ticket, Clinton ran a moderate campaign based on promises to reduce taxes on everyone except the very rich. In the midst of an economic slowdown, moreover, he did not want to threaten immediate, wrenching changes for employees of big insurance companies or for employees currently happy with health insurance packages arranged through their employers.

The third major alternative in 1991–92 was "play or pay," so labeled because it would require all employers either to offer and partially pay for health insurance for all employees or else pay a kind of "quit tax" to help subsidize expanded governmental coverage for all Americans not employed and insured by their employers. This approach had come to seem the most "pragmatic" road to national health insurance by the start of the 1992 presidential campaign.[20] Key Democratic senators sponsored proposals embodying play or pay.[21] The Pepper commission (officially the U.S. Bipartisan Commission on Comprehensive Health Care) and the National Leadership Coalition for Health Care Reform of big employers and unions also endorsed it in 1990.[22]

As Clinton sparred during the presidential primaries with Senators

Robert Kerrey and Paul Tsongas, he found he had to go beyond a general promise and outline what he would actually do about national health reform. Clinton's first move in January 1992 dallied with play or pay.[23] But this proved transitory. As President Bush attacked the payroll taxes and alleged antibusiness thrust of play-or-pay proposals identified with congressional Democrats, Clinton pulled back from that approach.[24] An intellectual conversion also occurred during the spring and summer, as Clinton talked with such advisers as John Garamendi, the insurance commissioner of California, Walter Zelman, and Paul Starr.[25] Building upon and modifying ideas from the economist Alain Enthoven (who advocated managed care and regulated competition among health insurance plans), these advisers convinced Clinton that it would be possible to use regional insurance purchasing agencies, various federal regulations, and very modest new tax subsidies to push the employer-based U.S. health care system simultaneously toward cost efficiency and universal coverage.[26]

This approach, which I will call inclusive managed competition with a budget, was just what Bill Clinton was looking for. It promised, at once, to satisfy the public's desire for affordable universal coverage and to slow cost growth as favored by powerful elites.[27] Managed competition would please big employers and large insurance companies, allowing the would-be president to court and work with these powerful interests, just as moderate southern Democratic governors had always done. This approach could presumably also be sold both to mainstream Democrats who care primarily about universal coverage and to "New Democrats" in the Democratic Leadership Council who want market-oriented reforms that minimize taxes and public spending.

Indeed, Clinton found the public finance features of inclusive managed competition with a budget particularly attractive. If he were to be elected president after a campaign promising deficit reduction without new taxes, he was going to have to devise a health care reform plan that did not include huge new taxes—and a plan with sufficient regulatory teeth to persuade Congressional Budget Office officials that future cost reductions would be forthcoming in medicaid and medicare. Competition within a budget might enable a new Clinton administration to do all of this, while still promising universal health security. The budgetary logic of the approach was irresistible to a moderate Democrat who wanted to cut the deficit and to free resources for new public investments.

In November 1992 Bill Clinton was elected president of the United States with 43 percent of the popular vote (and a much more commanding margin in the electoral college). The new president soon turned to working on economic reforms and budget cutting. Meanwhile, he convened a health reform task force under the leadership of his longtime friend, business consultant Ira Magaziner, and Hillary Rodham Clinton, the first lady. [28] Most of the work of the task force took place in a few frantic months from January to May 1993, but its report could not be completed until the end of the summer after President Clinton's budget emerged from a contentious Congress. During its life, the task force mobilized at least part-time participation from hundreds of government officials, health policy experts on loan to government, congressional staffers, and some state-level officials. Groups with a stake in the current U.S. health care system were not officially represented, but the task force held many hearings and consulted with hundreds of representatives of stakeholder groups. The purpose of such consultations was not to bargain but to elicit ideas and concerns that the task force could use as it helped the president to flesh out his overall approach to health reform.

Because the task force tried to maintain a modicum of confidentiality during its deliberations, it did not improve public understanding or generate broad support for the emerging Clinton reform plan.[29] Later on, once that plan came under attack for its alleged overreliance on governmental bureaucracy, the fact that a government-centered task force had fashioned it became an added liability—one more exhibit supporting demonization by the plan's opponents. Still, it is difficult to believe that the process followed by the task force was decisive in itself, apart from the actual contents of the Clinton Health Security plan and the political conflicts that unfolded after it was unveiled.

A Failure of D/democratic Communication

Analysts have placed the fatal wounding of comprehensive health reform at various times, ranging from the earliest months of the Clinton administration when the task force did its work, to the end of the summer of 1994 when Congress at last gave up trying to fashion a "mainstream" compromise that preserved some elements of what the president aimed to achieve. In my view, the critical period was the five months between the time of the president's late September speech and late February 1994—by which point concerted partisan campaigns against universal health reform had locked into place, and the support of elite and middle-class Americans for ambitious health reforms had begun its inexorable downhill slide. From then on, momentum toward inclusive reform was irretrievably lost.[30]

This view presumes, as I do, that it was never realistic to expect major stakeholders in the present system to keep bargaining over changes in the rules of the game, unless they saw that the voting public continued to want such changes. Nor could one expect the fractious Congress to fashion a difficult compromise, unless a majority of the U.S. public remained committed to some sort of presidentially sponsored comprehensive health care reform. President Clinton and his allies had to hold the public's interest and support as the details of their approach were spelled out, not because the president's bill had to be enacted unchanged, but simply to ensure that leaders in and out of Congress would remain willing to bargain. Favorable public opinion was essential to render some Republicans willing to flesh out the insufficient Democratic majority for passage of legislation in the filibuster-prone Senate, and also to give Democratic House and Senate leaders the leverage they needed to ride herd on competing committees and self-promoting colleagues.

By 1994 less than one-fourth of the American people believed the federal government would "do what is right" either "always" or "most of the time."[31] Against this backdrop, it is remarkable that the public received President Clinton's Health Security speech as well as it did and actually seemed for a time to be open to the idea that the federal government might be able to ensure health security for everyone. Given general skepticism about the capabilities of the contemporary federal government, the president and his advisers should have understood the vital need to follow up the introductory September speech with a persuasive vision of *how* new governmental regulations would actually work to deliver on the overall goals the president had articulated. But during the fall of 1993 the Clinton administration did *not* wage a successful campaign to explain the mechanisms of their proposed legislation.

There are some good reasons why the Clinton health reformers failed to do enough to sustain public support and deepen public understanding. First, as political scientists know well, presidents do not control their own agendas.[32] Soon after President Clinton introduced his health reform plan, events compelled him to turn his attention to other issues—the crisis in Somalia and the protracted public and congressional campaign to pass the North American Free Trade Agreement (NAFTA), an international treaty initiative that had been passed down to him from previous presidents. Given the reliance of his "economic recovery" plan on free trade, the president had to fight for NAFTA. But the impending NAFTA decision in Congress forced the president to wage an all-out campaign of public persuasion and congressional arm-twisting just when he should have been devoting his time to explaining health reform to the American people.

Another reason for not explaining the Health Security bill in detail was that its proponents took it for granted from the start that key elements (such as encompassing regional alliances and premium caps) might have to be bargained away.[33] During the summer 1993 budget battle, the media criticized the president as a "waffler" when he backed away from specific provisions he had originally presented. He and his advisers did not want to face such criticism again, should it prove necessary for the president to support an altered health reform bill. The Clinton administration drew up its detailed 1,342-page bill so that the Congressional Budget Office could estimate its costs as required by law. Yet the president proclaimed himself flexible about the mechanisms of his plan, allowing room for congressional modifications. Inadvertently, therefore, the president ended up outlining mechanisms that critics could attack while his administration was not mobilizing wholeheartedly on behalf of those mechanisms.

Looking at the situation more broadly, one can see that a U.S. president and allied policy promoters in the 1990s, especially if they are Democrats, have few means for forming strong alliances and communicating political arguments. The Democratic party no longer has a nationally widespread, locally rooted infrastructure of loyal local organizations and allied groups (such as labor unions) through which it can run grassroots political campaigns.[34] The conservative right now has such an infrastructure, in the form of local Christian fundamentalist groups and Rush Limbaugh-style talk radio stations. Democratic politicians, including a Democratic president, depend more exclusively than conservatives on pollsters, media consultants, and television to get messages out to the citizenry. Yet pollsters and political consultants—by the very nature of their skills, worldviews, and the means of communication open to their clients—tend to think in terms of appealing labels (Health Security) and advertising slogans ("security that can never be taken away") rather than in terms of explanatory discussions.

Given the way the national media operates, the president of the United States cannot be sure of getting television coverage to speak directly and at length to the American people. Had the president asked for more airtime, perhaps the networks would have refused to cover additional explanatory speeches soon after the September address. There is also the matter of how television and newspapers cover complicated and contro-versial issues such as national health care reform. As various observers have argued (and as a careful study by Kathleen Jamieson and her asso-ciates has documented for the 1993–94 health care debate), the media tend to focus not on the substance and adequacy of proposals, but on the "horse races" among conflicting politicians and interest groups.[35] They look at who is arguing with whom, giving at least equal weight to outrageous or extreme claims, while failing to help the public understand the details of proposals or to evaluate the validity of claims about them. To the degree that President Clinton had to rely only on media coverage to get his plan across to the American people, he was certain to face an erosion of sympathy and a steady increase of public disillusionment.

No doubt realizing that they could not rely on routine media coverage alone, the president's allies tried to construct a grass-roots campaign on behalf of health care reform.[36] During the summer of 1993, just as the Clinton plan was being formulated in the task force, an attempt was made to set up a nominally nonpartisan "National Health Care Cam-paign" designed to raise its own funds and use them to target messages to twenty-one states identified as keys to the ultimate passage of legisla-tion. Almost at once this project came under political attack as not really "nonpartisan," and the White House moved it under the auspices of the Democratic National Committee. This shift resulted in reduced funding and less capacity to mobilize coalitions that included groups that had to maintain nonpartisan identities. Much later, after the Clinton plan had been unveiled in the fall, Democratic Senator Jay Rockefeller initiated the Health Care Reform Project, a promotional coalition headed by John Rother of the American Association of Retired Persons. This well-organized effort had insufficient funds for a national media campaign, yet devoted itself to mobilizing support for "universal health care" in swing congressional districts. But it could not specifically promote—or explain—the president's bill as such, because some member groups, in-cluding Rother's AARP, had not endorsed the Clinton plan, only certain broad reform goals.

Throughout 1993–94, in fact, reform-minded politicians and groups in and around the Democratic party could not unite on even the most basic "how-to" features of health reform. Clinton's plan was not based on the major alternatives to which Democrats were loyal in 1992 and 1993, and the new president did not attract most Democrats to his specific approach. Democrats treated the president's bill as grist for pro-tracted bargaining over this or that provision and as fodder for infinitely complicated legislative maneuvering in five different House and Senate committees.[37] Persistent policy disagreements greatly undercut not only the explicability and credibility of Clinton's plan once it was officially announced, but also the possibilities for compromise in Congress.

Finally, there were problems inherent in the Clinton plan itself. The plan was intricate and called for daring leaps of innovative organization building. At the same time, its supporters were ambivalent about explicitly discussing the governmental mechanisms that would be involved in implementing the new arrangements.

Much of the complexity for which many commentators chided the Clinton plan was actually inherent in the existing private and public arrangements that the president wanted to modify, not revolutionize. In any event, sheer complexity was not the major difficulty. When medicare was debated and enacted in the mid-1960s, the legislation was very complicated, but its sponsors could build on widespread public understanding of and affection for the well-established social security program of contributory retirement insurance.[38] The core of public support was built on an analogy to a well-regarded earlier federal government program. The elderly, and many others in American society, appreciated the universal and non-means-tested nature of social security, and they had an operational image of how earmarked payroll taxes worked to fund federally administered benefits for individual elderly people. When he introduced his 1993 Health Security bill, President Clinton tried to invoke the social security precedent once again. This time, however, the analogy was purely rhetorical; it held only for the goal of universal, secure coverage. There was no relevant analogy to social security with regard to how governmental mechanisms in the proposed Clinton Health Security system would actually work.

The key mechanism in the new Health Security plan was the mandatory purchasing cooperative, something the Clintonites decided to label the "health care alliance." One or more of these new governmental institutions would be established in each state, and they would have all sorts of powers to collect revenues and data, to disburse information, and to regulate actions of employers, insurance companies, and individual citizens. Supporters of the proposed Clinton health plan never found any consistent examples of preexisting organizations that health alliances could be said to resemble. Sometimes alliances were likened to health purchasing cooperatives, such as the California Public Employees Retirement System, and sometimes they were said to resemble food co-ops or grain co-ops for farmers. Although one or another of these analogies may have resonated for particular audiences, no clear, convincing, well-understood, and popular federal program precedent could serve as social security did for medicare. Citizens were left to imagine the health alliances arising out of nowhere. Not surprisingly, in a poll taken in February 1994, only one in four Americans claimed to know what a "health alliance" might be.[39]

Promoters of the Clinton Health Security plan tried to avoid discussing the alliances as new sorts of *governmental* organizations. Instead of telling Americans as simply and clearly as possible why this kind of governmental endeavor would be effective and was desirable, and instead of explaining how the new regulations would work, they accommodated to the public's distrust of government by pretending that President Clinton was proposing a virtually government-free national health security plan. They portrayed alliances as giant voluntary groups.[40] Promoters operated like advertisers, using images of volunteerism and words about choice to prevent, or calm, Americans' fears about government takeovers or bungling in the health care system. Arguably, however, vague and evasive explanations of the new system merely left Americans prey to alternative descriptions purveyed by the plan's fiercest opponents. A portrayal of the Clinton plan as a vast set of voluntary associations simply was not plausible. If that was all the president had in mind, why did he need a 1,342-page bill?

An Ideal Foil for Antigovernment Countermobilization

Opponents determined to defeat or change President Clinton's proposal for national health reform swung into action even as the plan was unveiled. Many groups with an occupational or financial stake in the present U.S. health care system had already mobilized to present concerns to the White House. The minute the Clinton plan officially appeared, all of those groups could quickly decide how disappointed or angry they were with each relevant detail of the vast plan. Their leaders and staffs could immediately notify their own members across the country about threatening features of the plan, run press conferences, and lobby in Congress for changes. Well-endowed and vitally threatened groups, such as the Health Insurance Association of America, the association of smaller insurers who might have been put out of business had the Clinton plan passed, could also fund public relations campaigns designed to influence public opinion against the Clinton overhaul. In the end, according to a study by the Center for Public Integrity, health care reform would become "the most heavily lobbied legislative initiative in recent U.S. history." During 1993 and 1994, "hundreds of special interests cumulatively . . . [spent] in excess of $100 million to influence the outcome of this public policy issue."[41]

At first, the complaints of the many groups that had a stake in the existing health care system had little influence on public opinion or political observers. These complaints were understood to be opening gambits in bargaining over the details of legislation to be hammered out in Congress. President Clinton himself kept saying that he was prepared to make changes. Most early critiques of the Clinton plan were accompanied by disclaimers that their sponsors joined the president in wanting comprehensive reforms of some sort.

From very early on, however, hints of a much more hard-edged, total, and sincerely ideological opposition from the right wing of the Republican party were detectable. Soon after the president's September speech, House Republican Whip Newt Gingrich "promised an attack over costs and big-government inefficiency."[42] The October 13 issue of the *Wall Street Journal* carried a mocking letter from conservative Republican Dick Armey on "Your Future Health Plan."[43] According to Representative Armey, far from promoting a "streamlined and simpler system" as it promised, "the Clinton health plan would create fifty-nine new federal programs or bureaucracies, expand twenty others, impose seventy-nine new federal mandates, and make major changes in the tax code . . . [T]he Clinton plan is a bureaucratic nightmare that will ultimately result in higher taxes, reduced efficiency, restricted choice, longer lines, and a much, much bigger federal government." Cleverly, Armey accompanied his letter with a "flow chart" and "Clinton plan glossary" allegedly illustrating the hierarchical and ramified administrative leviathon that would hover over hapless "patients" should the Clinton plan be enacted. The Armey chart (or cousins to it) soon appeared on television, inspired cartoonists and editorialists, and became a staple of attacks on the Clinton plan.

Toward the end of 1993, right-wing Republicans realized that demonizing and then totally defeating the Clinton plan could splendidly serve their ideological fortunes within their own party, as well as the Republican partisan interest in weakening the Democrats as a prelude to winning control of Congress and the presidency. William Kristol of the Project for the Republican Future started to issue a steady stream of strategy memos urging all-out partisan warfare. Public support for the Clinton plan had begun to erode since September, Kristol pointed out, and "an aggressive and uncompromising counterstrategy" by the Republicans could ultimately kill the plan if it convinced middle-class Americans that there really was not a national health care crisis, after all. Noting that polls showed most Americans to be satisfied with their personal health care, Kristol argued that "Republicans should insistently convey the message that mandatory health alliances and government price controls will destroy the character, quality, and inventiveness of American health care."[44]

During 1994 the hard-line conservative attack on Clinton's Health Security plan brought together more and more allies and channeled resources and support toward antigovernment conservatives within the Republican Party. Ideologues and think tanks launched lurid attacks on Clinton's health reform plan.[45] The National Federation of Independent Businesses and other associations mobilized against the proposed "employer mandate."[46] Portrayals of the Clinton plan as a bureaucratic takeover by welfare-state liberals were regular grist for Rush Limbaugh and other right-wing hosts of hundreds of news-talk radio programs that reach tens of millions of listeners (indeed more than half of voters surveyed at polling places in the November 1994 election said they tuned to such shows, and the most frequent listeners voted Republican by a 3 to 1 ratio).[47]

Similarly, Christian Coalition groups, already attacking Bill and Hillary Clinton on cultural issues, began to devote substantial resources to the antihealth reform crusade. On February 15, 1994, Ralph Reed, the coalition's executive director, "announced that it was beginning a $1.4 million campaign to build grass-roots opposition to the Clinton plan," with tactics to "include 30 million postcards to Congress distributed to 60,000 churches; radio commercials in 40 congressional districts and print advertisements in 30 newspapers."[48] Moderate Republicans who had initially been inclined to work out some sort of compromise began to backpedal in the face of such antireform pressures from within their own party. And interest groups whose leaders had been prepared to bargain over reforms soon were pressured by constituents and Republican leaders to back off from cooperation with the Clinton administration or congressional Democrats.[49]

Despite all the resources—money, moral commitment, and grass-roots communication networks—that the conservative right could mobilize, the question remains why such attacks proved as influential as they did over the course of 1994. Middle-class Americans were (and remain) concerned about both the security of their access to affordable health care and the overall state of the nation's health financing system. Centrist Democrat Bill Clinton had done his best to define a market-oriented, minimally disruptive approach to national health care reform, and his plan was initially well received. Nevertheless, by midsummer 1994, and on through the November election, many middle-class citizens—not members of far-right groups, but independents, moderate Democrats and Republicans, and former Perot voters—had come to perceive the Clinton plan as a misconceived "big government" effort that might threaten the quality of U.S. health care for people like themselves.

Of course, 1994 is hardly the first time when political conservatives and business groups have used vivid antigovernment rhetoric to attack Democratically sponsored social programs. For example, back in the 1930s conservatives argued that the enactment of social security would end the American way of life. Congress passed it anyway. But while debating social security in the 1930s, Franklin D. Roosevelt and the Democrats faced a public mood and an overall governmental situation very different from those President Clinton faced as he fashioned and fought for his Health Security program. It is not just that Democrats enjoyed much greater electoral and congressional majorities in 1935—after all, many Democrats back then were southern conservatives who often opposed federal government initiatives. The more important differences between social security and health security have to do with the kinds of governmental activities they called for, and how their program designs related to stakeholders in the given policy area.

Some officials and experts involved in planning the social security legislation introduced in 1934 wanted to include a provision for health insurance, but President Roosevelt and his advisers wisely decided to set that aside. Because physicians and the American Medical Association were ideologically opposed to governmental social provision, and were organizationally present in every congressional district, Roosevelt feared that they might sink the entire social security bill if health insurance were included.[50] Instead, social security focused on unemployment and old-age insurance and on public assistance.

Parts of social security called for new payroll taxes, yet these taxes were tiny, and came when most U.S. employees paid few taxes and were worried mainly about getting or holding onto jobs. Of course, business leaders hated the new taxes; but in the midst of the Great Depression business opposition carried little weight with the public or elected officials and could be overridden. Beyond promising new insurance protections to the employed, social security also offered federal subsidies to public assistance programs that already existed, or were being enacted, by most of the states. Roosevelt administration policymakers wanted to accompany the new subsidies with a modicum of national administrative supervision, but Congress stripped most such prerogatives out of the bill before it became law. In the end, the Social Security Act mostly promised to distribute money. Citizens and state and local governments were wooed with promised benefits and not threatened with the reorganization of services to which they already felt accustomed.[51]

The contrast between the environment in which social security was enacted and that facing President Clinton's Health Security proposal could hardly be sharper. Clinton's plan was formulated during the "post-Reagan" political and governmental era, when taxes have been electorally anathema and public budgeting extraordinarily tight. Thus the proposed Health Security legislation was deliberately designed to offer little new federal revenue to most people or groups.[52] What is more, the U.S. health care system was already crowded with many institutional stakeholders with a large stake in the financing and delivery of health care. In addition, most middle-class employees already had health insurance coverage of some sort. Although the Clinton plan offered coverage to millions of uninsured, and promised increased security to the already insured, it also entailed a lot of new regulations that would push and prod insurance companies, health care providers, employers, state governments, and employees themselves. These new regulations were designed in an intricate and fairly tight way precisely in order to ensure that rising private and public health care costs really would come down. This was the rationale for including both caps on insurance premiums and mandatory regional purchasing alliances.

Historically, Americans have been perfectly happy to benefit from federal government spending and even to pay taxes to finance spending that is generous and benefits the privileged groups and citizens, not just the poor.[53] Such benefits are especially appealing if they flow in administratively streamlined and relatively automatic ways. But Americans dislike federal government regulations not accompanied by generous monetary payoffs. Ironically, precisely because Bill Clinton, a reformist Democrat, was working so hard to save money, he inadvertently ended up designing a health reform plan that appeared to promise lots of new regulations without widespread payoffs. Established participants in the current U.S. health care system became increasingly worried that the

Clinton plan might squeeze or reorganize customary ways of delivering, financing, or receiving health care. The right-wing critique of meddlesome governmental "bureaucracy" resonated so widely because it focused such worries.

A final feature of the situation in 1993–94 also helps to explain what may have happened to the Clinton plan in the eyes of average citizens. Not only did the Clinton plan end up provoking worries about federal regulations without payoffs, it also took on the baggage of whatever fears people had about the spread of "managed health care." The Clinton plan aimed to save public and private money in large part by using federal and state regulations of the insurance market to encourage the spread of high-quality managed care forms of health service delivery. Such delivery forms were already well established in a few states, but were hardly present in most, especially in the South and in many parts of the East.[54] When Clinton's Health Security plan was being formulated and launched in 1992 and 1993, many Americans remained "unenthusiastic" about the notion of controlling costs through managed care and managed competition.[55] Managed care was especially new and likely to be seen as worrisome by well-insured, upper-middle-class people in the East, and particularly in New York City, the heart of the nation's media empires and the nub of the constituency of Senate Finance Committee Chairman Daniel Patrick Moynihan. Journalists and other writers inflamed Americans' worries about managed care, falsely implying that low-cost and low-quality versions of such care was what President Clinton had in mind for everyone.[56]

From a broad historical perspective, in sum, Clinton's Health Security plan had many strikes against it from the start. The very societal and governmental contexts that originally made it quite rational for a centrist Democratic president to choose a reform approach emphasizing firmly regulated "competition within a budget" simultaneously made that approach ideal for political countermobilization by antigovernmental conservatives. The president and his allies could have done a better job than they did at explaining the regulatory mechanisms in their plan. But even if the Clinton administration had communicated more effectively, the Health Security plan launched so propitiously in September 1993 might still have gone down to a defeat that backfired badly against the Democrats. The bedrock fact is that the Clinton plan promised too much cost-cutting regulation and not enough payoffs to organized groups and middle-class citizens well treated by the existing U.S. health system.

Could They Have Done It Differently?

Defeat breeds contempt—and lots of Monday-morning quarterbacking. With unabashed arrogance, many have not hesitated to declare what President Clinton should have done differently. The alternatives most often invoked seem unworkable, however.

Adherents of the single-payer approach to health care reform are sure that the president should have championed their cause. The central ideas are easy to explain, they argue, because a single-payer plan reduces bureaucracy, cuts costs, and lets patients choose doctors and hospitals freely. I have long been sympathetic to single payer as a readily understandable way to finance health care for all. In retrospect, however, I do not find it plausible that President Clinton would or could have taken this route. Given his centrist-Democrat leanings and fear of raising taxes, I cannot conceive of Bill Clinton sincerely embracing a single-payer plan. What is more, the same restricted means of political communication that made it hard for the Clinton administration to tell the American public about its approach would have made it equally or more difficult to convey an accurate portrayal of single payer, which could easily have been caricatured as a "budget buster" and a "government takeover" of medical care.

Conservative Democrats and other self-styled "middle-of-the roaders" have been equally sure that Clinton was unwise to push for universal coverage. They think the president should have gone for incremental market reforms along the lines proposed by former Tennessee Representative Jim Cooper, supposedly cementing bipartisan support at the start.[57] But it makes no sense for a Democratic president to advocate changes in health insurance that leave many low-income workers in the cold. Likewise, it was (and is) dangerous for a Democrat to advocate minor regulatory changes in the existing private insurance market that may leave more and more middle-income Americans facing ever-higher premiums for the same, or less, coverage. I also question whether Democrats and moderate Republicans in Congress would have joined any specific presidentially sponsored plan in 1993, without lengthy debates over alternative schemes. Republican moderates were always under pressure not to undermine their party's interest in discrediting the Democratic president. Key congressional Democrats, moreover, were unlikely to join any disciplined collective endeavor, because many had health plans of their own or were committee chairs determined to have a piece of the legislative action.

In light of the analysis I have offered here, I see other retrospective possibilities. I offer them in a spirit of humility, for I am not at all sure that any course of action could have succeeded. Conceivably, President Clinton could have tried to spell out competition within a budget through a ten-to-twelve person bipartisan commission. Such a commission would have had to include key congressional players from both parties, experts willing to explain inclusive versions of managed competition, and carefully selected institutional actors (such as a big business executive, an insurance company leader, a physician, a union leader, and someone from the American Association of Retired Persons). The president could have given the commission a preliminary proposal to revise or otherwise structured its mandate and staffing to make it likely that the commission would report out something resembling the plan he ended up with—although a commission would probably have designed an approach emphasizing insurance regulations, health alliances for smaller businesses only, and some tax-financed subsidies for small business and low-income workers, but *not* mandatory health alliances for larger employers or premium caps for private insurance. Had such a commission succeeded, the president would have been able to claim a broader, even bipartisan, mandate from the start, perhaps educating public opinion and focusing congressional efforts more effectively.

But a commission approach might not have worked. How would the president have decided whom to include (and whom to leave out), while still keeping the commission to a workable size for actual deliberations? Key non-Democrats might well have refused to join, or the entire effort might have bogged down in intractable disagreements. Institutionally speaking, it is important to keep in mind that the United States is ill suited for corporate-style policy formulation.[58] Legislative procedures through which any commission recommendations must ultimately wend their way are so protracted and complex that dissenters have many opportunities to break apart, or get around, early bargains. And U.S. societal groups, including big business, are *not* organized into disciplined peak associations whose leaders can negotiate reliable bargains on behalf of all members. Thus President Clinton could have appointed a commission to work out a legislative plan, only to see a relatively consensual proposal emerge and later fall apart—as congressional committees dissected it and affected constituencies undercut the deals originally made by the institutional actors who served on the commission.

Another possibility is that Bill Clinton could have gone forward with the first approach he temporarily advocated during his presidential campaign, a version of play or pay that incorporated promises of eventual cost controls.[59] By 1992 some key congressional players and Democratic constituencies supported and understood play or pay, so it might have been easier to rally reform-advocates around it. Arguably, too, the president could more readily have explained the central mechanism of this approach to citizens—and to the employers and physicians who might, in turn, have signaled acceptance or tolerance to employees and patients. Every employer, the president could have declared, has to pitch in somehow, either by sharing costs or insurance with employees, or by paying a modest fee to help cover the uninsured. "Pay" fees for small businesses could have been set low early on, and low rates might have provoked less ideological countermobilization than a regulatory employer mandate (which was easily cast as "bureaucratic intrusion"). President Clinton could also have encouraged health purchasing cooperatives as voluntary cost-controlling mechanisms for business and public sector participants in the revised health system. He could, in short, have made a modest start at creating "health alliances," hoping that they would eventually come to be seen as familiar and desirable agents promoting lower costs and higher quality in a gradually transformed health care system.

Like the loose version of managed competition that might have emerged from a Clinton-appointed commission, this sort of play-or-pay approach (seasoned with voluntary health alliances) would have required the promise of greater federal revenues at the start. President Clinton would have had to sweeten the transition for insurance companies and all businesses, acknowledging that universal heath coverage costs money—something that the American public believed all along.[60] President Clinton would have had to give up the notion that comprehensive health care reform could be sold, up front, as a federal deficit-cutting measure. Back in the spring and summer of 1993, the Clinton administration thought it was impossible to put much new federal money into health care, and they were certainly obsessed with federal deficit cutting. That is why the Clinton task force worked out such an intricate and tightly regulated version of managed competition within a budget. But it would have been politically wiser to be initially less fiscally conservative—or else, to chop away parts of the existing federal budget to free up revenues for universal coverage.[61] Once all Americans were covered, however minimally, the president could have changed the emphasis to cost controls.

Conclusion

Very possibly, Americans who favor governmentally mediated universal health insurance have just had—and lost—their last opportunity for achieving it. Six times over the course of the twentieth century—in the late 1910s, during the 1930s, in the late 1940s, during the mid-1960s, during the 1970s, and in the early 1990s—reform-minded professionals pushed for government financing of health care for all, or large categories, of Americans. Again and again comprehensive plans for "rational" and "cost-efficient" reforms were drawn up, amidst considerable or great optimism that at last "the time was ripe" for the United States to join the rest of the civilized democratic-industrial world in providing broad health care coverage for its citizens.[62] Only once did such efforts succeed, during the mid-1960s, when medicare and medicaid were enacted at the height of the Great Society.[63]

Not only did that single success come at a juncture when liberal Democrats, very briefly, enjoyed the kind of ideological elan and congressional leverage that conservative Republicans enjoy in 1994, but the mid-1960s were also a time when Americans overwhelmingly trusted the federal government to do good and effective things, when Americans even briefly thought that the federal government might wage a winning "war on poverty." Perhaps even more important, this was a time when social security, a universal social insurance program, could serve as a positive model for *how* the federal government could extend nondemeaning health security to all of the elderly.

Health reformers searching for optimistic historical analogies often take heart in the example of President Harry S. Truman. After his campaign for universal health insurance was defeated in 1948–50, Truman and his allies devised an "incremental" strategy that eventually led to the enactment of medicare in 1965.[64] Reformers dream of doing this again, perhaps pushing toward universal health insurance by next focusing on extending coverage to all American children.[65] But today the policy legacies and governmental conditions are not as favorable as they were in the wake of Truman's presidency. Now a fully mature program, social security, has become since the 1980s an object of persistent criticism by fiscal conservatives in the Concord Coalition and beyond who consider its universalism to be "too expensive" for the federal government to preserve in the future.[66] Current struggles in Washington focus on how to cut taxes and federal spending, not on their gradual expansion, as was the case under moderate Republicans and Democrats during the 1950s and early 1960s. Democrats may look back wistfully to Harry Truman, cherishing his improbable electoral triumphs and the progressive legacies that grew even out of his policy failures. But Truman and his postwar era of U.S. governance are dead and gone.

As Henry Aaron explains in the introduction to this book, problems of receding coverage and rising costs will likely worsen during the coming years in the U.S. health care system. Conservative efforts to give more and more leverage to private insurance companies will, in my view, eventually lead to popular disillusionment. But even an issue like health security—central as it is for many Americans—will not, in itself, bring about a political revival for Democrats or a resurgence of faith in government. As the failure of President Clinton's courageous effort shows, the future of inclusive health reform depends on Americans' coming to believe that government can offer minimally intrusive solutions to the heartfelt needs of individuals and families. If progressives are actually to achieve universal health care coverage in America's future, it will be because new rationales for the role of government, and new majority political alliances, have been achieved first. I believe that such new rationales and alliances can be forged, because most Americans still want government to function efficiently, compassionately, and fairly on behalf of everyone. Yet the new rationales for government, as well as new majority political alliances, will necessarily have to be achieved on bases very different from the ones that prevailed in the aftermath of the New Deal.

Comments on Chapters 2 and 3

Margaret Weir: From the institutional and historical vantage point taken by Hugh Heclo and Theda Skocpol, the Clinton reform failed not because of any minor strategic or tactical error but from the weight of the institutional and political obstacles the administration confronted. My comments center on four aspects of the process, some of which the chapters address very persuasively. Others, I think, need more attention.

The first puzzle about the Clinton's health reform effort is why the administration undertook such an ambitious reform in the first place. After reading these two chapters, particularly Heclo's portrayal of the obstacles in the broad context of policy innovation in the United States, the inescapable question is why the administration with so few political and environmental resources undertook what seems, with hindsight, a tremendously risky task.

Heclo does not address this question directly but suggests that the decision to push comprehensive health reform extended the campaign mode into governing. Skocpol points to favorable public opinion polls, but it would be useful to know more of the administration's thinking about these polls. Did they overinterpret them or misread them as has been suggested by others at the conference, or was the administration more aware of the risks than the discussion here has given it credit for?

Missing from our discussion, and from these chapters to some extent, is an analysis of why the administration decided to take these risks. To understand this decision requires an examination of how health care reform fit into the broader political strategy of the administration. Central to that strategy was a conscious attempt to build a new Democratic majority by combining the support of the middle class and lower-income groups. Enacting policies that would benefit both groups was a key element of this strategy; health care was the most promising policy to achieve these political objectives. Health reform had many advantages: it did not evoke the racial divisions that have troubled the Democratic party since the 1960s, and it was an "economic issue," not a social issue, as Drew Altman notes in his comments.

Understanding how health reform fit into this political strategy is critical to understanding what the administration sought to achieve and why taking such a risk was plausible. Like Franklin D. Roosevelt, Clinton sought to use policy to consolidate a new political coalition.

The second puzzling aspect of the health care reform process is why the administration chose the particular plan that it did and what the political consequences of that choice were.

One of the most interesting arguments both Heclo and Skocpol make is that Clinton's efforts to anticipate political obstacles ironically left him with a plan and a process that made it very difficult to sustain either mass or elite political support. Skocpol begins and Heclo ends by pointing to a distinctive feature of the political process that characterized health care reform. The approach to reform adopted during the campaign—managed competition with cost controls—embodied a political compromise, namely, the desire to achieve universal coverage without big government and without taxes. Because it believed that this formula resolved major political contradictions, the administration assumed the job of showing that its ideas were technically sound and of selling them to the public. In so doing, it shortcircuited the political process.

These chapters suggest that the administration wedded itself to an approach that seemed to solve analytical problems but that tied its hands politically. Heclo points to the role of pollsters and likens the health care reform process to campaigning rather than public debate. Skocpol similarly argues that the plan tied the administration's hands at the public level because the policy could not be explained simply. She stresses that there were no available analogies to the mechanisms the administration proposed and argues that the administration ended up simply advertising its plan, rather than promoting genuine public discussion. I believe her characterization of public reasoning as one of finding plausible analogies better describes public deliberation than does the rational process laid out in the Yankelovich chapter. After all, Roosevelt did not explain that social security was a generational transfer in which citizens had to give up current income. He said it was like having your own savings account.

Again, a broader perspective on Clinton's version of new Democratic strategy is helpful in understanding why these mechanisms were selected. At its most ambitious, this strategy sought to overcome the recurring left-right divisions that had blocked major Democratic social policy initiatives since the 1960s. The aim was to shift the axes of debate to allow movement. Clinton's new Democratic strategy had three components: to counter distrust of federal government, policy would work through market mechanisms or the states, and it would "reinvent" government; to counter such "wedge" social issues as crime, race, and family values, policy would set clear expectations for individual responsibility and impose sanctions on bad behavior; to counter arguments that social interventions were too costly, policy would highlight the long-term benefits of "investing" in people.

This set of ideas had problems when it hit political reality.

The first problem was that public aversion to taxes and elite concern about the deficit forced the immediate abandonment of the investment strategy. In health care, as both chapters note, this retreat deprived Democrats of the ability to provide sweeteners to ease the transition to their system. In this regard, Heclo stresses the fundamental difference between policy fields that are already crowded with institutional attachments and entrenched interests. "Big bangs" of policy innovation, such as social insurance for the aged, come in policy areas in which the federal government does not have to contend with interests already attached to a particular way of doing things.

A second problem posed by this new Democratic approach is the difficulty that the president had in articulating what reinvented government would mean in specific policy areas. The administration seemed more intent on avoiding the tag of "big government" than in articulating and defending its distinctive approach to government. As Skocpol notes, in the health care debate the administration never really defended the regulatory approach that was central to its plan.

In sum, Clinton's strategy sought to achieve Democratic political and substantive goals in a new setting hostile to "old Democratic" methods. But because these ideas could not easily be translated into policy instruments, they created their own problems.

The third aspect of the political process that bears examination is the effects of the institutions through which the public and elite debate had to proceed. Heclo and Skocpol make an important contribution by framing the public and the elite debate in terms of the institutions, organizations, and social networks through which debate occurs. Skocpol points out that grass-roots communication is dominated by right wing groups opposed to the health plan. The virtual disappearance of locally based party organizations and the weakness of organized labor handicapped a Democratic president with an activist agenda in his efforts at shaping the public debate.

Neither chapter says enough about one central institution, Congress, although each raises questions about the congressional role. Skocpol needs to distinguish the problems that were a product of the institutional fragmentation in Congress from those that stemmed from ideological differences with the president. In retrospect, it seems that there were centrist Democrats and there were old Democrats, but no new Democrats of Clinton's stripe in Congress. The story of intraparty ideological differences needs to be told, along with that of the institutional fragmentation of Congress.

Heclo argues that the gestation period for health care was too short: the ideas that became central to Clinton's plan were not part of a prolonged period of sorting out. He contrasts the early 1990s with the 1950s, when Congress worked through the issues in many policy innovations later adopted in the 1960s. But this comparison raises the question, why were the 1980s not a similar period in which policy alternatives could be worked out? How have changes in Congress affected the prospects for such gestation periods? Did more extreme partisanship in Congress prevent such policy discussion or did the complacency of congressional Democrats (to which both chapters refer) block debate? Another possibility is that the more plebiscitary nature of presidential politics has disconnected presidential politics from policy debates in Congress.

A fourth and final point concerns the broader ideological and partisan context within which health care reform took place. Neither chapter articulates this context with sufficient precision. From a historical perspective, the current political period resembles the 1930s more than it does any era since. As in the 1930s, two sharply different organizing views about the role of government in the economy and society are vying with each other. Put simply, the antigovernment, promarket ideology, always strong in the Republican party, has grown stronger since 1980. In contrast, the Democratic party remains attached to the belief that government can and should correct problems that emerge in the market, although Democrats have not always been forthright about articulating this view. Among such problems are growing economic inequality and insecurity.

Such fundamental ideological disagreement raises doubts about the possibility for rational discussion and political compromise among elites. Perhaps there was a window of opportunity for building a bipartisan consensus among moderates, but I think the quiescence of the antigovernment elements in the Republican party early in the health care debate should not be taken for powerlessness or willingness to go along. Their concerted effort to discredit and destroy the administration's health plan once it became vulnerable, through grass-roots mobilizing and reverse lobbying, suggests that they would have strongly resisted any "middle-of-the road" reform.

In the political context of intense ideological conflict, health care reform assumed greater significance than it would have carried in another setting. Even modest health care reform would not have been just an incremental reform but rather a political victory for a distinctive view of government's role.

James J. Mongan: The chapters by Hugh Heclo and Theda Skocpol seemed to me very solid and comprehensive reviews of last year's debate. Both offered a thorough analysis of many substantive and political factors that led to the demise of health reform. And both are well rooted in the history of past legislative struggles.

But, in a sense, the strength of these chapters may also be their weakness. In their comprehensiveness they gloss over, or fail to focus on, what I believe to be the root cause of failure.

Before continuing my critique and analysis, I will say a word about my background, bias, and perspective. I do not possess any academic credentials in this area. I have, however, worked on this issue for twenty-five years. I have had three opportunities to see and participate in this debate from a front row seat—first as a staffer for the Senate Finance Committee when Congress debated the Nixon health insurance proposal in 1974, then as a White House staff person when the Carter proposal was debated in 1980, and finally as moderator and faculty coordinator for the Senate Finance Committee weekend health care retreat last March.

The key lesson I learned during these twenty-five years is that the health reform debate, in Congress at least, is not now, and never has been, primarily about health care—it is about the *financing* of health care. It is about who pays. Here I disagree with Heclo. The debate has never centered on benefits, or alliances, or cost controls, or markets. The debate has always started and ended on financing—who pays. This is where health reform died last year. The most important cause of the death of health reform was that avoiding tax increases and their thinly veiled cousin, employer mandates, took priority over expanding coverage.

Having seen this dynamic play out in 1974 and 1980, I prepared at the start of this round of debates in mid-1993 a chart that displays how the deterioration of the drive for universal coverage would play out. It describes in detail the elaborate congressional dance away from any hint of taxes or mandates.

In 1974 and 1980 this dance played out in executive and legislative back rooms generally outside of public view. In 1994 we watched it play out on the front page of the newspaper.

President Clinton started—as had Presidents Nixon and Carter before him—with a proposal to achieve universal coverage financed primarily through an employer mandate. My chart, constructed in September 1993, shows the various compromises that were to be put forth in an attempt to assemble a majority in favor of an employer mandate: first, limiting the benefits and thereby the costs of a mandate, then excluding small employers from the mandate, then extending the phase-in period for the mandate, and, finally, making the mandate conditional upon future circumstances (figure 3-1, part A).

Even with these compromises it was predictably impossible to assemble a majority, and thus the employer mandate was abandoned. That led to a brief flirtation with a moderate Republican option, an individual mandate. But the individual mandate predictably failed because it required large subsidies, which required large tax increases.

So my assumption, well before the debate began, was that Congress

Figure 3-1. *Slippery Slope from Universality to Diminished Coverage*

Part A

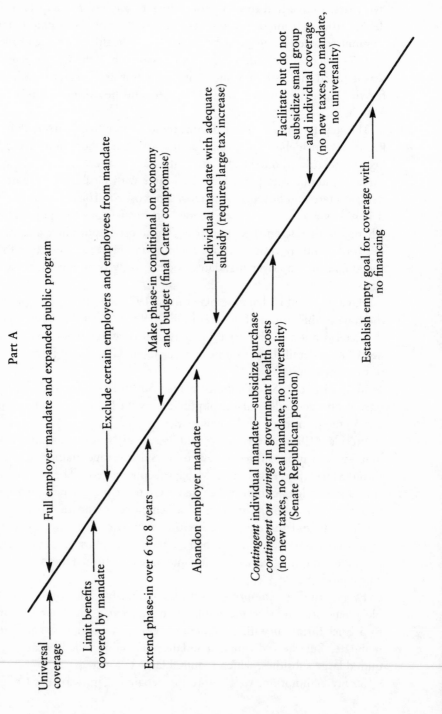

Universal coverage

Full employer mandate and expanded public program

Limit benefits covered by mandate

Exclude certain employers and employees from mandate

Extend phase-in over 6 to 8 years

Make phase-in conditional on economy and budget (final Carter compromise)

Abandon employer mandate

Individual mandate with adequate subsidy (requires large tax increase)

Contingent individual mandate—subsidize purchase *contingent on savings* in government health costs (no new taxes, no real mandate, no universality) (Senate Republican position)

Facilitate but do not subsidize small group and individual coverage (no new taxes, no mandate, no universality)

Establish empty goal for coverage with no financing

Part B

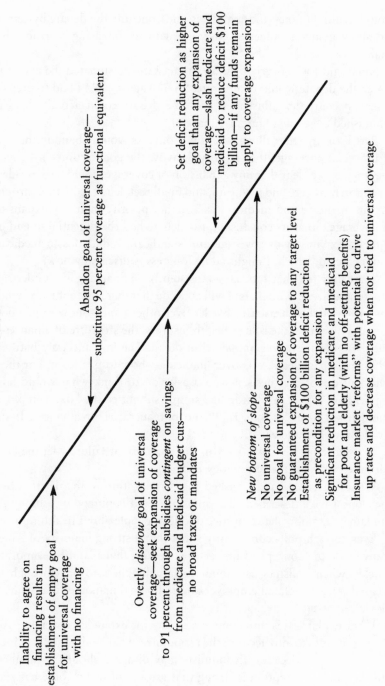

Inability to agree on
financing results in
establishment of empty goal
for universal coverage
with no financing

Overtly *disavow* goal of universal
coverage—seek expansion of coverage
to 91 percent through subsidies *contingent* on savings
from medicare and medicaid budget cuts—
no broad taxes or mandates

Abandon goal of universal coverage—
substitute 95 percent coverage as functional equivalent

Set deficit reduction as higher
goal than any expansion of
coverage—slash medicare and
medicaid to reduce deficit $100
billion—if any funds remain
apply to coverage expansion

New bottom of slope
No universal coverage
No goal for universal coverage
No guaranteed expansion of coverage to any target level
Establishment of $100 billion deficit reduction
  as precondition for any expansion
Significant reduction in medicare and medicaid
  for poor and elderly (with no off-setting benefits)
Insurance market "reforms" with potential to drive
up rates and decrease coverage when not tied to universal coverage

Source: James J. Mongan, M.D., part A, September 1993; part B, August 1994.

would avoid all taxes and mandates and conclude the debate by setting an empty goal for universal coverage with no financing to reach that goal.

Some said I was overly cynical. In fact I underestimated the extent to which the debate would deteriorate. So in August 1994 I had to prepare a second chart that illustrated how the debate could actually lead to diminished coverage (figure 3-1, part B).

Part B of my chart illustrates how Congress would abandon the goal of universal coverage, then overtly disavow the goal of universal coverage, then make clear that any expansion of coverage would be dependent on cuts in medicare and medicaid, and finally set deficit reduction through cuts in medicare and medicaid as a higher priority than any expansion of coverage. So at its conclusion, the debate had the potential to end up with no expansion of coverage and significant reductions in medicare and medicaid, which, I might add, Congress is discussing now.

Some may feel that I focus too insistently on financing and understate the complexity of the debate. I will concede that there undoubtedly would have been pitched legislative battles over other issues—how to pay doctors and hospitals, the role of health insurers, the structure of alliances—but these debates never happened in detail. The first and only battle in 1994, as in past years, was over financing—how to pay for it. For those who still doubt my thesis, I would ask you to think what would have happened if President Clinton had simply submitted the Nixon employer mandate—150 pages, not 1,500, no bureaucracies or alliances. It still would have been defeated.

In a sense my chart shows you the anatomy of failure—let me close with the causes or the physiology of failure.

What "invisible hand" pushed the deterioration of the debate down the slope I have described? The invisible hand is purely and simply the fundamental ambivalence of the American people about health reform.

Even though polls consistently show that a strong majority of Americans favor the concept of universal coverage, that majority evaporates quickly when pollsters ask about their willingness to pay through increased taxes or related employer and individual mandates that come to be viewed as the equivalent of taxes.

What explains this unwillingness to pay for expanded coverage? Any answer must take into account the economic, social, and political context of the past two decades. Economists may disagree about the numbers, but the public perception is strong that growth of real income has stagnated—that families are working harder to stay even. The social context is that people tend to take for granted the progress achieved through social insurance programs like medicare and social security; they perceive little progress or achievement from welfare expenditures targeted to low-income people. Politically, and this is very important, politicians from the courthouse to the White House have played to an antitax sentiment and have convinced Americans and American business that they are staggering under oppressive taxation that saps most productive effort. Although there is little evidence, in comparison with other countries, to support this belief, it is widely and deeply held.

This economic, social, and political climate fosters a self-centered-ness—a focus on the individual's needs rather than the community's needs. Some liberals might use a harsher, more grating word—selfish-ness—to describe this state of mind. But many conservatives would use the phrase "rugged individualism" to describe it and defend the concept with pride.

I am not a philosopher. I do not pretend to know at what point rugged individualism becomes self-centeredness or self-centeredness becomes selfishness, or what the difference between those terms may really be. But I believe that somewhere in here is where health reform died.

And I further believe that until we as a nation make the right diagnosis and begin an honest dialogue about our national values, about the balance between self-interest and community interest, we will not see our nation join almost all others in guaranteeing health coverage to all of our people.

Notes

1. Quotations in this paragraph from the president's speech come from the prepared text, as reprinted in Erik Eckholm, ed., *Solving America's Health-Care Crisis* (Times Books, 1993), p. 302.

2. Paul Starr, "What Happened to Health Care Reform?" *American Prospect*, no. 20 (Winter 1995), pp. 20–31; Lawrence R. Jacobs and Robert Y. Shapiro, "Don't Blame the Public for Failed Health Care Reform," *Journal of Health Politics, Policy and Law*, vol. 20 (Summer 1995), p. 418, table 3; and Adam Clymer, "The Clinton Health Plan Is Alive on Arrival," *New York Times*, October 3, 1993, p. E3.

3. Clymer, "The Clinton Plan."

4. *Contract with America: The Bold Plan by Rep. Newt Gingrich, Rep. Dick Armey and the House Republicans to Change the Nation*, edited by Ed Gillespie and Bob Shellhas (New York Times Books, Random House, 1994). For the outlook from which current initiatives flow, see Newt Gingrich, *Window of*

Opportunity: A Blueprint for the Future (New York: Tom Doherty Associates, 1984), especially chaps. 4–6; and Newt Gingrich, *To Renew America* (Harper Collins, 1995).

5. Polling and focus group data supporting this appear in Stanley B. Greenberg and others, *Third Force: Why Independents Turned Against Democrats—and How to Win Them Back* (Washington: Democratic Leadership Council, November 1994), p. 6.

6. "National Election Night Survey," news release (Menlo Park, Calif.: Henry J. Kaiser Family Foundation, November 15, 1994).

7. Robert J. Blendon and Karen Donelan, "Public Opinion and Efforts to Reform the U.S. Health Care System: Confronting Issues of Cost-Containment and Access to Care," *Stanford Law and Policy Review*, vol. 3 (Fall 1991), pp. 146–54. The authors add, "Since 1989, nine national and statewide surveys indicate that between 60 and 72% of Americans favor such a plan. Some of these figures indicate that current public enthusiasm for a comprehensive national health insurance program exceeds the level of popular support for Medicare in the year prior to its enactment. In fact, a recent Roper Organization . . . survey indicates that 69% of Americans surveyed approve extending Medicare coverage to all citizens."

8. Dale Russakoff, "How Wofford Rode Health Care to Washington," *Washington Post National Weekly Edition*, November 25–December 1, 1991, pp. 14–15; and Robert J. Blendon and others, "The 1991 Pennsylvania Senate Race and National Health Insurance," *Journal of American Health Policy*, vol. 2 (January–February 1992), pp. 21–24.

9. Blendon and Donelan, "Public Opinion and Efforts to Reform," p. 147.

10. A list of "Proposals for Universal Health Coverage Introduced in the 102nd Congress Through August 2, 1991, and Selected Recent Bills" appears in Robert J. Blendon, Jennifer N. Edwards, and Andrew L. Hyams, "Making the Critical Choices," *Journal of the American Medical Association*, vol. 267 (May 13, 1992), pp. 2514–16, table 6. See also Mark A. Peterson, "Momentum toward Health Care Reform in the U.S. Senate," *Journal of Health Politics, Policy and Law*, vol. 17 (Fall 1992), pp. 553–73.

11. A selection of such proposals is outlined in Blendon, Edwards, and Hyams, "Critical Choices," pp. 2512–13, table 5.

12. American Medical Association, *Health Access America: The AMA Proposal to Improve Access to Affordable, Quality Health Care* (Chicago, Ill.: AMA, 1990); and James F. Todd and others, "Health Access America—Strengthening the U.S. Health Care System," *Journal of the American Medical Association*, vol. 265 (May 15, 1991), pp. 2503–06.

13. Blendon, Edwards, and Hyams, "Critical Choices," p. 2509.

14. Lawrence R. Jacobs and Robert Y. Shapiro, "Public Opinion's Tilt Against Private Enterprise," *Health Affairs*, vol. 13 (Spring I 1994), pp. 285–98.

15. The plans being discussed in the late winter, early spring of 1992 by Democratic presidential contenders Bill Clinton, Bob Kerrey, and Paul Tsongas are outlined in Blendon, Edwards, and Hyams, "Critical Choices," p. 2511, table 4.

16. Republican incremental proposals, and criticisms of them, are discussed

in Richard A. Knox, "Health Care Leaps to Top of Political Agenda," *Boston Globe*, December 29, 1991, pp. 1, 16.

17. For versions of single payer, see Kevin Grumbach and others, "Liberal Benefits, Conservative Spending: Physicians for a National Health Program," *Journal of the American Medical Association*, vol. 265 (May 15, 1991), pp. 2549–54; and Robert Kerrey, *Health USA Act of 1991* (Washington: U.S. Senate, 1991), which is explained in Robert Kerrey, "Why America Will Adopt Comprehensive Health Care Reform," *American Prospect*, no. 6 (Summer 1991), pp. 81–91.

18. Theodore R. Marmor and Jerry L. Mashaw, "Canada's Health Insurance and Ours: The Real Lessons, the Big Choices," *American Prospect*, no. 3 (Fall 1990), pp. 18–29.

19. An engaging story about Bill Clinton's brief consideration and quick rejection of single payer in November 1991 appears in Tom Hamburger, Ted Marmor, and Jon Meacham, "What the Death of Health Reform Teaches Us about the Press," *Washington Monthly* (November 1994), pp. 35–41.

20. For a cogent explication of the approach and its practical rationale, see Ronald Pollack and Phyllis Torda, "The Pragmatic Road Toward National Health Insurance," *American Prospect*, no. 6 (Summer 1991), pp. 92–100.

21. Peterson, "Momentum in Senate."

22. The Pepper Commission, *A Call for Action: Final Report* (Washington: U.S. Bipartisan Commission on Comprehensive Health Care, 1990), as explained in John D. Rockefeller IV, "A Call for Action: The Pepper Commission's Blueprint for Health Care Reform," *Journal of the American Medical Association*, vol. 265 (May 1991), pp. 2507–10; and in Judith Feder, "The Pepper Commission's Proposals," *Social Insurance Issues for the Nineties*, proceedings of the Third Conference of the National Academy of Social Insurance, edited by Paul N. Van de Water (Dubuque, Iowa: Kendall/Hunt, 1992), pp. 53–58. On the National Leadership Coalition, see Susan B. Garland, "Already, Big Business' Health Plan Isn't Feeling So Hot," *Business Week* , November 18, 1991, p. 48.

23. Bill Clinton for President Committee, "Bill Clinton's American Health Care Plan: National Health Insurance Reform to Cut Costs and Cover Everybody," typescript, January 1992. My copy of this statement, which I received from Clinton headquarters in April 1992, does not have a date. The original was produced in January 1992 during the New Hampshire primary according to Jacob Steward Hacker, "Setting the Health Reform Agenda: The Ascendance of Managed Competition," senior honors thesis, Harvard College, Committee on Degrees in Social Studies, November 1993, p. 111. My account of Clinton's embrace of managed competition during the presidential campaign draws insights from chapter 4 of this thesis, which is currently being revised for publication by Princeton University Press.

24. Hacker, "Setting the Agenda," pp. 111–12.

25. For overviews of the relevant ideas, see Alain Enthoven and Richard Kronick, "A Consumer-Choice Health Plan for the 1990s," *New England Journal of Medicine*, vol. 320 (January 5, 1989), pp. 29–37; John Garamendi, "California Health Care in the 21st Century: A Vision for Reform," Department of Insurance, State of California, February 1992; and Paul Starr and Walter A. Zelman, "A

Bridge to Compromise: Competition under Budget," *Health Affairs*, vol. 12 (Supplement 1993), pp. 7–23.

26. Cogent discussions of the practical and intellectual steps through which a "liberal synthesis" version of managed competition was worked out appear in Hacker, "Setting the Agenda," chaps. 2 and 3; and in the preface to Paul Starr, *The Logic of Health-Care Reform: Why and How the President's Plan Will Work*, revised and enlarged edition (Whittle Books, in association with Penguin Books, 1994).

27. Ordinary Americans care most about attaining secure protection and keeping their own insurance payments low, while experts and institutional leaders such as employers and politicians are obsessed with spending less overall and having each major organizational sector spend less on health care. See Robert J. Blendon, Tracey Stelzer Hyams, and John M. Benson, "Bridging the Gap between Expert and Public Views on Health Care Reform," *Journal of the American Medical Association*, vol. 269 (May 19, 1993), pp. 2573–78.

28. On Magaziner, see Robert Pear, "An Idealist's New Task: To Revamp Health Care," *New York Times*, February 25, 1993, p. A14.

29. The reasons why task force leaders said little to the media, and the problems this caused, are cogently discussed in James Fallows, "A Triumph of Misinformation," *Atlantic Monthly*, vol. 275 (January 1995), pp. 26–37.

30. Media concentration on the arcane Whitewater scandal made things worse in 1994, especially because trust in President Clinton and Hillary Clinton was undercut, and everyone was distracted from rational discussion of health care reform (on this point, see Kathleen Hall Jamieson, "Health Care Drowns in Whitewater," *Philadelphia Inquirer*, April 9, 1994, p. A7). But I do not believe that Whitewater was the principal cause of the erosion of public faith in the Health Security plan.

31. A time-line of the percentage of Americans, from 1958 to 1994, answering "always" or "most of the time" to the question "How much of the time . . . can you trust the government to do what is right?" appears in Everett Carl Ladd, ed., *America at the Polls, 1994* (University of Connecticut, Roper Center, 1995), p. 33.

32. Charles O. Jones, *The Presidency in a Separated System* (Brookings, 1994), chap. 5, pp. 147–81.

33. Interviews with Ira C. Magaziner, March 1, and May 3, 1995; confidential interview with a political adviser to the White House.

34. David R. Mayhew, *Placing Parties in American Politics: Organization, Electoral Settings, and Government Activity in the Twentieth Century* (Princeton University Press, 1986), pp. 308–32; and Marshall Ganz, "Voters in the Crosshairs: How Technology and the Market are Destroying Politics," *American Prospect*, no. 16 (Winter 1994), pp. 100–09.

35. Hamburger, Marmor, and Meacham, "What the Death of Reform Teaches Us about the Press"; Kathleen Hall Jamieson and Joseph Cappella, "Newspaper and Television Coverage of the Health Care Reform Debate, January 16–July 25, 1994," a report by the Annenberg Public Policy Center, funded by the Robert Wood Johnson Foundation, Philadelphia, Pa., August 12, 1994; and Joseph N. Cappella and Kathleen Hall Jamieson, "Public Cynicism and News Coverage in Campaigns

and Policy Debates: Three Field Experiments," p. 5, paper presented at the 1994 annual meeting of the American Political Science Association.

36. The account in this paragraph is based on an interview with Heather Booth, health care outreach coordinator at the Democratic National Committee. She was involved in the 1993–94 health reform campaign.

37. An excellent account of congressional maneuverings appears in Allen Schick, "How a Bill Didn't Become a Law," in *Intensive Care: How Congress Shapes Health Policy*, edited by Thomas E. Mann and Norman J. Ornstein (Brookings, 1995), pp. 227–72.

38. Lawrence R. Jacobs, *The Health of Nations: Public Opinion and the Making of American and British Health Policy* (Cornell University Press, 1993), chap. 9.

39. Blendon, Hyams, and Benson, "American Public and Critical Choices," p. 1543.

40. As, for example, in the explanatory pamphlet "Health Security: the President's Health Care Plan," which was distributed by the Clinton administration starting in the fall of 1993. Pages 8 and 9 of the pamphlet discuss "The System after Reform," describing health alliances as "groups of individuals, families, and local businesses who use their combined purchasing power to negotiate for high-quality, affordable health care." The word CHOICE appears like a mantra throughout the pamphlet. We are assured that "the President specifically rejected a government-run health care system and broad based taxes" and that the "U.S. Government will create a framework for reform and then get out of the way." We do not learn *how* the framework will be created.

41. Center for Public Integrity, *Well-Healed: Inside Lobbying for Health Care Reform* (Washington, 1994), p. 1.

42. Clymer, "Clinton Plan Alive," p. E3.

43. Dick Armey, "Your Future Health Plan," *Wall Street Journal*, October 13, 1993, p. A22.

44. William Kristol, "Defeating President Clinton's Health Care Proposal," typescript, Washington, Project for the Republican Future, December 2, 1993, pp. 1–4. See also Adam Meyerson, "Kristol Ball: William Kristol Looks at the Future of the GOP," *Policy Review*, no. 67 (Winter 1994), p. 15.

45. For the Heritage Foundation's attack, see Robert E. Moffit, "Clinton's Frankenstein: The Gory Details of the President's Health Plan," *Policy Review*, no. 67 (Winter 1994), pp. 4–12. See also "No Exit," *New Republic*, February 7, 1994, pp. 21–25, by Manhattan Institute John M. Olin Fellow Elizabeth Mc-Caughey, who was soon to be elected lieutenant governor in New York on the Republican ticket.

46. Center for Public Integrity, *Well-Healed*, p. 33.

47. These facts come from Timothy Egan, "Triumph Leaves Talk Radio Pondering Its Next Targets," *New York Times*, January 1, 1995, pp. 1, 22. For a sense of how Rush Limbaugh discussed the Clinton plan, see his *See, I Told You So* (Pocket Star Books, 1993), especially pp. 167–74, where ridicule of Hillary Rodham Clinton is a running theme.

48. Robin Toner, "Hillary Clinton Opens Campaign to Answer Critics of Health Plan," *New York Times*, February 16, 1994, p. A11.

49. Such pressures are discussed in Graham K. Wilson, "Interest Groups in the Health Care Debate," in this volume.

50. Daniel S. Hirschfield, *The Lost Reform: The Campaign for Compulsory Health Insurance in the United States from 1932 to 1943* (Harvard University Press, 1970), chap. 2.

51. The one new national program enacted in 1935, contributory retirement insurance, came in an area where state governments had not previously legislated. What is more, the few corporate pensions plans that had been developed during the 1920s mostly collapsed during the Great Depression. What we today call "social security" was thus fashioned on uncluttered terrain.

52. It is true that the task force incorporated certain sweeteners for key interests into the Health Security bill. The elderly (and the American Association of Retired Persons) were to get prescription drug benefits and contributions to long-term care expenses, and General Motors and other large corporations with generous health plans were to get government subsidization of early retirees. But these sweeteners were fairly minor in the overall scheme, and even their intended beneficiaries doubted that they would survive congressional deliberations. Fiscal constraints operated on Congress as well as the president, making it difficult for any group to be given—or reliably promised—federal subsidies.

53. This argument is enveloped in Theda Skocpol, "Targeting within Universalism: Politically Viable Policies to Combat Poverty in the United States," in Christopher Jencks and Paul E. Peterson, eds., *The Urban Underclass*, (Brookings, 1991), pp. 411–36; also reprinted as chapter 8 in Theda Skocpol, *Social Policy in the United States: Future Possibilities in Historical Perspective* (Princeton University Press, 1995).

54. Maggie Mahar, "What Clinton's Health Plan Would Mean to You," *New York*, April 26, 1993, p. 31.

55. Blendon, Hyams, and Benson, "Bridging the Gap," p. 2576.

56. The *New Republic*, for example, stoked fears about managed care in McCaughey, "No Exit," and in a steady stream of editorials. See also Ralph Kinney Bennett, "Your Risk under the Clinton Health Plan," *Readers Digest*, March 1994, pp. 127–32. During the 1994 health reform debate, best-selling author (Doctor) Robin Cook published *Fatal Cure* (G. P. Putnam's Sons, 1994), a medical horror story about the arrival of managed care in a small Vermont town. The direct villains in the novel are hospital administrators and capitalists, but every few pages we are reminded that governmental regulations are pushing these villains to cut costs and murder patients. The paperback version of the novel carries a quote from the *Detroit News* calling it "a hair-raising, cautionary tale about the possible pitfalls of impending health-care reform in America."

57. On the Cooper plan, see Hilary Stout and David Rogers, "Tennessee Democrat's Rival Health-Care Plan Inspires Industry Support, Administration Wrath," *Wall Street Journal*, December 3, 1993, p. A14; and Trudy Lieberman, "The Selling of 'Clinton Lite,'" *Columbia Journalism Review* (March–April 1994), pp. 20–22. Problems with the Cooper plan are well explained in Joseph White, *Competing Solutions: American Health Care Proposals and International Experiences* (Brookings, 1995), chap. 8.

58. Robert H. Salisbury, "Why No Corporatism in America?" in Philippe C. Schmitter and Gerhard Lehmbruch, eds., *Patterns of Corporatist Policymaking*, (Beverly Hills, Calif.: Sage Publications, 1982), pp. 213–30.

59. See note 23.

60. On the public's view about taxing and financing, see Robert J. Blendon, Mollyann Brodie, and John Benson, "What Happened to Americans' Support of the Clinton Plan," *Health Affairs*, vol. 14 (Summer 1995), pp. 16–17.

61. Now, in the wake of the 1994 congressional elections, the Clinton administration is doing such chopping, and the American people might well wonder: If they can do it now, why couldn't they do it then? The answer is that back then the president had to deal with a Democratic Congress with vested interests in every piece of the federal bureaucracy. Still, the president might well have captured the public imagination, and very broad voter support, had he proposed in 1993 huge cuts in the federal government, in exchange for money to pay for universal health care coverage. And this approach might have brought him considerable leverage in Congress, after it became apparent that the public approved.

62. See Paul Starr, *The Social Transformation of American Medicine* (Basic Books, 1982), book two, chaps. 1, 4; and Theda Skocpol, "Is the Time Finally Ripe? Health Insurance Reforms in the 1990s," *Journal of Health Politics, Policy and Law*, vol. 18 (Fall 1993), pp. 531–50.

63. Jacobs, *Health of Nations*, chap. 9; and Theodore R. Marmor, *The Politics of Medicare* (Aldine, 1973).

64. Monte M. Poen, *Harry S. Truman Versus the Medical Lobby: The Genesis of Medicare* (University of Missouri Press, 1978).

65. See the call for such an approach by the editorial board of the *New York Times* in "Anybody Home?" *New York Times*, January 8, 1995, p. E18.

66. See Peter G. Peterson, *Facing Up: How to Rescue the Economy from Crushing Debt and Restore the American Dream* (Simon and Schuster, 1993). I discuss the attacks on "entitlements" in "Remaking U.S. Social Policies for the 21st Century," the conclusion to *Social Policy in the United States*.

CHAPTER FOUR

The Debate That Wasn't
The Public and the Clinton
Health Care Plan

Daniel Yankelovich

IN JULY 1988 Congress passed a bill capping out-of-pocket costs for catastrophic health care at $2,000. The bill's supporters in Congress had cited opinion polls showing that 69 percent of older Americans were worried about paying their hospital bills in the event of catastrophic illness and strongly supported action to address this concern.

Astonishingly, a year and a half later, a humiliated Congress was obliged to reverse itself and repeal the bill. Fierce protests from older Americans whom the bill was designed to help shocked Congress. These older people, especially the well-to-do, had refused to accept the higher medicare premiums needed to defray the costs of the cap.

In 1994, a few short years later, supporters of the Clinton health care bill suffered an even worse defeat, one that hurt the administration's political fortunes and also failed to win badly needed reforms of the health care system.

What is it about health care reform that causes America's political leadership to stumble so badly? Why does public support for reform, so strong at some stages of the reform process, vanish and even turn against the reformers? Is the public fickle? Perverse? Manipulable by those with the deepest pockets to pay for negative advertising? Or are other factors at work that explain the miscalculations of our political leaders?

A Cornucopia of Causes

It is not easy to pinpoint the precise causes of the Clinton plan's failure. Ironically, the difficulty is an overabundance of choices. The outcome, various observers urge, would have been different if the plan had been less grandiose and had not sought to reform one-seventh of the economy all at once; if the plan had put more emphasis on reducing costs and less on expanding insurance coverage; if the plan had been less complicated; if there had been fewer starts and stops in developing and presenting the plan to the nation, thereby fatally slowing its momentum; if those who opposed the plan had told the truth and not distorted its contents so badly; if a more bipartisan approach had been taken from the outset; if the president had not locked himself into an unrealistic commitment to universal coverage; if the administration had taken a more incremental approach; if the administration had been more aggressive in developing countermeasures against its critics, for example, by fighting the Harry and Louise ads with its own commercials; if big business had not reneged on its support for an employer mandate; if the political climate had been less hostile to modest tax increases and government supervision to ensure that costs were kept under control; if the plan's friends were as ardent in their support as its enemies were in their opposition; and if the many vested interests opposed to the plan had not been able to outspend the plan's supporters.

This list does not exhaust the possible causes of failure. Moreover, in varying degrees there is some truth to all of them. Unfortunately, having too many explanations is as unhelpful as having none. Since they all point in different directions, it becomes exceedingly difficult to draw the lessons that must be learned if failure is to be avoided in the future.

A Failure of Deliberation

Since all complex phenomena have multiple causes, the question of which one to highlight depends on one's purpose. Mine is twofold: to help avoid failure in the future and to show how to get health care reform back on track. With these purposes in mind, it is illuminating to see the defeat of the Clinton reform package in 1994 as reflecting a *massive failure of public deliberation*. The failure of health care reform is one consequence of a serious disconnect between the electorate and the nation's leadership class, which includes the leaders of medicine, industry, education, the legal profession, science, religion, and journalism as well as national and community political leaders. The public and this broad leadership class do not seem able to converse with one another in a way that makes productive public deliberation possible. Instead, they talk at each other across a void of misunderstanding and misinterpretation. The nation's leadership and the public are carrying out a bizarre dialogue of the deaf, with health care reform a victim of its destructive effects. The nation's elites have little trouble talking with one another. But when it comes to engaging the public, elites talk down to the public, failing to connect with them. Mechanisms of top-down communication—public relations, punditry, advertising, speechifying, spin-doctoring, and so-called public education—abound. But the absence of plain give-and-take between leaders and public is remarkable. The disconcerting truth is that most leaders do not know how to talk to the public.

The president's reform plan was not shaped by discussion with citizens about rising health care costs and what to do about them but by experts and experts alone. Technical experts designed it. Special interests argued it. Political leaders sold it. Journalists more interested in its political ramifications than its contents kibitzed it. And advertising attacked it. The public served merely as confused spectators who never became knowledgeable about the specifics of the plan and its implications for their lives.

The political reality is that Americans were not prepared to deliberate and did not, in fact, deliberate on the nature and scope of the reforms the Clinton plan proposed. Whether the reforms were the right ones— some were, some were not—the public did not directly engage any of them.

Nor is health care reform the only victim of the disconnect between leaders and public. Crime, immigration, welfare reform, education reform, racial politics, and other urgent issues also elude solution because of this strange defect at the heart of our democratic political system. But no other issue dramatizes it so well as the failure of the president's health care reform, which unfolds with the inexorability of Greek tragedy. First, we watch the administration respond to opinion polls and other political signals that persuade it that health care reform is the public's top priority and seduce it into believing that the public supports its reform proposals. Then, as the administration climbs further and further out on a limb of commitment to its plan of reform, we witness public support mysteriously fade away. We watch with fascination as this weakening of support makes it fatally easy for the opposition to cut off the limb. The administration falls bitterly into the dust of defeat, without ever really understanding what happened. The spectacle makes compelling drama and good partisan politics. But defeats of this sort deepen public cynicism and weaken the fabric of American life.

The blame for this failure of public deliberation lies squarely at the feet of the American leadership class, which is what makes this post-mortem of the Clinton plan so important.

In the early stages of deliberating any issue, average citizens will know few specifics. The purpose of debate and deliberation is to give people time to understand the costs and benefits of alternative choices and, if there are tough choices as in health care, the opportunity to mull them over. Admittedly, the word "deliberate" is too rationalistic in its overtones. (More often than not, the so-called debate is informal and messy, charged with irrational and emotional elements. Yet somehow it takes place and the public's work gets done).

When a reform fails to win public support, it is either because the proposal is out of tune with the public's perceptions and desires or because deliberation did not take place. Both failures marked the debate on health care reform. When people don't have the chance to work through the meaning of proposed changes to their lives, fear of change itself takes over and people settle for the status quo, however unsatisfactory, preferring it to change they do not understand and have not seriously considered.

What about the Clinton health care plan? Suppose the administration had given the public a much better opportunity to absorb, digest, and consider the plan carefully. Would the outcome have been different?

My interpretation is that on a take-it-or-leave-it basis the public would have ultimately rejected the Clinton plan because it did not match well with public concerns and values.[1] But the essence of public deliberation precludes a take-it-or-leave-it approach. Opening a policy to deliberation also opens it to the possibilities of revision. Deliberating is not the same as being sold or persuaded. The president fully, if belatedly, accepted this reality in his dealings with Congress. He initially declared his plan negotiable except for universal coverage, but in the end he was willing to negotiate about this element as well.

But the opportunity to deliberate and negotiate was not available to the public. The American people seriously want health care reform. If the reform plan had been critiqued and revised through give-and-take with the public, the United States would, in my judgment, now have a health care reform package. It would be incremental, to be sure, but it would be a plan that could evolve gradually and in tune with the public's priorities.

The Clinton plan's loss of public support occurred not because a majority of voters rejected the plan on its merits but because its opponents found it easy to raise the public's fears about reforms people did not understand. To fill the vacuum, opponents conjured up a nightmare: the prospect of ever more impersonal "cattle car" care, regulated by the federal government, with higher out-of-pocket costs for medical care, higher taxes, less choice, lower wages, and increased unemployment.

Public deliberation is not a technical matter of devoting more time and money to public education, salesmanship, and public relations. It is the process of shaping public policy through genuine interaction between the public and experts, and it requires that the views of the public count in shaping policy.

From the point of view of organized interests—the insurance industry, the pharmaceutical companies, the trade unions, the business corporations, the medical profession—there may have been a debate. From the point of view of warring factions in Congress, there may have been a debate. From the point of view of the administration, its friends and opponents, there may have been a debate. But from the point of view of the public, there never was an opportunity to deliberate alternative choices and to engage the plan in all of its virtues and shortcomings. As far as the public is concerned, the great health care debate of 1994 never took place.

The Unmaking of a Consensus

In light of the intense discussion of health care reform in the last several years in Congress, the media, and the health care professions, the proposition that there was not much public deliberation seems to defy common sense—especially to the casual observer. From the presidential election of 1992 to mid-1994, citizens could not escape the flood of newspaper articles, public opinion polls, political speeches, and television ads on health care reform. The president and the first lady made this issue the centerpiece of their legislative plan. Several congressional committees made it their special preserve, struggling for months to reach compromises a majority could support. Few issues interested the public more intensively. And the public did, after all, change its mind about the Clinton health care plan. In what sense, then, did the public fail to deliberate the president's plan?

To see why the public rejected the Clinton health care plan without ever having seriously deliberated it, one should understand the mind set of the public before the president's presentation of his plan, and what happened subsequently.

The Public's State of Mind Prior to the Clinton Plan

When President Clinton formally introduced his plan for health care reform in September 1993, the public had been waiting for a long time and held high expectations for it. Nor were they disappointed by the president's speech announcing his plan. Concern with rising health care costs had been growing. People had long traded horror stories about $7 aspirins, "minor" outpatient surgery that cost tens of thousands of dollars, and insurance companies that canceled insurance just when it was most needed. The public was also mindful that many Americans had no health insurance whatever, and a majority felt this was wrong and should be corrected. To average Americans, the appeal of health insurance that can never be taken away and of achieving universal coverage while simultaneously controlling health care costs was enormous.

The speech heightened expectations that were already unrealistically high. Polls several weeks after the president's speech showed plurality approval of the plan (43 percent favorable to 36 percent opposed).[2] Yet by July 1994, nine months after the announcement, the public's favorable endorsement of the plan had eroded and the favorable-unfavorable ratio had flip-flopped.[3]

To comprehend what happened in this brief span of months, one needs to understand the strong preconceptions that shaped public reaction. These preconceptions shaped the initial positive reaction and the subsequent disillusionment. This mind-set made inevitable the plan's loss of support:

HEALTH CARE AS A RIGHT. The belief that health care is a right is deeply ingrained in the American consciousness. This belief includes the government's obligation to ensure health care for those who are too poor to pay for it. When any benefit is regarded as a right, Americans automatically assume it is the government's responsibility to honor it.

The public has held this preconception for more than half a century. A 1938 Gallup poll reported that 81 percent of adults nationwide subscribed to the view that "government should be responsible for medical care for people who can't afford it." Fifty-three years later in 1991, the number was 80 percent—a remarkably stable conviction.[4] A Harris poll found almost universal agreement (91 percent) with the idea that "everybody should have the right to get the best possible care—as good as the treatment a millionaire gets."[5]

HIGH PERSONAL SATISFACTION. Although polls vary somewhat, all show the overwhelming majority of Americans report high levels of satisfaction with the medical care they and their families receive. A Yankelovich Partners survey, conducted in the same month the president's plan was revealed, reported an 80 percent level of satisfaction.[6] A 1993 Roper survey showed only modest decline over a twenty-year period in people's satisfaction with their quality of medical care—from 83 percent to 73 percent—and no erosion in the "availability of medical care you get when you need it"—75 percent in 1973 and 74 percent in 1993.[7]

MOUNTING CONCERN ABOUT THE STATE OF THE AMERICAN HEALTH CARE SYSTEM. Though personally satisfied with quality and availability, most people nonetheless felt that the medical system was troubled. One poll reported that the fraction of the public convinced that the nation should "overhaul the entire system" rose steeply from 25 percent in 1983 to 55 percent a decade later.[8] Another showed that eight out of ten Americans (79 percent) believe that "we are headed toward a crisis in the health care system."[9] A 1991 Gallup poll records a whopping 91 percent believe that "there is a crisis in the health care system."[10] Every year since 1982, the Harris poll has asked whether people believe the health care system needs only minor changes, fundamental changes, or a complete overhaul because so many things are wrong with it. In 1992, a presidential election year, a majority opted for completely rebuilding the system.[11]

PINNING THE BLAME ON THE PROFESSION. Why the public feels the health care system is in deep trouble goes a long way toward explaining the later reaction to the Clinton plan. Above all, the public is unhappy about ballooning health care costs.

Asked in a 1993 Gallup poll about the "main problem facing health care in the US today," 74 percent named rising costs—nine times the 8 percent who cited problems with access, and nineteen times as many as cited problems with quality (4 percent).[12] In an earlier Gallup poll in 1991, in response to an open-end question, 42 percent of adults nationwide volunteered that "the biggest problem with health care in the US today is cost."[13] In another 1991 poll, three out of four Americans said they felt the cost of health care was "much higher than it should be."[14]

And a Roper poll found that almost two-thirds of Americans feel "the cost of the medical care (they) receive is unreasonable." Most of them feel it is *very* unreasonable. Gallup reports that four out of ten people say they have put off going to a doctor because of high cost.[15]

The public squarely blames hospitals, lawyers, physicians, and drug companies for rising costs. Asked to identify who or what is most responsible for higher health care costs, the vast majority in a 1991 *Time/CNN* poll cited hospital costs (83 percent), awards in malpractice suits (75 percent), physician fees (73 percent), fraud and abuse in the health care system (72 percent), and the costs of medications (70 percent).[16] Small wonder, then, that public confidence in medicine as a profession has been eroding for decades. In the 1960s the level of confidence in the medical profession was almost twice that of all other institutions (73 percent to 40 percent). But by 1993 American confidence in medicine fell to a dismal 22 percent, lower for the first time than confidence in other institutions such as law and education.[17]

On the causes of rising costs the public is on a collision course with most experts who attribute rising costs mostly to new technology and the aging population. The majority of the public brushes aside both of these explanations. People believe that technology does not raise costs but lowers them, and they emotionally resist the idea that an aging population adds significantly to costs. (A typical response: "The costs go up more because of malpractice than because of the number of older people.") Only 20 percent of adults nationwide endorse the idea that the explosion of health care costs should place "limits on what health care is available to the average person." An impressive 77 percent majority insists that "the cure to rising health care costs is . . . to cut the waste, high profits, and fraud in medicine."[18] Quite naturally, the public that holds these views rejects calls for sacrifice and change of behavior, on the assumption that if the medical profession is to blame for rising costs, it should take the hit, not the innocent public.

LACK OF REALISM. Since most Americans attribute the rising costs of health care to waste, fraud, greed, and inefficiency, they assume that the money saved from curbing such venality and waste will fully pay for added health care benefits. This is what most Americans mean by reform. The wish list of the majority of Americans at the time President Clinton presented his plan is impressive in its breadth and lack of realism. The public wanted to "limit the price of prescription drugs" (86 percent); "retain quality by reducing waste and greed-driven costs" (84 percent);

"make health insurance portable" (83 percent); "limit doctor and hospital fees" (82 percent); "include mental illness to the same extent as physical illness" (82 percent); "limit rates on private insurance" (81 percent); "reduce the cost of malpractice" (74 percent); and "provide universal coverage without increasing costs" (55 percent).[19]

A DRIVING SENSE OF URGENCY. In the last two years of the Bush presidency, the economic recession frightened many middle- and lower-income Americans. Hourly wages had been stagnant for years. Even dual-income households were having difficulty making ends meet. Workers were growing progressively more worried about losing their jobs, and their nervousness spilled over to concern about their health care. Their reasoning: "We can cope if we lose our jobs (or one of us does), but if we also lose our health care insurance, we won't be able to cope." Polls in 1991 and 1992 showed concern with health care in the number one or two spot in public priorities.

Growing Reservations

When President Clinton announced his plan in late September 1993, the public listened with high hopes and unrealistic expectations. They expected government to ensure that the quality of health care to all Americans would remain high, that all workers could retain health insurance even if they lost their job or had some pre-existing condition, that costs would be controlled or reduced so that insurance premiums did not keep rising, that the miracles of modern technology would be encouraged, and that all this would be paid for by wringing waste and greed out of the system so that taxes would not have to be raised. The point about higher taxes was particularly sensitive. The president had recently raised taxes, and the public was fiercely resistant to any added increase.

This mind-set explains the mainly positive reaction to the president's speech. His reassurance that, aside from modest sin taxes on tobacco or liquor, no general tax increase would be needed to pay for the reforms the public desired, gave the initial impression that the administration had met all the public's wishes.

But a closer look at the quality of the public's support gave warning of the erosion that was to come. In the week following the president's address to the nation, people were asked how much they knew about the plan. That only 21 percent said they knew a lot about it is not surprising because the plan was new and the specifics were not clear.[20] But the following month, even fewer people (17 percent) felt they knew a lot about the plan.[21] By November only 13 percent felt they knew a lot about the plan.[22]

The public's lack of confidence in its own knowledge about the specifics of health care reform persisted throughout the congressional debate. By August 1994 a Harris poll showed only 13–15 percent of Americans felt they were very well informed about the debate and how the various proposals for reform would help them and their families. This lack of knowledge did not reflect lack of interest: most people felt it very important to them personally that they understand the proposals for reform and how they would be affected by them. Significantly, only 5 percent felt that television and other news media did an excellent job in explaining the reform proposals to them, while 64 percent rated the media's explanations as only fair or downright poor.[23]

The little that people did know about the plan aroused their anxieties. In response to a *Washington Post* poll a month after the plan was announced, 34 percent responded that the plan would worsen the quality of the health care they received, while only 19 percent felt it would improve care.[24] From the outset, then, people were apprehensive about how well they personally would fare under the plan. This undercurrent of public nervousness made it easy for the plan's opponents to nourish the seeds of doubt. In the months that followed, people's reservations grew ever more serious. The reasons are manifold. Three stand out as contributing most to the public's growing rejection of the plan.

NONNEGOTIABLE UNIVERSALITY. The first had to do with the president's commitment to universal health insurance as a moral principle on which he would not compromise. The impression of solid public support encouraged the president in this commitment. In thirteen different national polls an average of 72 percent said they supported universal health insurance.[25] Unfortunately for the fate of the president's plan, however, when most people say they support universal coverage they really mean: "We don't believe anybody should be deprived of care because of money. We support the President's goal of insurance for all that can never be taken away but only if the nation can afford it and it doesn't limit choice of doctors or raise taxes or cause employers to cut jobs."[26]

As Congress scrutinized the cost of the reform plan, people began to suspect that maybe extending generous health care benefits to the 39 million Americans who lacked insurance would be too costly, especially when employers began to balk about footing the bill. Americans may share the president's *desire* to extend health care coverage, but not at their expense.

TECHNOLOGY. Overall levels of satisfaction with quality and access plus public enthusiasm for the miracles of technology make people apprehensive about health system overhaul. Public dissatisfaction is sharply focused on rising costs, not on the health care system overall. As the plan's opponents raised people's fears about the complexity of the plan, the public did not feel it knew enough about it to endorse such sweeping changes.

ANTIGOVERNMENT SENTIMENT. Antigovernment resentment has intensified since President Clinton was elected in 1992. The 1994 midterm elections made clear that Americans blame big government for many of the nation's problems. Opponents successfully labeled the Clinton health care plan as a big government plan, adding yet another nail to its coffin.

Evidence of the Absence of Serious Deliberation

The essence of the deliberative process is that people come to grips with reality. The persistence of wishful thinking and the failure to wrestle with hard choices are sure signs that deliberation has *not* occurred.

The public's continuing belief that they can have it all—quality *and* convenience *and* high-tech medicine *and* lower costs—shows that people have not yet confronted reality and worked through the hard choices that must sooner or later be made. People avoid making hard choices by hiding behind the mantra of "cutting waste, fraud and abuse."

At one level of consciousness, they know better. But at the level of policy deliberation, the administration failed to disabuse people that the no-free-lunch law of economics had not miraculously been suspended for health care reform. The polling data clearly show that Americans do not understand the causes of rising health care spending to which the habits and demands of the public itself contribute to cost escalation. They do not realize the extent to which an aging population, scientific advances, and the existence of a cost system that systematically hides the total costs of health care from consumers are, among other forces, important drivers of health care costs. They do not understand what their choices are and what sacrifices and benefits each choice entails, let alone the need to make sacrifices. The closer one looks, the less evidence one sees of serious public deliberation.

UNRECOGNIZED CONSEQUENCES. The public's failure to fully grasp the consequences of its own opinions is a sure sign of lack of public deliberation. Polling data on health care are replete with evidence that people do not accept the consequences of implementing their wish list of expanded health care benefits. In a CBS/*New York Times* poll, 55 percent of the public admitted to being worried that the quality of their own health care will suffer if health insurance is provided to everyone.[27] In a Gallup poll, by a margin of four to one (52 percent to 13 percent) people expressed the fear that health care reform featuring universal coverage will increase the total amount of money they would have to pay for medical care.[28] A DYG, Inc., deliberative poll showed that endorsement of universal coverage withered when people directly confronted the cost consequences of providing health insurance to everyone. Whether or not a reform is seen to add to personal costs is the single most important predictor of lack of public support.[29]

When views are volatile and people fail to confront the consequences of their own opinions the public is said to be in a state of "raw opinion."[30] As people deliberate an issue, their views gradually evolve from raw opinion to more thoughtful judgment. As deliberation progresses, they begin to feel more knowledgeable, their opinions grow firmer, less volatile (they do not shift their views with every slight change in the wording of poll questions), less contradictory, and, above all, realistic choicemaking replaces wishful thinking. The surest sign that people have reached genuine deliberative judgment is when they are fully cognizant of the consequences of their opinions and take responsibility for them. I call the end product of this deliberative process "public judgment" to contrast it with raw opinion.

In two analyses of public opinion published several years ago, I presented evidence that public opinion on health care had not progressed much beyond the raw opinion stage.[31] At that time health care reform had not yet been the subject of the massive publicity that it received in 1993 and 1994. It is sobering to realize that, following an unprecedented amount of debate among leadership groups, public deliberation had made so little progress.

The Failure of Elites

If the disconnect crippling our democratic process merely reflects an inability of leaders to converse with the public, it should be easy to fix.

After all, conversation is a skill that all of us practice every day of our lives. Something else must be going on beneath the surface that is eluding us and that accounts for the failure.

There *is* something else going on beneath the surface. The failure of public deliberation is not merely a matter of leaders saying, "Oops, we forgot to talk with our constituents. Maybe we'd better give them a little more attention." Most leaders know full well that they had better pay more attention to their constituents, but they are still failing to carry on a genuine dialogue. What is this hidden obstacle?

It relates to the inappropriate attitudes and skills associated with the dominant one-way, top-down model of communication that is part and parcel of our culture.

One way of describing the attitudes associated with the dominant culture of professionalism comes from noted anthropologist Clifford Geertz. Geertz writes that anthropology has long been dominated by a "me-anthropologist-you-native" outlook, a professional attitude that un-wittingly and automatically converts the subject of study into an *object* of study, depersonalizing the relationship in the process. Similar attitudes dominate other professions. For example, "me-journalist-you-Joe-six-pack," or "me-surgeon-you-broken-hip-in-room-360," or "me-teacher-you-ignorant-parent," or "me-Senator-you-blue-collar-vote."

Professionals automatically take for granted that a certain distance separates them from their subjects, with the professionals in the superior position because they have specialized knowledge. These attitudes of experts, professionals, and leaders create an invisible barrier between them and average citizens. Leaders come to see themselves as elites who "do things for" the people. And "the people" are placed in the role of those for whom things are done.

This attitude is bad for both sides. It creates a new class system, with class distinctions based on the expertise that comes with professionalism. Responding to the new "upper class" of professional leaders, average citizens who are the objects of their "services" grow passive and unreal-istically demanding, abdicating their responsibility for their own lives. The relationship between leaders and citizens inevitably deteriorates, with citizens constantly nagging government about their rights, while government officials, tiring of the unreasonableness of incessant public demands, respond by becoming more secretive, more cunning, and more manipulative.

The new leadership attitudes embrace a theory of communication that reinforces the identity of leaders as professionals in possession of superior knowledge, some tiny fraction of which they may from time to time wish to impart to the public. Their preferred method of communication with the public is top down, expert driven, and information based. It is designed primarily to raise public awareness of information that leaders believe the public ought to know.

This model of communication wrongly assumes that the public is a *tabula rasa* on which one can write whatever message one wishes to convey. In fact, people come to an issue like health care armed with a lifetime of prejudices, convictions, personal experience, information, and misinformation. People's reactions to leadership diverge wildly from the intentions of those conducting the public's so-called education.

Policymakers rarely, if ever, use this model to communicate among themselves. With each other, they try to gain mutual understanding, develop and criticize policy choices, and take ample time to grasp pros and cons and likely consequences. On complex issues, this process often takes years.

In communicating with the public, however, experts no longer engage in the give-and-take of dialogue and the probing of choices. They do not spend the time to gain mutual understanding and to take consequences into account. Rather, they stress "education campaigns" of limited duration, mass media, and telecommunications from leaders to public. It is not unusual to hear leaders speak blithely of the need for "education campaigns" to cause the public to grasp virtually overnight what they themselves took years to digest in briefings, readings, and discussions with other leaders and experts.

It should now be clearer why conversation between leaders and the public has grown so troubled in recent years. Leaders resort to monologue, not dialogue, with feedback from the public gained only from opinion polls, talk radio, mail from constituents, and other imperfect devices.

The skills needed to communicate with the public through dialogue are very different from the ability to read opinion polls. Leaders must have the skills to engage a worried citizenry on how to allocate limited resources among health care and other pressing goals. And they must discuss these matters with the public as equals, not as superior professionals imparting a fraction of their expert knowledge to an ignorant public. This exchange must occur before proposals are cast in stone, so that the public's responses shape what leaders propose.

Moreover, the dialogue must be genuine, in Martin Buber's sense of an encounter between I and Thou, in which both sides change in fundamental ways. The techniques that work most poorly are the lawyerlike debates that take place in Congress, the undigested packages of policy-linked information whose consequences for the public are not clearly spelled out, as in the Ira Magaziner health care proposals that formed the basis for the Clinton health care plan, and media-based campaigns of public education that fail to take into account the public's need to reconcile conflicting values.

When Public Deliberation Is Indispensable

Not all issues require public deliberation. Congress passes many laws without public deliberation or resistance. But for several reasons, health care reform and issues of equal importance require a serious deliberative effort.

The reasons are almost self-evident. Public deliberation is required when an issue meets one or more of three criteria.

It is important to people's lives. Health care certainly passes this test. Because most Americans are satisfied with their own health care they will resist change. Deliberation of reform proposals is therefore essential, or public support will crack as soon as proposals for change are attacked.

The reform calls for sacrifice. Public deliberation is essential when proposed reforms cost money, cause inconvenience, make people modify their behavior, or compromise values important to them. When legislation calls for sacrifice, voters will automatically oppose the reforms unless they have a say in its formulation. This is what happened to catastrophic health care for the elderly in 1988 as well as to the Clinton plan.

Special interests oppose the reforms. Special interests exert their greatest power when the public is indifferent or fearful of change. It takes a strong shove from the public to give political leaders the courage to stand up to wealthy and powerful special interests capable of mobilizing their constituencies over night and pouring resources into efforts to defeat members of Congress who oppose them.

Any one of these reasons would be enough to make a public deliberation indispensable. That all three apply so cogently to health care reform is compelling evidence that deliberation is indispensable for success.

Making Deliberation Happen

Merely announcing that a public debate will take place on health care, as the Clinton administration did, does not make it so. To achieve genuine public debate, a skillful strategy must be devised to deal with the public's wishful thinking and with leadership's blind spots. A successful strategy must address both the *sequence* of health care reforms and the public deliberation *process*.

The Sequence of Reforms

The reality that leadership is most prone to overlook—at its peril—relates to timing. The public will not support far-reaching reforms until it is mentally and emotionally ready. It takes at least three to five years to conduct a genuine deliberative process.

Leaders are so absorbed in solving technical obstacles to health care reform that they pay scant attention to the political reality that the American people must play a key role in reforming the health care system, which must ultimately reflect the deepest values of our society. Perhaps Americans really are willing to consume a far larger proportion of our GDP on health care than other nations are. Maybe Americans are prepared to sacrifice other good things to try to save the lives of "preemies" and to follow every possible technological lead for every patient at public expense. But we will never know what we truly value until we face the reality that ever-increasing medical care may mean abandoning other values of equal or greater importance to our society.

No health care reforms will endure that do not conform to our society's core values. And there is no way to design such reforms other than through giving citizens the opportunity to deliberate the hard choices that each one involves. But the hard choices cannot be dumped on the public all at once, willy nilly, which is what the Clinton plan did because its authors were not concerned with the sequence of reforms from a *citizen* point of view.

What choices is the public prepared to deliberate at the present time and in what sequence?

In the aftermath of the Clinton plan's defeat, several reform ideas continue to float around. The public is ready to accept reforms that will make it easier for people to carry their health insurance from job to job and more difficult for insurance companies to blackball people with preexisting conditions. It is also ready to encourage individual states to experiment more freely with various reform packages and curb some of the legal excesses that cause physicians to practice costly defensive medicine.

None of these demands require major sacrifice on the part of the public or large changes in behavior and so do not need further public deliberation. And they can be accomplished without having to repair the larger disconnect between leaders and public.

Public deliberation is urgently needed for those reforms that do require the public to make sacrifices. Public sacrifices are inevitable because the American people demand more medical care than they are willing to pay for. Ordinarily, the constraints of a market economy accommodate these kinds of strains. The desires of the public for, say, bigger, better, and nicer houses would be insatiable were it not for the discipline of the market. If price were no object and the best possible housing were considered a sacred right to which every American was entitled regardless of ability to pay, the cost of housing would also zoom out of control.

Health ethicist Will Gaylin puts the matter cogently:

> Most of the experts and policy makers in Washington have been focusing on the deficiencies and failures of modern medicine: greedy pharmaceutical and insurance companies (not to mention physicians); unnecessary procedures; bureaucratic inefficiency and paperwork; expensive technologies; and so forth. . . . Opposed to this group are those, myself included, who acknowledge that although there is waste in the system, it is incidental to the basic forces driving up costs. I would argue, in fact, that the greatest part of the increase in health-care costs can best be understood as the result not of the failures of medicine but of its successes. The relentless increase in costs is actually a product of the expanding capabilities of medicine. Implicit in this view is the assumption that controlling waste will save money only in the short haul, and that we had best use the limited time such a strategy will buy to figure out a way to confront the deeper and more challenging reasons for escalating health costs: our unbridled appetite for health care and our continuing expansion of the definition of what constitutes health.[32]

As Americans age and as technology expands the capabilities of medicine, the desire of people for all of the benefits that modern health care offers intensifies. The central issue in health care reform, therefore, is how best to manage insatiable public demand for the growing supply of health care benefits that technology is creating for us. Which aspects of health care should fall under the rules of the market where people get only what they pay for, and which aspects should fall under the rules of entitlement where people receive health care benefits as a matter of right whether or not they can pay for them?

I believe we can confront these issues best by debating them in a sequence proposed by two research organizations that have long been studying the public's relation to health care.

The Public Agenda–Kettering Plan

The Public Agenda and Kettering Foundations have proposed a sequence of subjects for health care reform arranged in ascending order of difficulty from the public's perspective. Their research has led them to conclude that the public has yet to confront three major dilemmas of health care reform.

PRESERVING BENEFITS VERSUS CONTROLLING COSTS. The first is how to retain (and if possible improve) the health care benefits of those who are now insured, while controlling public costs. Although Americans would like to expand health insurance coverage to everyone, most citizens are more concerned with holding onto existing benefits while at the same time cutting taxes, reducing the federal budget deficit, and keeping their employers prosperous. The dilemma is how to maintain or increase the benefits now provided by employers and government without financially overburdening employers or taxpayers. Almost every large employer is currently confronting this dilemma. The result is tense labor negotiations and movement toward managed care. The debate is moving fast to Congress.

CONTROLLING COSTS VERSUS RAPID TECHNOLOGICAL ADVANCE. The second dilemma requires the public to confront the conflict between its desire to curb the growth of health care costs and its thirst for the benefits of state-of-the-art, high-tech medicine. With less than 5 percent of the world's population, the United States has half of the world's CAT scanners and two-thirds of the world's MRIs. Since World War II, Americans have enjoyed the world's most advanced and sophisticated medical care and have been largely shielded from awareness that they are paying for it. Experts in the field are accustomed to debating such issues as whether to use tissue plasminogen activator (TPA) at a dosage cost of $2,000 or the slightly less effective streptokinase at a cost of $200 to dissolve blood clots that cause heart damage. Yet few such debates have filtered down to the general public, who remain unready to wrestle with these kinds of decisions. It will take several years, much skill, and special effort on the part of leaders to encourage a deliberative process whereby people are willing to face such dilemmas head-on.

THE BALANCING OF BENEFITS AND COSTS. The third dilemma is one that Americans are least ready to confront. It is the conflict between reducing costs and doing everything possible to save lives. Americans fiercely resist dealing with conflicts between heroic medicine that exhausts all technical means for prolonging life and curbing costs. In one well-publicized case, Siamese twins were separated in a Philadelphia hospital where, as expected, one twin died right after the surgery and the other was given only a 1 percent chance to live. The cost: hundreds of thousands of dollars in public money (the parents had no resources) just for the surgery and intensive neonatal care, and even larger sums for long-term care, should the surviving twin outlive her infancy. Americans are currently ill-equipped, mentally and psychologically, to participate in decisions that mean rationing in these kinds of life-and-death decisions. It will take a long time (at least three or four years)—and great leadership skill—to engage public deliberation on this inescapable aspect of health care.

The outcome of a successful deliberative process on all three of these dilemmas, considered in sequence, is unlikely to be confined to laws and government regulations. Nor need they force average citizens to make life-and-death decisions for their loved ones routinely under circumstances charged with anxiety and feelings of incompetence and helplessness. In these arenas, the private sector rather than government, and the medical profession rather than individuals will assume most of the responsibility. But the public must participate in these and other difficult decisions—as consumers, employees, and citizens. The government is also obliged to play an important role in those aspects of health care deemed to be rights that cannot be decided solely on the basis of ability to pay.

A Different Model of Public Communication

Leaders cannot rely solely on top-down communication if they are to confront these three dilemmas effectively. Incidentally, the new skills needed to stimulate public deliberation on health care reform will serve well also in overcoming the larger disconnect between leaders and public.

I propose a new communication model to accomplish these objectives.[33] The model, which I refer to as the Public Judgment Model (PJM), defines three stages through which public opinion must evolve on complex issues such as health care: consciousness raising, working through, and resolution. Each stage is divided into substages, adding to a total of seven steps in the entire process. For complex issues like health care, the journey from the raw opinion characteristic of step 1 to the considered judgment at journey's end at step 7 is an arduous one.

The seven steps are (1) awareness; (2) developing a sense of urgency; (3) reacting to "trial balloons"; (4) confronting one's own wishful thinking and other forms of resistance; (5) "choicework": deliberating the pros and cons of the hard choices, weighing trade-offs and clarifying priorities; (6) reaching a provisional decision; and (7) coming to full deliberative judgment.

In practice, the life cycle from raw awareness to mature judgment of an issue such as health care is not an orderly process. But extensive research shows that such issues sooner or later pass through all of these stages of public deliberation. Even under ideal conditions making the journey though all seven steps takes years. More often than not, people get stalled at the resistance stage (step 4) or the choicework stage (step 5) and can remain stalled for decades. (The problem of rising health care costs is almost thirty years old.)

Our mass media and policymaking institutions do an outstanding job in the early steps—helping the public to create awareness of issues, drumming up a sense of urgency, and floating trial balloons to elicit people's early reactions. Sad to say, however, they do a remarkably bad job in helping the public navigate the middle and late steps.

Where does health care reform stand in relation to this seven-step model? Through what steps has it already progressed? What comes next?

—*Awareness.* Americans had their consciousness raised about swelling health care costs way back in the mid-seventies two decades ago! From the mid-seventies to the early 1990s, awareness grew slowly, always lagging behind an ever-worsening situation.

—*Urgency.* The upset senatorial victory of Democrat Harris Wofford in Pennsylvania in November 1991 (Wofford ran and won on health care) gave the issue strong political urgency. Abruptly, it seized the center of the political stage.

—*Trial balloons.* It was not until the presidential election of 1992 that people began seriously to heed specific proposals for reforming the health care system. In an October 1992 *Fortune* article, I concluded that health care had clearly arrived at step 2, the stage of rising urgency, and had just begun to advance into step 3 but had not yet reached step 4 among the broad public.[34]

—*Resistance*. This is the critical stage and the least understood. At this stage the public confronts its own wishful thinking and begins to acknowledge that attacking waste and greed will not magically pay the cost of guaranteeing quality medical care for all. Only after people confront specific policy ideas are their emotional resistances fully mobilized. President Clinton's proposal to guarantee health insurance that can never be taken away has helped to flush these resistances into the open where, in the future, people can work them through and thereby open the way ultimately to a more thoughtful and realistic solution to the health care dilemmas described above. My interpretation is that the American public is today in the early stages of step 4—confronting its resistance to being realistic about health care costs and choices.

—*Choicework*. People will remain stalled until they work through their resistances. Only then can they do the hard work of wrestling with the difficult choices and trade-offs involved in the various health care dilemmas. The public has not yet reached this stage on any important reforms in health care policy that require citizens to make sacrifices or accept real change.

—*Cognitive Stand*. After the choicework comes a sixth step when people reach tentative conclusions, largely cognitive in character. For example, people may agree intellectually on the need to curb heroic medicine, without realizing emotionally that they may have to forgo high-tech interventions to prolong life for a loved one.

—*Judgment*. In the seventh and final step, people add strong elements of emotional and moral conviction to their cognitive conclusions. If, in the example above, people did confront the decision on whether or not to pull the plug on a loved one and fully accepted all of the practical, emotional, and moral consequences of their decisions, they would have reached full deliberative judgment. The public is years from this stage.

Summary and Conclusion

The Clinton health care plan fell victim to the larger disconnect between our nation's leaders and its citizens. If the public had been more directly engaged in the health care debate of the last few years, instead of a crashing defeat, something positive might have been salvaged: out of the give-and-take between public and leaders, a viable plan of incremental reform might have emerged. Even now only the most limited short-term reforms are likely to succeed, because long-term reform will require Americans to make sacrifices and hard choices that they will not make unless the larger disconnect is addressed.

I propose for further discussion a strategy for stimulating a five-year process of public deliberation on health care. The strategy that will work best for health care reform will also help to repair the larger disconnect between political leaders and the public. The leadership skills needed for discussing health care reform with the public are the same as those required to deal with crime, education reform, welfare reform, race relations, and other important issues. If we are able to resolve our health care dilemmas and fix the larger disconnect at the same time, our democratic process will be the winner.

Comments

Drew E. Altman: I am in substantial agreement with Daniel Yankelovich and believe strongly that the Washington policy world has to do a better job of informing and engaging the public on big policy issues like health reform, welfare reform, or budget policy. The Kaiser Family Foundation has directed a major share of its work to this challenge. I also readily admit that I have made most of the mistakes in doing polling and in interpreting public opinion that Daniel Yankelovich describes. However, I do not necessarily think the outcome of the health reform debate would have been changed with better public deliberation, because the obstacles to public support for such reforms are more fundamental than lack of information and poor communications. I believe that even if the nation moved smoothly and sequentially through Yankelovich's "seven stages to public judgment," it would be a long time until the public arrived at that all important "stage eight." That is the stage when people are ready to say, "I want Congress to change *my* medical care, and I'm ready to pay more in taxes."

No amount of deliberation or better communication is likely to quickly change some of the broader, underlying trends. The most important trend public opinion analysts see in the surveys over the last many years is a decline in concern about social issues and social welfare and a rise in concern about economic issues and, most especially, increased distrust and frustration with government and Washington. Topical issues come and go, the Persian Gulf war and the war on drugs, for example, but if one steps back and analyzes the surveys, the longer-term trend persists. One can debate the depth of antigovernment feeling, the degree to which it is engineered for political advantage, and whether it translates into a genuine mandate for Republicans or just represents the latest episode of channel surfing by an angry public, but I think virtually everyone would agree that the rise of antigovernment feeling is real.

The health reform debate contributed to and was affected by these broad, underlying trends. It was the most visible example people took with them to the polls of failed government and of a government in Washington they viewed as just not able to get its act together. The antigovernment sentiment also, obviously, contributed to the demise of health reform.

Against this backdrop, the Clinton plan—and virtually any comprehensive reform plan—was easy to characterize as a big government program and as a social rather than economic one. What made health care a first-tier issue in recent years and caused President Clinton to seize on it as a top priority was the transformation of health care from a social to an economic issue. In 1994 health care was redefined, again, as a social problem. What Harris Wofford had accomplished in Pennsylvania— making health care a focal point for people's economic insecurities—was lost.

Reformers have always dealt with the bedrock reality that when it comes to the public and health reform, people want reform as long as they do not have to change their own medical arrangements and do not have to pay more in taxes to get it. The Clinton plan proposed not just to solve defined problems—for example, insurance reform or even coverage for 38 million uninsured Americans—but rather to change the way most Americans get their health care and their health insurance. The plan also implied a redistribution of income, from the insured to the uninsured, though every effort was made to hide the transfer through cross subsidies built into health alliances. Because the Clinton plan exceeded the public mandate, it was easy for opponents to frighten people that the cure (the plan) would be worse than the disease (continuation of the status quo).

Nothing is wrong with exceeding the public mandate and pushing the public to do things that may be right but require some sacrifices. In a different time, we called this "leadership." Leaders should not be, and, by definition, are not, slaves to the daily public opinion poll in a representative democracy. But having pushed beyond the mandate, the administration had to get everything else right—the politics, the public relations, and the timing. Without repeating the experience we observed and lived through in 1994, that obviously did not happen. That failure, however, was not confined to Washington, because the very same thing happened in most states. It is hard to imagine having a broader public debate on health reform than occurred in Vermont or Oregon. Vermont's plan was killed in the state senate, and in Oregon, even though the architect of the plan is now governor, the employer mandate that was proposed to move to broader coverage is dead.

My view is that it might have been possible to sell a major reform plan if the plan had been different and if the politics and the timing had been handled differently as well. Clearly by the time it became apparent that the Clinton plan would not fly, too much time had elapsed, and it was too close to the election and too late to fashion a compromise in the face of the intensifying partisan politics that always comes in an election season.

I do not think that the interest groups defeated health reform. I have been quoted as saying, "The problem was not Harry and Louise. The problem was us."[35] By that comment I did not deny that the interest groups played a significant role but rather that they had a better fix on where the public was and took better advantage of it than did the advocates of reform. But, most significant, I think we saw a development of historic importance in this debate.

That development is that business and insurance companies and other "monied interests" now believe they can do more than operate behind the scenes: they can shift public opinion on big issues or at least make sure that the political agenda does not go against their interests. They can do this by using the tools of political campaigns for private purposes on a scale never seen before—polls, focus groups, grass-roots organizing, and especially negative media ads. I expect that these techniques will become regular features of the policy process on big national issues. Although such practices are not entirely new, the scale is new, and it is a development worthy of close scrutiny.

Conservatives may well enjoy an advantage in using these methods. Our surveys are showing that conservatives are now more politically active than liberals and independents. This activism gives conservative interest groups a base for mobilization. Members of Congress say that during the health reform debate they heard constantly in their districts from antireform groups but almost never from the advocates of reform. Perhaps this behavior reflects the classic case of concentrated costs for interest groups and diffused benefits for the public. The concentrated costs mobilize opposition; the diffuse (and debatable) benefits fail to mobilize support. The former Speaker of the House in Vermont captured the essential point perfectly, "Eighty-five percent of Vermonters have health insurance or don't care about it. If the public can't be engaged, a citizen legislature without the public education capacity to counter Harry and Louise is doomed."[36]

I agree with Yankelovich that observers have to be a lot smarter about how they read the polls. However, the problem is not polling—an otherwise entirely respectable and important enterprise—but politicians and others who give polling a bad name by paying too much attention to it and using it for their own narrow purposes.

In 1994 polls indicated the distinct unpopularity of anything called the Clinton plan.[37] The very next day the entire Democratic leadership stood up together and recited in unison, 'This is not the Clinton plan.' It was probably not a wrong strategic judgment, but it was also a powerful reminder of the influence that polling has on elected officials today.

Polls are most useful for uncovering people's underlying values and beliefs. They are less useful for identifying reliably where the public stands on specific policy options, because personal policy preferences change with events, with media coverage, and most especially, with the popularity of the public officials putting various policies forward. Unfortunately, polls are also useful for showing elected officials how to market their ideas, rather than how to genuinely engage the public in an effort to convince them of the rightness of their views.

The media face a major challenge. They must decide whether they are simply in the business of covering the news or whether they indeed have a broader obligation to educate and engage the public and to correct misstatements and distortions of the facts when they arise.

Where is public opinion going on health reform? For starters, health reform will not be the big health policy issue on the agenda. The big issue will be the budget and entitlement debate, which brings with it the potential for absolutely historic changes in our largest public programs in health and a huge challenge to inform and engage the public. A Kaiser poll recently showed that more Americans picked foreign aid and welfare as the items receiving the largest share in the federal budget.[38] These preconceptions, incorrect though they may be, are important. As long as people think that we can salvage the federal budget and reduce the federal deficit simply by cutting programs for foreigners and welfare recipients, they will never understand arguments made by elected officials that tougher choices need to be made. More important, they will get angrier and angrier at elected officials who they believe are proposing distasteful choices when the public believes there is an easier way out.

If the health reform debate resurfaces, the polls show that the public, though no longer supportive of comprehensive reform, would still strongly support a more modest Republican or conservative Democratic plan as long as it does not significantly expand government control of the health system. The most popular idea with the American people for an incremental plan is the "Kids First" idea—beginning by covering uninsured children.

Make no mistake, the mandate for health reform is not as strong as it was. But there is an opportunity for Republicans to move forward with a plan consistent with their own ideology and views that expands or protects coverage. Such a step can be taken, of course, only if there is enough money left in medicare and medicaid after the budget entitlement fight to help finance a modest, say $10 billion, Kids First insurance expansion without new taxes. Will the leadership in Congress choose to put a health proposal forward? Will the money be there? These are two very big questions. But there would be substantial public support for a modest health reform plan, and putting a proposal forward could be a big winner for many in Congress.

In summary, an ideal world might have an opportunity for better deliberation and real public judgment. In the world we are stuck with, it is very hard to plan for "seven steps to public judgment." Efforts to influence public opinion are concentrated around elections, and big decisions in Congress and windows of opportunity come rarely, and if they are missed they are gone. The challenge to educate the public about health reform is huge, but historians studying President Clinton's failed efforts or future leaders planning the next generation of reforms should not kid themselves that better communication and information would have necessarily produced a different public judgment on health reform in 1994.

Karlyn H. Bowman: I am not as critical as Daniel Yankelovich is about the health care debate that took place in 1993 and 1994. I would not call it, as Yankelovich does, a "debate that wasn't." The debate was incomplete and imperfect, but we learned much about public beliefs that should serve future reformers well. Although Americans have not confronted the health care dilemmas that Yankelovich identifies as requiring sacrifices and hard choices, they did render a clear negative verdict on the *approach* the Clinton administration proposed. They rejected the approach not because health care experts and interest groups who opposed the Clinton plan found it easy to raise doubts about the plan—they did—but because the plan violated core beliefs Americans held in this area. We now know in broad brush strokes what Americans do not want. Perhaps Yankelovich's deliberate model can help us learn what they do want in areas where difficult choices must be made.

What did we learn from this imperfect debate? We learned that Americans bring clear predispositions to their thinking about health care and that they will evaluate any reforms in the context of these. The Bush administration appeared to ignore many concerns and the Clinton administration misread them. The public's mind-set and a powerful contemporary critique of federal government performance combined to sink the bill. Yankelovich's discussion of Americans' core beliefs is compelling.

First, as he points out, Americans expect the federal government to play a major role in the provision of health care. In many policy areas today, including possibly welfare reform, the public prefers the states to take the lead. The belief that the federal government should be responsible for providing medical care for those who cannot pay for it themselves has not changed in fifty years. Second, Americans profess, as they have for many years, high satisfaction with the quality of the health care they receive and with their access to care.

Yankelovich identified a third theme of "mounting concerns about the state of the health care system" (particularly its cost) driven in large part by surface economic anxiety in 1992 and 1993 and subterranean anxiety in 1994. In 1992 many Americans believed that the Bush administration was ignoring this concern. Although I believe the public found the "crisis" formulation used by so many policymakers and pollsters a meaningless one and therefore gave wildly conflicting responses to questions that used it, they nonetheless wanted Washington to take their concerns seriously, as recent polls confirm. A January 1995 ABC News/*Washington Post* poll found that 45 percent of Americans thought that it was absolutely critical to reform health care as soon as possible, while 39 percent said it was important but not critical.[39] Only cutting the deficit produced higher overall numbers.

Although Americans expressed a strong desire for action throughout the 1993–94 debate, solid majorities said toward the end of the congressional deliberations that they were "relieved" and not "angry" that Congress had not passed a health care bill. These two superficially contradictory responses make perfect sense when one understands what the "do something tomorrow/crisis" responses really mean. Polls urging action are frequently admonitions to leaders to "pay attention." They should not be read as timetables for action. The data today appear to suggest that Americans would be satisfied with modest health care reforms in the near future. When 45 percent of Americans put health care on the critical list as they did in the January 1995 ABC/*Post* poll, they are not answering the question literally.[40] They are simply saying to decisionmakers, "Don't ignore my concerns." Throughout the debate, Americans believed that Bill Clinton was taking their concerns seriously. In the end, however, they disagreed with his approach to reform.

Yankelovich believes Americans rejected the plan for three reasons, and I agree with his assessment. A superficial reading of polls convinced the president that the public was as committed to universal coverage as he was. Universal coverage is an important goal for the public. But other goals are important too, and they trump universal coverage. The Gallup Organization posed a revealing battery of questions in January 1994 on this point. In response to the first question, Americans voiced strong support for a health care package that guarantees every American health insurance that cannot be taken away. The next question revealed high support for the president if he vetoed a bill that did not guarantee universal coverage. The conviction seemed to strengthen when Americans answered the third question in this series. Slightly over seven in ten supported universal coverage even if their taxes would go up to pay for it. But the final question raised the possibility that universal coverage might cause the availability of health services to be limited. Opinion turned decisely against universal coverage. Support for universal coverage withers, Yankelovich says, "when people [are] directly confronted [with] the cost consequences of providing health insurance to everyone." Many people, including the architects of the Clinton plan, should be aware of this response now.

Yankelovich also identifies a second reason for the failure of the Clinton plan—that Americans did not like its apparent complexity. This concern is related to the sentiment that, Yankelovich suggests, put the final nail in the coffin for the administration's plan—growing anti-Washington sentiment. Both the plan's complexity and the idea that it would enhance the reach of an already problem-causing federal behemoth worked powerfully to turn public opinion against the plan.

I would add another item—the perception that the plan would restrict choices in the provision of health care. One of the most powerful currents in our democracy is the importance of individual choice. The sentiment comes up in response to questions about abortion, smoking, or even suicide. It may seem anachronistic to talk about the freedom to choose one's own doctor when this option is no longer available to many Americans, but the public worries when it perceives that choices will be restricted further.

The tide of opinion not only turned against the Clinton health plan but also affected perceptions of the Democrats. In most polls today, Democrats maintain their historic advantage as the party better able to handle health care, but that edge has diminished. The advantage Democrats had as being more compassionate about the issue is swamped by the advantage Republicans have as being seen as more opposed to a bigger federal government. In the last thirty years, polls have produced much evidence that suggests Americans are deeply ambivalent about the proper role of the federal government. On the one hand, Americans believe that government should do many things in a country as rich and powerful as our own. They believe also that government causes problems and is wasteful, inefficient, and intrusive. The weight of public opinion today is clearly that government is a problem-causer, and this sentiment undergirds negative reaction to a health plan the public thought would increase government's role.

The Clinton administration, having misread the survey data on universal coverage, also misread the polls showing support for the plan when it was announced. The so-called "support" was not support at all. What the public approved instead was a strong speech on a subject of great concern to them. Bill Clinton, unlike George Bush before him, appeared to be paying attention. The public knew little about the details—something that should have raised red flags for journalists and pollsters that "support" was not what it seemed. The public indicated throughout the debate that it did not know much about the plan.

Today Americans tell their leaders in Washington that this issue (like welfare reform and crime, to mention just two others) is important. Solid majorities continue to tell the pollsters they are satisfied with the quality and availability of their health care. Most say they can meet routine medical expenses, but they worry about rising costs and about their ability to deal with catastrophic illnesses. In large part because of the way the debate took place in 1993 and 1994, the public seems inclined to modest reforms. Yankelovich agrees that a consensus exists about some of these, particularly insurance reforms. I conclude that a debate did take place—albeit an incomplete one. The debate that took place, however, did not move the United States very far toward mature public judgment.

Yankelovich also raises some lesser issues that are worth mentioning. I share his concerns about the reliance policymakers put on polls. Polls are blunt instruments, and, as the Clinton administration's experience illustrates, even the most sophisticated analysts can misread them. Yankelovich says that journalists performed a useful service early in the debate by raising awareness of health care as an issue, but that they then "kibitzed" the issue. I, too, would give the media high marks for trying to initiate a discussion on important health care dilemmas, but they then dropped the ball and covered the issue in a familiar campaign mode—whether the president was winning or losing, up or down. The way the press covered the issue spilled over into the way pollsters polled on it. The media pollsters covered the health care debate as if it were a political campaign too, with Clinton up early on and losing ground thereafter. These polls were virtually useless from a policy standpoint.

Polls are invaluable in the formation of policy in the kind of work Yankelovich has pioneered at the Public Agenda Foundation. The in-depth focus groups Public Agenda conducts often in conjunction with national polls are enormously useful for policymakers. Over and over again in Public Agenda reports on health care issues, Americans expressed concerns about more federal involvement in health care. These concerns were not manufactured by interest groups; they were spontaneous. When experts and interest groups later raised the specter of increased federal government involvement in health care under the Clinton plan, they found a receptive audience. If officials had paid attention to the concerns identified in these focus groups and polls, I doubt the administration would ever have advanced the reforms they did.

Analyzing what happened is considerably easier than charting a new course. Yankelovich provides a detailed playbook on a public deliberation model that he believes will serve policymakers well. There are many serious obstacles to its implementation, and he discusses some of them. One of these is the disposition of leaders who will need to be involved.

Many polls reinforce the perception of a profound distance between leaders and the public, and like Daniel Yankelovich I worry about the consequences of this situation for the democratic process. Leaders are removed from the public not only by their education and income but also by their professional training. The gulf between leaders and the public will be hard to bridge, especially when professional culture reinforces it. I wish Yankelovich had said more about how leaders can break out of the debilitating straightjacket to become involved in the health care debate in the future.

Leaders have work to do, but so does the public, and I am not confident the public will rise to the challenges set out in Yankelovich's paper. It is not because Americans do not think these issues are important—they do—or because they resist the hard work that will be needed to resolve difficult conflicts—they do not. Instead, Americans are reluctant to participate in large measure because the debates are so complex and there are so many competing demands on their time. Yankelovich says that full public deliberation could take years to complete and that the final stages—resistance and choicework—where Americans confront their own wishful thinking are especially difficult. With both parents working in many families and not enough time to spend with children, families may well stay on the sidelines, settling for the kind of imperfect debate that occurred last year.

Beyond the concerns about whether leaders will change to engage in this kind of dialogue and the public will embrace it, I have some practical question about Yankelovich's model. How would the process of deliberation start? Would the media play a central role? Although Yankelovich lauds the media for their contribution to the early stages of public deliberation, he argues that they did not carry out the more complex and demanding communication tasks needed at later stages of the debate. Did the media not try or did the limitations of print and television make this time-consuming task impossible to carry out? Realistically, how many Americans can be expected to get involved? If the forum for the exercise is to be television, my guess is that the audience will be small and unrepresentative.

A final concern I have is related to the priority health care will be given when other issues warrant this kind of debate. Although health care is clearly important, Yankelovich says that there are many other issue that demand this kind of intensive effort. An obvious one is environmental protection. How much risk are Americans willing to take? How clean is clean enough? If the public cannot institute genuine deliberation—and I believe the obstacles are great—more reliance on the kind of work Yankelovich has designed, and Public Agenda has carried out over the years, can serve policymakers well.

Uwe Reinhardt: Daniel Yankelovich argues that this nation's recent attempt at health reform failed largely because the American public failed to "deliberate" properly on the issue. By "deliberation" Yankelovich means "mulling over" the costs and benefits of alternative choices and making tough choices, all in a serious "give and take" with the nation's "leadership class." Yankelovich blames the public's failure to "deliberate" properly squarely on the shoulders of the "leadership class" which, according to him, deliberated only within its own ranks. "The disconcerting truth is that most of them [the leaders] do not know how to talk to the public."

Embedded in Yankelovich's grand thesis are three subhypotheses that warrant closer scrutiny. These are the leadership class itself had properly "deliberated" on health reform but failed to communicate the product of that "deliberation" to the public; channels of communication exist through which the leadership class could, if it wished, engage in a "give and take" with the public; and the public is intellectually and temperamentally predisposed to "deliberate" sincerely on complex issues of public policy and to make the requisite tough choices in a lengthy conversation with the nation's leaders.

I believe each of these subhypotheses is utopian, as is Yankelovich's strategy for fixing the "disconnect" between leaders and the public.

Deliberation within the Leadership Class

When America's "leadership class" sets out to debate health policy, its members invariably preface their "deliberations" with the mantra, "We all want the same things in health care. We are merely arguing over the means to that end." This is utter nonsense.

The great health reform debate of 1993–94 was not just a technical dispute over alternative means of reaching widely shared goals. It was a fierce ideological battle over the goal itself. The nation's leadership class was and remains deeply divided over the ethical precepts that should govern the distribution of health care.

At one end of the ideological spectrum are the pure egalitarians who would like to see health care made equally available to all members of society regardless of the individual's ability to pay for it. Adherents to this school of thought would like to see health care financed collectively, through mandatory contributions that vary strictly with ability to pay but certainly not according to the health status of the household's members.

At the other end of the ideological spectrum is what one may dub the "food people," who are puzzled why anyone would distinguish between health care and other basic, private consumption goods, such as food and housing. As Representative Dick Armey, leader of the House of

Representatives put it to the *Wall Street Journal* in his inimitably blunt style: "Health care is just a commodity, just like bread, and just like housing and everything else."[41] The food people regard the procurement and financing of health care as chiefly the responsibility of the individual whose own behavior is thought to be a major determinant of his or her health status. To be sure, the members of this school of thought do admit that external factors may cause illness, and they are prepared to guarantee the poor and near poor at least a basic ration of critically needed health care. At the same time, however, they see nothing wrong with a health system in which the quantity, timeliness, and quality of the health care received by American families vary systematically and positively with household income. If one believes, as adherents of this school of thought tend to believe, that the American economy is the closest approximation worldwide to a true meritocracy, then an income-based health system is much more defensible on ethical grounds than would be a purely egalitarian one.

In the great health reform battle of 1993–94, the food people won squarely, although perhaps not fairly. One may question the fairness of the battle, because it was never fought openly, in the blunt language favored by Congressman Armey. Instead, much of the action was camouflaged behind such soothing code words as "empowerment," "personal responsibility," and the "freedom to chose whether or not to be insured," words all adding up to the proposition that well-to-do Americans should be empowered to allocate their income to health care and other commodities as they see fit, and that poor and low-income households should be empowered to do likewise with their much more meager budgets.

With the victory of the food people the U.S. Congress has all but officially sanctioned an income-based health system with the following three tiers.

First, for poor or near-poor uninsured Americans—chiefly families of people who work full time at low wages and salaries—we shall reserve and perhaps expand our current patchwork of public hospitals and clinics. These publicly financed institutions will be sorely underfunded, as they always have been, and suffer from severely limited physical capacity. Such limits, in turn, will beget the long queues that have always been the classic instrument of rationing. Lack of funding will also limit the medical technology available to the physicians working in these public institutions. The uninsured will increasingly be driven to these public facilities, as government programs and private managed care systems eat ever more deeply into the profit margins of private hospitals, thereby reducing the capacity of these institutions to act as insurers of last resort.

Second, the employed broad middle class will increasingly enroll in capitated health plans, such as health maintenance organizations. These plans will be budgeted prospectively, on a per capita basis, through competitively bid premiums. To control their outlays, the plans necessarily must limit the patient's choice of doctor and hospital at time of illness. Furthermore, these health plans will inevitably come to withhold some care that patients and their physicians might judge desirable, but that the management of the capitated plan and the clinical experts advising them may find too expensive relative to the expected medical benefits.

Finally, well-to-do Americans will continue to enjoy an open-ended, free-choice, fee-for-service health system without rationing of any form, even when additional care is of dubious clinical or economic merit. Well-to-do Americans will demand no less, and they will have it. Furthermore, they will continue to have it on a fully tax-deductible basis, a tax preference to the rich that no economist would ever defend, but that no politician would dare to remove.

Though congressional sanction for this three-tiered health system is now a *fait accompli*, no consensus among the "leadership class" supports it. In Yankelovich's sense of the term, that class did not "deliberate" properly on the matter either. But even if there had been a forthright deliberation and there had been a consensus on the disability of a three-tiered health system, exploring that idea in an open "give-and-take" with the general public would have been an extremely delicate task, with large segments of the public finding themselves at the short end of this arrangement, Furthermore, what channels exist for the conduct of such a "conversation"?

The Media as a Channel of Communication

Yankelovich takes the by now almost obligatory swipe at the media with his assertion that journalists were more interested in the political ramifications of the Clinton health plan than with its contents. Although there is something to that proposition, his indictment is much too broad. At the very least, a distinction should be made between the television media and the print media.

Television may one day become a medium through which policymakers communicate with the general public in an informative "give-and-take." So far, however, that medium has not been structured to facilitate such an exchange. Both C-span and the public television stations do allow the public to observe experts in the act of "deliberation," but that is not a conversation with the public. The remainder of the television industry has not been able to facilitate even a coherent one-way, top-down communication with the general public, aside from a bewildering scatter of sound bites.

The producers of television programs devoted to public policy invariably feel compelled to pack these program with a variety of opposing views. By the time they have accommodated this dictate of "fairness" and the imperative of commercials, any one person's role on the program is limited to a few minutes of air time. Producers decisively nix even the thought of using a simple graph or table to amplify a point in such discussions as too intellectually taxing for the general public. In fact, almost every anchor on whose television program I have appeared has apologized in advance for the necessary brevity and superficiality of the proceedings.

The print media offer a better potential. Indeed, the staff reporters of the major newspapers deserve high marks for their ceaseless efforts at digging out the relevant facts on the Clinton or other health reform plans. They also deserve high marks for their skill in presenting these facts to the public in well-structured articles. Unfortunately, this channel is best suited for the one-way, top-down communication Yankelovich decries. Furthermore, it is not clear that the general public had the patience to digest the lengthier, excellent articles on health reform in the major dailies.

To the extent that the print media did improperly *politicize* the recent health reform debate, as Yankelovich suggests, one must lay the blame on the leaders of the industry, not on the rank and file. A concrete case can serve to illustrate this assertion.

In a commentary dramatically entitled, "The Clintons' Lethal Paternalism," and published in the widely read weekly Newsweek, syndicated columnist George Will flatly asserted that, under the Clinton plan, "there would be 15-year jail terms for people driven to bribery for care they feel they need but the government does not deem 'necessary.'"[42] To the best of my knowledge, this statement is a documentable falsehood. The Health Security Act clearly states: "Nothing in this Act shall be construed as prohibiting the following: (1) An individual from purchasing any health care services. (2) An individual from purchasing supplemental insurance (offered consistent with this Act) to cover health care services not included within the comprehensive benefit package."[43] Indeed it would be truly astounding to see an American president advocate fifteen-year jail terms for anyone seeking to purchase health services the government deems unnecessary (and therefore excludes from the mandated benefit package). Accordingly, I requested in correspondence with George Will that he pinpoint the paragraph in the *Health Security Act* that calls for the alleged penalty. He has not been able to do that, and I doubt that he ever will.[44] One must wonder whether any senior editor of Newsweek at the time ever challenged him on this point, as he ought to have been.

It is entirely proper for a syndicated columnist to refract policy recommendations through the prism of his or her own ideology and to judge them on that basis. It is another matter entirely, however, when syndicated columnists use the extraordinary privilege granted them by the media to proffer their own ideology in the guise of synthetic "facts" that the general public is likely to accept as reliable. Senior editors of op-ed pages who passively accept fantasy masquerading as fact shortchange not only their own conscientious staff reporters but the general public. They allow a potentially useful channel of communication to be polluted with disinformation and thereby make it all the more difficult for conscientious leaders to communicate with the public. The recent debacle of health reform offers the leaders of the media an opportunity for some soul-searching on this point.

Deliberation by the Public

Suppose that America's leadership class had deliberated properly on health reform, and suppose the leaders of the print media had acted responsibly, carefully checking the veracity of whatever was presented as fact in their publications. Would this happy circumstance then have led to a productive "give-and-take" between the leadership class and the general public, and would this happy circumstance have triggered the proper "deliberation" within the general public?

One wishes it were so. Alas, Yankelovich's own paper is anything but reassuring on this question. He deplores the American public's habit of "blaming the system rather than itself," its "lack of realism," its "persistence of wishful thinking and [its] failure to wrestle with hard choices," and its "continuing belief that [the public] can have it all-quality and convenience and high-tech medicine and lower costs." "Polling data on health care," he writes, "are replete with evidence that people neither understand nor accept the consequences of implementing their wish list of expanded health care benefits."

If one had to distill Yankelovich's description of American public opinion on health reform into one adjective, it would be "adolescent." This eternal adolescence of the plebs is, of course, by no means confined to health policy, nor is it a uniquely American trait. Of the Roman plebs, for example, that era's great poet Juvenal wrote, in the first century A.D., "Duas tantum res anxius optat, panem et circenses."[45] (Its anxious longing is confined to but two things—bread and circus games.) Yankelovich's chapter suggests that not much has changed in the ensuing millennia. Although, unlike their peers in other nations, America's "leadership class" seems unduly anxious to pay homage to the legendary perspicacity of the grass roots, Yankelovich's survey of public opinion in his paper leads one to wonder whether politicians' habitual praise of the grass roots really is more than an expedient courtesy.

Indeed, Yankelovich's paper leads one to wonder whether the American public is intellectually or temperamentally inclined ever to engage in the protracted, sincere "public deliberation" of complex public policies called for by the optimistic author. If successful health reform must await the day when the public musters the patience to deliberate carefully on the hard choices beforeit, at the price of abandoning the endless latter day "circus games" that engage the public's mind, then we may have to wait for a very long time.

I certainly do not mean to be disrespectful of a basically admirable people. Nor am I persuaded, however, that the American public somehow stands out among its counterparts elsewhere in the world in its willingness and ability to "deliberate" seriously on serious issues of public policy. My observation of this nation during the past thirty years persuades me that, in almost all cases, successful major initiatives in public policy occurred when the leadership class had reached a broad consensus on the matter and then simply told the plebs what was good for it. President Reagan's "supply-side economics" was enacted on that basis, and so was the quite revolutionary tax act of 1986. In either case, the general public had only the dimmest idea of what these policies entailed; it simply took the leadership's assurances on faith.

Given the general public's age-old preoccupation with panem and circenses it will generally go along passively with its leadership, unless that leadership makes obvious and egregious mistakes or unless that leadership is evidently divided. Thus we start wars, thus we bomb whomever our leadership has decided to bomb, thus we end wars, thus we pass tax laws and civil rights laws, thus we allow the leadership (along with leaders of sundry special interests) to regulate and sometimes to deregulate the conduct of the plebs, and thus, perhaps one day, we shall undertake a major reform of our health insurance system. Perhaps.

Notes

1. Americans age 65 and older were initially the most resistant age group in the population to all health care reforms when they first heard about them. But unlike younger Americans, they were the only group whose support for reform actually *increased* after they had wrestled with the trade-offs that reform would entail. DYG, Inc., for the American Association of Retired Persons, *Health Care Reform in America: Where The Public Stands* (Washington, March 1992).

2. Yankelovich Partners for *Time*/CNN, October 1993.

3. Ibid., July 1994.

4. *Gallup Poll Monthly*, no. 311 (August 1991), p. 6.

5. Louis Harris and Associates, April–May 1987.

6. Louis Harris and Associates, September 1993. See also Karlyn H. Bowman, "The 1993–1994 Debate on Health Care Reform: Are the Polls Misleading the Policy Makers?" Washington, American Enterprise Institute for Public Policy Research, 1994, p. 3.

7. Roper Search Worldwide, Inc., New York, 1973, 1993.

8. *Wall Street Journal*/NBC, September 1993.

9. CBS/*New York Times*, August 1991.

10. *Gallup Poll Monthly*, no. 311 (August 1991), p. 4.

11. See "The Public Decides on Health Care Reform," *Public Perspective*, vol. 5 (September–October 1994), pp. 23–28.

12. Ibid.

13. Forty-two percent is a huge open-end response. *Gallup Poll Monthly*, no. 311 (August 1991), p. 8.

14. *Time*/CNN, August 1991.

15. Gallup poll, June 26–29, 1991.

16. Yankelovich Clancy Shulman for *Time*/CNN, August 27, 28, 1991.

17. Robert J. Blendon, Tracey S. Hyams, and John M. Benson, "Bridging the Gap between Expert and Public Views on Health Care Reform," *Journal of the American Medical Association*, vol. 269 (May 19, 1993), pp. 2573–78.

18. Julie Kosterlitz, "What the Public Prefers . . . We're Demanding It All—except the Bill," *Washington Post*, February 14, 1993, p. C3.

19. Harvard School of Public Health and Martilla and Kiley for the Robert Wood Johnson Foundation. See "A Survey of American Attitudes toward Health Care Reform" (N.J.: Robert Wood Johnson Foundation, June 1993); and *Wall Street Journal*/NBC, September 1993.

20. *Los Angeles Times*, September 1993, pp. 25–28.

21. Robert J. Samuelson, "Don't Be Afraid of the Health Debate," *Washington Post*, October 20, 1993, p. A29.

22. ABC News/*Washington Post*, November 1993.

23. Louis Harris and Associates for the Robert Wood Johnson Foundation, August 1994.

24. *Washington Post*, October 7–10, 1993.

25. This result was obtained from a search of the archives of the Roper Center for Public Opinion Research at the University of Connecticut at Storrs using the database POLL.

26. For additional interpretation see Daniel Yankelovich, "What Polls Say— and What They Mean," *New York Times*, September 17, 1994, p. 23.

27. "The Public Decides."

28. *Gallup Poll Monthly*, no. 347 (August 1994), p. 52, conducted by the Gallup organization for CNN and *USA Today*.

29. DYG, Inc., for AARP, March 1992.

30. See Daniel Yankelovich, *Coming to Public Judgment: Making Democracy Work in a Complex World* (Syracuse University Press, 1991).

31. Ibid.; and Daniel Yankelovich, "How Public Opinion Really Works," *Fortune*, October 5, 1992, pp. 102–08.

32. Willard Gaylin, "Faulty Diagnosis: Why Clinton's Health-care Plan Won't Cure What Ails Us," *Harper's Magazine*, October 1993, pp. 57–64, quotation on p. 58.

33. Yankelovich, *Coming to Public Judgment*.

34. See Yankelovich, "How Public Opinion Really Works." I summarized the situation in October 1992 as follows: "People feel a sense of urgency about changing the health care system but haven't even begun to confront realistically the hard choices that need to be made. Unfortunately, policymakers are largely unaware of the depth and intensity of the public's resistance, for the simple reason that the bulk of it has not yet made itself felt—voters have not yet focused on the hard choices."

35. Adam Clymer, Robert Pear, Robin Toner, "The Health Care Debate: What Went Wrong?" *New York Times*, August 29, 1994, p. A1.

36. *States of Health*, vol. 5 (January 1995), p. 5.

37. Robert J. Blendon, Maryann Brodie, and John Benson, "What Happened to America's Support of the Clinton Plan?" *Health Affairs*, vol. 14 (Summer 1995), pp. 7–24.

38. Kaiser/Harvard Survey on Welfare and the Budget, January 1995; and Kaiser/Harvard Election Eve Survey, November 15, 1994.

39. ABC News/*Washington Post* poll, January 1995.

40. Ibid.

41. Rick Wartzman, "Economy: Linking of Universal Health Coverage to Cost Containment Endures Scrutiny," *Wall Street Journal*, November 23, 1993, p. A2.

42. George F. Will, "The Clintons' Lethal Paternalism," *Newsweek*, February 7, 1994; p. 64.

43. Title I, section 1003, page 15, of the *Health Security Act* as presented to Congress on October 27, 1993. (Reprinted by the Commerce Clearing House, Inc, Chicago, Ill., 1993.)

44. Because I had apprised Mr. Will in my first letter that I would like to share the correspondence with others, I feel at liberty to offer anyone interested in it copies of that correspondence.

45. Juvenal, *Satires*, sec. viii, p. 83.

CHAPTER FIVE

Interest Groups in the Health Care Debate

Graham K. Wilson

W HO KILLED health care reform? The list of heroes or villains (depending on one's point of view) is lengthy, including both White House policy "wonks" who allegedly thought about everything but the politics of the issue and Republican congressional leaders determined to deny the Clinton administration a major victory. For many Americans, however, interest groups are the explanation for the failure of the Clintons' health plan. When the *New York Times*/*CBS* pollsters presented respondents with a list of explanations for the stalemate over health care reform, "the respondents pointed most frequently to special interests and lobbyists."[1] Hillary Rodham Clinton seemed to share this view at least partially, telling the press that "she was not prepared for the amount of resources that were readily available to the opposition."[2] She suggested that political resources were balanced heavily against reform, estimating that between $120 million and $300 million was spent against the plan compared with only $12 million to $15 million spent for it by the Democratic National Committee. The widespread suspicion that "the special interests" have the resources to block any meaningful reform has been an important element in contemporary American political argument. Was the failure of the Clinton plan just another, though particularly important, example? If so, what were the broader implications of the failure for the state of American democracy?

I am grateful to Bob Turner and Virginia Sapiro for invaluable assistance and advice; all judgments, interpretations, and errors remain my responsibility.

Danger Signs

Two trends might have prepared Hillary Clinton for the scale of the mobilization against the administration's health care proposal that apparently so surprised her: the increasing vigor of interest group politics and the unfortunate results of previous attempts to reform health care financing.

Interest Groups

The activity of interest groups in Washington, D.C., has increased massively in the past thirty years. The number of lobbyists in Washington has increased considerably. New forms of interest group activity have emerged, such as political action committees, Washington law firms, and the new profession of contract lobbyists. Groups such as consumers or environmentalists conspicuously absent from the interest group system thirty years ago are conspicuously present today. Interests long represented in Washington engage in more political activity employing more lobbyists and making more contributions through their PACs than ever before. Thus increased activity by interest groups represents both the growth of existing interest groups and the creation of new organizations; a single issue of the *National Journal* in 1993 recorded the opening of D.C. offices by groups as diverse as the Women's Mining Coalition, the Society of Manufacturing Engineers, and the National Telecommuting and Telework Association.

The increase in interest group activity continued during the Clinton years, aided among other things by the debate over health care. Health industry groups increased their political contributions from $6.6 million in 1991 to $8.4 million in the first ten months of 1993.[3] A huge demand existed for lobbyists to work on health care, especially if they had any contacts with the Clintons. One trade association, the Pharmaceutical Manufacturers' Association, spent $7 million on public relations by September 1993, and a single firm, Porter Novelli, reported having received $1.5 million of business related to the Clinton plan by the same date.[4] Although the health care debate was not the only reason, it is an important factor explaining why the number of registered lobbyists in Washington increased by 234 in 1994 from 7,633 during the Bush administration.

The growth of interest group activity often represents disaggregation within sectors, including health. Interests that once felt adequately represented by a single organization such as a trade association covering an entire industry now feel the need to represent themselves directly. In the pharmaceutical industry, for example, the major manufacturer, Merck, now has twice as many representatives in Washington, D.C., as the Pharmaceutical Manufacturers' Association.[5] The trend toward lobbyists representing individual universities is another example. Ever more and ever narrower interests are developing a permanent lobbying capacity.

Thus we see a trend toward a greater variety of interests to be represented in Washington in the interest group system and also for interests already represented to fragment into smaller units. The increased variety and the fragmentation of interest representation make securing agreement on policy proposals even more difficult than in the past. Yet the increased resources and sophistication of interest groups have simultaneously made more severe the penalties that interest groups can exact if politicians do not reach agreement with them.

Past Attempts at Health Care Reform

That every major health care reform in the past had been accompanied by considerable interest group conflict might have prepared the administration for the onslaught of interest groups. The most famous of all these conflicts was the dispute between the American Medical Association (AMA) and a liberal coalition led by the American Federation of Labor-Congress of Industrial Organizations (AFL-CIO) over the adoption of government-funded health care schemes, including medicare.[6] Interest groups were highly visible actors, but they did not play a decisive role largely because powerful groups counteracted each other. A well-funded and organized campaign against medicare by the AMA was matched by a well-funded and organized campaign in favor led by the AFL-CIO. Theodore Marmor suggested that any future attempt to reform the health care system extensively would prompt the reappearance of fierce conflict between what he described as "remarkably stable" coalitions of liberal and conservative interest groups. "The federal government's role in the financing of personal health services is one of the small class of public issues which can be counted on to activate deep, emotional and bitter cleavages between what political commentators call 'liberal' and 'conservative' pressure groups."[7]

Interest Group Preferences

The administration showed some signs that it had partially realized the inevitability of conflict among interest groups on the issue. A January 1993 memo from Ira Magaziner to Hillary Clinton had anticipated the arguments that groups such as insurance companies and small business would advance against the administration's plan while failing to foresee—as he admitted later—the resources and intensity of effort of their opposition.[8]

But was Magaziner correct that interest groups have stable preferences that policymakers can do little to alter? It is common to assume that interest groups always immediately know what constitutes the interest they exist to protect. In practice, interest group preferences are constructed in a process that is influenced by their ideology, the needs of the organization itself, the groups' understanding of policy problems, policy problems and alternatives, and the incentives rooted in the structure of the decisionmaking process.

It is an error to suppose that there is a single obvious "interest" for an interest group to pursue. For example, the conservative ideology of the American Farm Bureau Federation long led it to reject farm subsidy programs that seemed to others (such as the National Farmers' Union) clearly in the "interest" of farmers.[9] Marmor's analysis of the politics of medicare suggested that the AMA long opposed proposals for federal financing of medical care for the elderly that contributed to physicians' "interests."[10] David Vogel argued that American business executives have displayed a chronic suspicion of state involvement in solutions to their problems, even when solutions involving state action seemed to serve their "interests."[11]

Interest groups also have organizational needs of their own that can influence the position that they take on policy issues. James Q. Wilson has provided a brilliant analysis of how organizational needs such as recruiting and retaining members can shape interest group strategy.[12] Interest groups adopt policies and pursue strategies not only to try to influence public policy. They also need to convince members or potential members that they provide "selective incentives" (individualized reasons) to join. Selective incentives may be opportunities for material gain. They may also be the means of obtaining psychological benefits such as a way to express rage about politics or policy or simply to enjoy the satisfaction of belonging. American interest groups operate in a highly competitive environment, in which nearly always several groups are claiming to represent the same section of society. Giving the members (and potential members) the impression that they get value for money can lead groups to adopt visible and even strident policies, even if these strategies are not the most likely to influence the outcome of legislation. Interest groups that enjoy a monopoly or that dominate a sector have more opportunities to make compromises than those that are competing for members. Statesmanship is hard to display when competitors are likely to tell your members that you have "gone soft," "become part of the Washington establishment," or to use the phrase popular with my generation in the 1960s, "sold out."

Even were these influences absent, a bill's content alone does not automatically translate into interest group opinions about it. Interest groups often struggle (frequently with limited research capacity) to understand how proposed legislation will affect their members. The difficulty of this calculation occurs partly because of the challenge (shared with all other political actors) of understanding its purposes and, if possible, its unintended consequences. The implementation of a bill may be much different than its framers' intent, creating further uncertainty for interests groups. The notorious length of the Health Security bill and its complexity made understanding its implications for any interest group a difficult and often uncertain process. Further complexity resulted from differences that might exist between a group's short- and long-term interests. In more prosaic terms, a group might be persuaded to settle for something it dislikes if it is convinced that something worse will otherwise happen tomorrow.

Finally, interest groups' policies are also dictated by the institutional situation in which they operate. At the very least, interest groups want adequate opportunity to present their concerns and needs. Beyond that, as institutional analysis rooted in game theory has emphasized, the way in which decisionmaking is structured has a profound impact on what its reactions will be to any given proposal. Interest groups might accept that they will have a policy somewhat contrary to their interests if they know that all similar interests are "losing" similarly; a group is unlikely to accept arguments for making sacrifices if it cannot be sure that all similar groups will be obliged to do the same. For example, a union is less likely to accept a wage freeze (no matter how strong the arguments that this will increase workers' future incomes) or a corporation an environmental regulation (no matter how strong the evidence that there is a problem that must be addressed) if it thinks that other unions or corporations will not be required to make the same sacrifice.

Policymakers in stable democracies such as the United States might seem to have few opportunities to change either the underlying ideologies of interest groups or the structure of decisionmaking. A Democratic administration is unlikely to imbue the National Federation of Independent Businesses (NFIB) with liberalism; no one seriously expects the U.S. Constitution to be amended significantly. Policies can be presented in a variety of ways, increasing or diminishing the degree to which they conflict with interest groups' core ideologies. Skilled political packaging, seen, for example, in President Lyndon Johnson's presentation of initiatives such as the War on Poverty as a continuation of the American tradition of opportunity, can help to avoid intense opposition. Political skills can also be brought to bear in deciding how policy is made in practice. Policymaking structures are not mere legal entities but political practices that also contain less formally and explicitly defined procedures. These procedures can be varied in ways that either increase or diminish the force of opposition to the decisions that are made. Interest groups are likely to be concerned that policy is made only after they have had adequate opportunities to state their case and that competing interests have been given no procedural advantages.

In short, if policymakers want the leaders of an interest group to compromise with them, they need to consider not only the content of their policy but how it is presented and developed. Politically sensitive packaging and decisionmaking matter as well as content. In a policy sphere such as health care, where interest group activitiy will be intense and considerable, astute political management consists not merely of predicting the original attitudes of interest groups but of developing a strategy for manipulating them. Such manipulation certainly includes changing the content of the policy to appeal to an interest group. It also includes shaping the presentation of a policy to fit a group's ideology and choosing decision procedures that maximize cooperation.

The Clinton Administration's Opportunity

Historical analysis would have prompted the Clinton administration to expect considerable and predictable opposition from some interest groups and support from others.[13] A survey of interest groups concerned with health care suggests, however, that the administration faced interest groups that were more open to persuasion than ever before and more internally divided, opening the prospects for alliances with interest groups that once would have been unreachable.

No group illustrates the opportunities for disrupting the well-established interest group alliances on health care better than the AMA, the bedrock of opposition to medicare. Since the fight over medicare, the

AMA had declined as an organization. By the early 1990s, it represented only 41 percent of American doctors.[14] Who were the AMA's political friends and enemies was no longer clear. Whereas doctors had long feared that under "socialized medicine" the government would take away their professional freedom, they now found that insurance companies were doing the same. As market forces and insurance companies pushed doctors into health maintenance organizations (HMOs) and other forms of managed care that competed for business by offering discounted rates to employers, and as insurance companies insisted on approving costly procedures in advance, the idea that the choice was between an expanded role for the government or "freedom to practice" became anachronistic.

The AMA and its former political allies, the insurance companies, clashed publicly.[15] In consequence, the AMA was divided. The head of the AMA's Chicago office headquarters, Vice President John B. Crosby, favored the Clintons' plan. The head of the Washington office, Lee J. Stillwell, who had worked previously for a conservative business group, was strongly opposed.[16] In consequence, the political situation within the AMA was highly fluid. The AMA early supported a central but controversial feature of the Clintons' plan, employer mandates. But then House Republican Whip Newt Gingrich and fifty of his party members wrote to all 450 members of the AMA House of Delegates attacking the position the AMA leaders had taken.[17] Nonetheless, the possibility remained from the administration's point of view of taking the AMA out of the opposition coalition, a move that in terms of the past politics of health care would have been equivalent to sacking the quarterback.

Equally alluring for the Clinton team was the possibility of securing support of business, the faithful ally of the AMA in earlier health wars.[18] This possibility arose from two sources.

The first was the heavy burden on corporations purchasing health insurance for employees, especially those in traditionally unionized sectors such as steel and automobile manufacturing. Health care insurance had become a significant element in the cost of U.S. manufacturing, believed by many to impede competition with imports and with nonunionized companies. By the late 1980s, health insurance was an issue in a majority of strikes in the United States.[19] Many employers were already contributing to the costs of the health care system in general more than they would under any of the major plans for reform. Employers pay 86 percent of private health insurance costs, but these costs are divided very unevenly.[20] The highest medical costs fall on utilities, which spend $3,924 per worker, while the lowest costs fall on the retail sector, averaging $1,044 per worker.[21] Many large corporations that provided comprehensive health insurance for their workers had a powerful reason to support reform. Other employers in sectors where benefits were low would have fared less well under the Clintons' plan.

The reflexive opposition among business executives to medicare had given way to an acceptance of an expanded role of government. Joel Cantor and others found that 80 percent of the *Fortune 500* executives they interviewed believed that "fundamental changes are needed to make it [the health care system] work better" and a majority supported employer mandates.[22] In her impressive study, Cathie Jo Martin also found that a small majority of business executives (54 percent) were in favor of employer mandates while another 18 percent had mixed views.[23]

The second feature of business politics that seemed to increase the prospects for the Clintons' plan was the moderation of the main business groups on the issue. The Business Roundtable had been created in the 1970s in response to the feeling in large corporations that existing business groups were too ideological and too attached to general conservative causes to represent business interests effectively.[24] In the 1990s the Chamber of Commerce, one of the organizations most open to this criticism, had moved to the center politically. The promotion of William T. Archey within the chamber seemed both to reflect and cause this change. Archey believed that the chamber needed to make clear that it represented business, not the Republican party or conservatives in general. Much criticized by conservatives such as columnists Roland Evans and Robert Novak and *Human Events* magazine, Archey replied that "the far right wing considers the Chamber to be its bastion, its home away from home, its mouthpiece."[25] The chamber initially accepted employer mandates, prompting a fierce attack on its leadership by congressional Republicans. Perhaps illustrating Archey's comment that the right believed it owned the Chamber of Commerce the then-House Republican leader Robert H. Michel wrote a letter to the president of the chamber, Richard Lesher, telling him, "Your current posture is unacceptable."[26] Finally, business groups that were prepared to compromise, such as the Chamber of Commerce, found themselves menaced in the competition for members by the National Federation of Independent Businesses (NFIB), a group that promised total opposition to any expanded federal role in health care. The NFIB showed no interest in any compromises and refused to testify before the task force led by Hillary Clinton.[27] This was entirely in line with the NFIB's style. The NFIB had found a niche in the business interest group market by being more obdurate than any other group.

NFIB President Jack Faris commented on its relations with the Clinton administration, "We're not going to make our decisions just to get invited to lunch at the White House or to a meeting in the Oval Office."[28] Faris previously was an employee of the Republican party. How seriously competition from NFIB was hurting the Chamber of Commerce is a matter of dispute. The chamber's revenues had dropped from $71.7 million in 1989 to $65.8 million in 1991, whereas NFIB revenues had grown from $52.3 million to $58.4 million in the same period. However, much of the chamber's loss was reduced advertising revenue in its journals owing to the recession. Chamber membership actually increased from 185,000 to 215,000 in the fifteen months before April 1993.[29] Nonetheless, competition from the NFIB was a major constraint on the ability of the Chamber of Commerce to maintain its compromises with the administration on health care reform.

In the period following the defeat of the Clintons' plan, no industry seemed more responsible than the insurance industry, and no interest group seemed to have played a larger role than the Health Insurance Association of America (HIAA).

Again, however, the situation was more malleable than most accounts suggested. For a start, the insurance industry was divided between the largest five companies on the one hand and smaller companies on the other. The larger companies were prepared to operate in the brave new world of managed competition and were busily acquiring HMOs to do so. Smaller companies were less sure that they could make the transition.[30] By 1993 nearly all the largest companies such as Aetna had left the HIAA and had chosen to represent their own interests directly; the last of the big five companies, Prudential, left in December 1993.

The HIAA still faced major difficulties internally in agreeing on its policy. The twelve largest remaining corporations were thought capable of surviving if the Clintons' plan was modified slightly. The others were not. HIAA members hoped that the Clinton administration might solve their internal problems by announcing a proposal for health reform they could accept. HIAA representatives met the Clinton transition team in Little Rock to convey the HIAA's willingness to compromise. As a gesture of good faith, the HIAA retreated from its traditional total opposition to a larger federal role in health insurance. Only after it had concluded that its chances of influencing those responsible for developing the plan were close to negligible did the HIAA launch the expensive and famous commercials featuring Harry and Louise. Even then, major insurers such as

Blue Cross/Blue Shield distanced themselves from the HIAA's political position.[31]

Not all the developments in interest group politics were as promising for the administration. If the growing complexity of health care had reduced the unity of groups once solid in their opposton to medicare, it had similarly broken the ranks of supporters such as the AFL-CIO. Unions did commit $10 million to promote the Clintons' health plan,[32] the largest amount they had ever committed to a single issue. Yet everyone knew that the unions' first preference had been a Canadian single-payer plan, and that their members worried about losing their often very desirable existing plans.[33] Moreover, unions had lost members and political influence since the fight over medicare, and their support was worth less than in the past.

Strategy toward Interest Groups

By April 1994 all the important potential converts to the cause of reform—the Chamber of Commerce, the Business Roundtable, the AMA—had retreated from their earlier support for the politically difficult but crucial aspects of the Clintons' plan, notably employer mandates.

The Clintons' plan was not lost because of their strategy toward interest groups alone. Other errors such as the creation of a plan too difficult to explain to the public or long delays that frittered away impetus created by presidential speeches may have been more important. But, as the opponents of the plan realized, cultivating interest groups was important.

The Republican leadership realized that the attitudes of major interest groups toward health care reform were highly malleable. Representatives Michel and Gingrich worked hard to prevent crucial wavering groups such as the AMA or the Chamber of Commerce from defecting to the cause of reform.

The administration also realized to some degree the possibility of winning over interest groups. The administration's plan was in part designed to appeal to a broader constituency. The decision to emphasize managed competition was influenced by the a belief that it would be easier to sell business an approach with a heavy market element than to persuade them to support a "single-payer" approach. Moreover, the administration's plan, as noted above, provided a very profitable future for the largest insurance companies. Indeed, Sidney Wolfe and Sara Nichols of Public Citizen denounced the Clintons' plan for giving the largest insurance companies "the deal of the century."[34] Hillary Clinton complained after the plan was lost that it was "an opening offer, 'constructed to be deconstructed,'" that "was described as an ultimatum by our opponents and therefore used to undermine the process of reaching agreement."[35] Whatever Hillary Clinton had intended, her strategy had not seemed so geared to compromise to the groups most involved. In the end, the administration did not come across as willing to deal or compromise.

Several different sections of the administration shared responsibility for consulting and persuading interest groups. Hillary Clinton and the staff running her task force handled the early phases. The White House Office of Public Liaison, the lead organization in all dealings between the administration and interest groups, managed the later stages. Misperceptions and misunderstandings characterized both stages.

The work of the task force itself was a case in point. Although some interest groups—notably the NFIB—were determined to resist anything that the task force might produce, the task force's mode of action gave wavering groups the sense that they were denied the opportunity to influence decisions while other groups had privileged access. Most of the groups allowed to parade before the task force were forced to give their reactions in incredibly condensed form. More than sixty witnesses from interest groups testified before the task force in a thirteen-hour session in late March 1993.[36] The administration's refusal to announce the membership of the task force and its staff prompted doubts among interest groups about whether they had a real opportunity to make their case. This secrecy caused one group, the Association of American Physicians and Surgeons (AAPS), to bring an irritating law suit about the legality of the task force.[37] The association claimed that among the hundreds of private individuals working for the task force were many who had close ties to other groups.[38]

Nor did Hillary Clinton's style compensate for these difficulties. Although she believed that she was ready to compromise with groups, the groups felt otherwise. The story of her dealings with the HIAA, which was to play such a crucial role in the campaign against the Clintons' plan, is a case in point. Before launching the Harry and Louise commercials, the HIAA requested a meeting with Hillary Clinton. A date that was unsuitable was offered, and Hillary Clinton's office never offered an alternative. The group did meet Ira Magaziner, who scarcely mollified the HIAA by telling them that the administration needed an interest group to campaign against, and they were the obvious choice.[39] One comment by Hillary Clinton illustrates the problem. In May 1994 she said, "I'm looking forward to intensive consultations in the next several weeks *over the details.*"[40] Interest groups were expecting more than consultations over details. Though Hillary Clinton was described as having had serious discussions with groups such as "the AFL-CIO, nurses' associations and Indian leaders,"[41] the AMA felt that it "had token consultation" and felt its expertise was neglected.[42]

Meanwhile, leaks from the task force antagonized interest groups. Reports that caps on premiums were imminent frightened insurance companies. Reports of plans for short-term caps on hospital charges disturbed hospitals. And reports that health benefits would be taxed angered union leaders.[43] Although the final plan contained none of these provisions, these rumors undermined prospects for agreement.

In the end, although Hillary Clinton felt that she was exuding a willingness to compromise, all others saw it differently. As Representative Pete Stark, chair of the health subcommittee of the House Committee on Ways and Means, put it, "They came over and saw us all the time but ignored what we said."[44] The *Washington Post* reported, "Key players from the American Medical Association to the scientific research community were alternately wooed and dissed [sic]. White House political experts never materialized. 'They never asked the question: Where is the consensus? Instead it was: How can we redesign the system? We have the magic formula, says Michael Bromberg, chief of the Federation of Health Systems."[45] Even Paul Starr, one of the principal architects of the plan, conceded that "the real problem was that time was spent developing a plan that should have been spent negotiating it. . . . Those who felt shut out responded predictably."[46]

Two alternative strategies might have worked better. Administration officials, many of whom knew the political scene much better than the task force members, could have engaged in exhaustive consultation. Alternatively, the planning process could have been genuinely inclusive by involving all interest groups, particularly those that were wavering and that the administration needed to win over. The task force was an unsatisfactory compromise between the two.

After the task force ended its work, the Office of Public Liaison took over the job of working with interest groups, and in particular of keeping business groups happy. Accounts of general competence of this office vary. The *New York Times* in what appears to have been a "puff piece" based largely on the Office's own self portrait, wrote that Alexis M.

Herman, director of the office, "is credited with the deft management of a number of delicate relationships especially between the White House and the Congressional Black Caucus or the traditionally Republican business community."[47] In contrast, political scientist Cathy Jo Martin reported that business interest groups were unimpressed with the performance of Herman's team. Martin claims that the Office of Public Liaison under Herman has operated on the basis that consultation has to be earned and that groups that criticize lose access. Martin quoted one of her interviewees from a business organization as saying, "Outreach to them means access to those who have been with them from the beginning and shutting out everyone else."[48]

Whether through the ineffectiveness of the Office of Public Liason or through a failure to control the strategy followed by other parts of the administration (notably Hillary Clinton), a crucial failing emerged in the administration's handling of business organizations.

The administration had banked on obtaining the support of business groups for its plan, a plausible strategy as both the Business Roundtable and the Chamber of Commerce had favored employer mandates. Now, however, the administration took a crucial step that was guaranteed to turn their support into neutrality. That step was to search for a villain to attack. The administration believed that only with a villain to attack could the battle for public opinion be waged effectively. This was Hillary Clinton's interpretation of some of the Clintons' triumphs in Arkansas.[49] Julie Kosterlitz wrote in January 1994 that the Clintons wanted an enemy to run against,[50] a view that Ira Magaziner himself confirmed in his statement to the HIAA. As Cathie Jo Martin summarizes the administration's thinking, "In the area of health care the administration decided that doctors were too powerful to be the villains but that drug companies and insurers were perfect for the part."[51] Unfortunately for the administration, it had failed to understand that in the world of business politics, these sectors alone could rip away the support of business interest groups on whose support it had set such stock. The administration had failed to appreciate that organizations such as the Business Roundtable or the Chamber of Commerce are not majoritarian organizations. No private organization ever can be entirely, for the "exit" option is always open to a minority that feels that its interests or opinions have been neglected. In the highly competitive American business interest group system, where groups such as the NFIB are waiting to snap up disaffected members from the Chamber or other business organizations, the risks for an interest group of failing to placate a minority are very high indeed.

Administration strategy toward interest groups was therefore inconsistent. The strategy of seeking popular support by attacking villains in the insurance and pharmaceutical industries undermined the strategy of coopting interest groups that might have been expected to oppose health care reform. Then, ironically, the administration undermined its own plans to wage a popular crusade for health reform by belated attempts to compromise in the summer of 1994 when it described its floundering plan as merely an opening offer subject to amendment. Even the American Association for Retired People (AARP), which the administration hoped would campaign hard for health reform, backed away from a public campaign when the AARP became uneasy that the administration would safeguard AARP's vital interests.[52] Once again, the administration's inconsistent strategy toward interest groups ended whatever chances of success might have existed.

Interest Group Strategy

Interest groups exist to exert pressure, however, and they did indeed so. The most frequently discussed aspects of interest group strategy have been advertising and campaign contributions. The Annenberg School for Communication has estimated that interest groups spent more on commercials about the health care reform in 1993 than the total spent by presidential candidates in 1992.[53] Political action committee (PAC) contributions by interest groups associated with health care averaged more than $2 million a month in 1994, $26.4 million between January 1993 and May 1994,[54] a 40 percent increase in contributions by these groups.[55] A significant proportion of this ($8,240,694) went to members of the five congressional committees most concerned with health care.[56]

Besides such public and publicized aspects of interest group strategy, quiet lobbying also increased. In addition to the lobbyists regularly employed by interest groups in the health sector, ninety-seven lobbying firms were hired to influence the debate, and eighty former members of Congress or executive branch officials were employed to lobby on the issue. Of these, twelve left Congress and eleven the executive branch in 1993 or 1994 to work for health interest groups. Firms of political consultants can form the center of a temporary coalition of interest groups created to support or oppose a particular measure. Several of these coalitions such as the Health Care Leadership Council formed during the fight over the Clintons' plan.

As with the German fleet, which influenced the World War I without ever leaving port, the largest interest groups, such as the Chamber of Commerce or the AMA, exercised a powerful influence on the strategy of protagonists although they never mounted a full-scale campaign. The administration framed its proposal to deflect anticipated all-out opposition from these groups.

It has been common in discussions of interest group strategy to contrast "insider" and "outsider" strategies. Insider strategies of quiet persuasion based on long-established and close ties to decisionmakers (cemented by PAC contributions) have been thought for many decades to be incompatible with "outsider" campaigns based on extensive mobilization.[57] In general, groups were thought to prefer an insider strategy when possible, perhaps because it cost less and made fewer political enemies. The HIAA's strategy might seem to be an example. The HIAA adopted an adversarial and public strategy built around the Harry and Louise commercials only after its insider strategy failed.

Contemporary interest group strategy is best understood as a blend of insider and outsider strategies. Just as presidents have been tempted to "go public" more frequently in order to increase their influence within Washington, so interest groups have placed increased emphasis on public campaigning and on mobilizing support at the "grass roots" in order to bolster their lobbying in Washington.

The Harry and Louise campaign of the HIAA is a case in point. Although remembered as a series of commercials that changed public opinion, the commercials were in fact shown in only eleven media centers with a disproportionate emphasis on Washington, D.C., itself.[58] The campaign was intended not to change public opinion in general but to change public opinion in enough locations to influence decisionmakers. One of the most successful campaigns was that of the Health Care Leadership Council, which blended skillfully elements of insider and outsider strategies in destroying one of the original planks of health care reform, cost containment. They used large campaign contributions together with commercials produced by the Ridley Group, an organization run by a one-time aide to Senator Lautenberg. A firm that specializes in grassroots campaigning, Bonner and Associates, was also hired to stimulate grass-roots opposition by radio advertisements. Bonner "patched" telephone calls from suitably outraged members of the public through to members of Congress. The firm also employed experienced campaign organizers to campaign in seventy "swing" congressional districts.[59] This mixture of insider and outsider campaigns was also totally successful.

The Impact of Interest Groups

Many critics charged the press with being too focused on the horse race questions of who won and lost rather than focusing on the substantive issues involved. Although the question of who won and who lost is popular, it is difficult to answer for several reasons.

First, the major interest groups were not sure or consistent in defining what constituted their interest. Powerful groups such as the AMA, the Business Roundtable, and the Chamber of Commerce shifted their positions during the debate not only on whether they supported the Clintons' plan in general but also on their attitude to crucial issues such as employer mandates. Even the HIAA was much less certain of its position than most would suppose.

The second difficulty in deciding who won and who lost flows from ambiguity in defining what was at issue. The overwhelming majority of interest groups entered the debate dissatisfied with the status quo and yet ended up with the status quo unchanged and, because of the defeat of the Clintons' plan, unlikely to be changed in the near future. Doctors faced increasingly irksome constraints from insurance companies, and corporations faced rapidly rising health insurance costs. Even the members of the HIAA faced a bleak future as market forces threatened to do what the administration could not—put them out of business as HMOs (often owned by their large competitors) win their markets. It is tempting to conclude that the interest group system, like the market in classical economics, brings about the socially optimal outcome, but this view is untenable for the overwhelming majority of interest groups. Perhaps only the NFIB, which opposed all government-managed solutions to the problems of the nation's health care system, could claim to be a winner.

The third problem in assessing who won and who lost is that interest groups are not the only actors. Critics of congressional campaign contributions and of expensive lobbying by health groups seem to believe that if such activities did not go on, the outcome would have been very different. This assumption is highly debatable. Significant resources were available to both opponents and supporters of the Clintons' plan. The political fire power deployed by groups such as the HIAA was significant, but it was balanced by the opposition of other interest groups, including unions, which as late as 1994 were planning to spend $10 million on promoting the Clinton plan.[60] Finally, interest groups who opposed the Clintons' plan were not merely working in partnership with other political actors but were mobilized by them. In primitive accounts it is interest groups who are the mainspring of politics, pressuring politicians to adopt a certain position. In fact, crucial strategy decisions by interest groups were the result of lobbying by Republican *politicians*, reversing the usual flow. For better or worse, Republicans, not interest groups, led in killing the Clintons' plan.

In two areas interest groups may well have made an important contribution: in shaping Republican party and public opinion. Republican leaders influenced interest groups, but several interest groups also influenced the Republican leadership. It is easy to forget at this point how essential it seemed in 1993 and 1994 for the Republicans to adopt a positive attitude to health care reform. The failings of the old system—the 35 million uninsured Americans, the risk of losing coverage with unemployment, the costs to corporations and the economy in general of a system that consumed almost 14 percent of gross domestic product—were so obvious that many believed Republicans could not afford a purely negative response to the Clinton proposal. Following Clinton's September 1993 speech on health care, the *Washington Post* reported "the readiness of Senate Minority Leader, Robert J. Dole (Republican of Kansas), Clinton's most effective foe in the first seven months of his presidency, to line up GOP support for a measure that incorporates some of the key elements of Clinton's bill—gives hope to administration supporters."[61] William McInturff, who advised the Republicans on public opinion on health care, thought as late as October 1993 that Republicans "have to be perceived as supporting dramatic change in today's health care system."[62] The activities of interest groups implacably opposed to the Clintons' plan such as the NFIB and, later, the HIAA showed the Republican leaders that viable ways existed to oppose what had seemed initially a popular response to an obviously pressing problem.

The determined efforts of groups such as the NFIB and the HIAA deserve some of the responsibility for the collapse in support for the Clintons' plan (from 59 percent approving and 33 percent disapproving in September 1993 to 40 percent approving and 55 percent disapproving in mid July 1994).[63] In contrast, no effective campaign was mounted in favor of the Clintons' plan. The precipitous decline in the strength of organized labor in the United States, such an important source of support for the passage of medicare in the 1960s, is one explanation. Moreover, perhaps the Clintons' plan was very much a second choice for the unions, which had favored strongly the "single-payer" or "Canadian" approach. The AARP, the largest interest group in the United States, failed to provide the administration with anticipated support, perhaps because of the administration's strategic miscalculations. Finally, the character of the Clintons' plan made it easier to oppose than support. Whereas the AARP had to train speakers to understand the plan, opponents could simply ridicule its length and complexity.

Evaluating Interest Groups from Society's Perspective

Political scientists have long assessed the performance of interest groups not only in terms of which group won and how, but also in terms of how their activities have affected the wider polity. At least since Alexis de Tocqueville's *Democracy in America* writers have argued that interest groups have improved the performance of the American polity and the quality of American society in four ways. First, interest groups increase opportunities for participation. Second, interest groups are a training ground for an active citizenry, providing experience in the practice of democracy. Third, interest groups provide decisionmakers with information, drawing on a knowledge of technical problems often beyond the capacity of government itself to provide. Fourth, interest groups are problem solvers, not only identifying problems or potential solutions but providing practical solutions to them by working in partnership with government agencies or running their own programs as an alternative to government ones.

Other writers have criticized the interest group system, denouncing its bias toward the wealthy and powerful, neglect of the general or public interest in favor of narrow or "special" interests, and use of such parts of the political system as congressional committees to produce gridlock. American interest groups, typically more fragmented than their counterparts in other democracies, may represent many viewpoints but, say their critics, impede the solution of problems: in a competitive interest group system, any group leader who displays a statesmanlike willingness to compromise risks losing members to a group that takes a tougher, more intransigent position.[64]

How did the American interest group system perform from the viewpoint of society as a whole on the health care issue?

Increasing Participation and Training in Citizenship

The tactics used by the most determined opponents of health care reform included a major effort to arouse the public against the Clintons' plan. The HIAA and NFIB were in the vanguard in spreading debate on the issue to the level of the mass public. Commercials and grassroots campaigning effectively increased the number of people involved in the health care debate. Mobilization in favor of the Clintons' plan was less effective and less enthusiastic. The group created by the Democratic National Committee under the leadership of a former governor of Ohio, Richard Celeste, never really got off the ground. The $10 million that unions planned to spend campaigning for the plan was little more than the HIAA alone spent. In general, however, it cannot be denied that interest groups helped increase popular participation.

It is less clear that interest groups contributed to a higher quality *of citizenship*. Tocqueville's enthusiasm for interest groups was based largely on his belief that they provided a forum within which citizens could deliberate about their concerns. Much of the participation sparked by the "grass-roots" campaigning of groups such as the NFIB and the HIAA was designed not to inspire deliberation, informed participation, or even increased knowledge of the issues but to hit "hot buttons," sparking a spasm of rage sufficient to prompt a telephone call on an 800 toll-free line provided by a public relations firm that would "patch" it through to a legislator's office. Not surprisingly, a campaign that focused on anecdotes did little to increase public understanding of the fundamental issues. Indeed, a study by the Kaiser Foundation concluded that public understanding declined during the campaign. The percentage of people who knew that the Clintons' plan was designed to ensure universal coverage fell; after being read a lengthy description of what an employer mandate was, nearly 40 percent of respondents could not identify a single health care reform proposal that contained it.[65] Claims that interest groups performed an educational function cannot be sustained.

Providing Ideas, Solving Problems

Did interest groups contribute to governance by providing information, ideas, and solutions? Even to ask the question after the preceding analysis seems redundant. The primary involvement of interest groups was negative, opposing the Clintons' plan but playing little part in improving the plan or developing any alternative to it.

The more difficult question to answer is whose fault this was. Interest group officials would probably blame the administration. Locked out of the development of the Clintons' plan by the supposed secrecy of the task force's process, groups such as the HIAA adopted a negative, defensive strategy. If only, interest groups argue, they had been allowed to play a more constructive part, they would have been sure to do so.

Yet this (hypothetical) defense from interest group officials is unconvincing. Major interest groups such as the AMA and Chamber of Commerce had opportunities to deal and negotiate after the task force had completed its work in spring 1993. Whatever the image of his wife might be, President Clinton is not thought of as a leader who defends his policies or beliefs obdurately. Political scientist Richard F. Fenno Jr. criticized President Clinton for being too willing to give ground: "Even before you say trick or treat, you get the candy."[66] It is difficult to believe that the president would have refused to compromise in exchange for a credible offer of support from key constituencies. The congressional process also offered numerous opportunities for constructive amendments to the Clintons' plan. The major interest groups did not take these opportunities. The administration can be criticized for failing to seek compromise but so can interest groups. Crucial interest groups such as the AMA, the Business Roundtable, and the Chamber of Commerce chose to listen to Republican leaders and retreat from their earlier constructive engagement with reform.

Perhaps it is deep ideological antipathy to any solution that involved an expansion of government power that explains this lack of statesmanship on the part of interest group leaders. David Vogel has argued that American business executives—and, we might add, doctors—react emotionally and viscerally against extensions of state power even when, as in the health care sector, the private sector seems to be failing.[67] Vogel's interpretation would certainly fit the health care debate. The leaders of major interest groups such as the Chamber of Commerce accepted crucial aspects of the Clintons' plan, such as employer mandates, then, under appeals from Republican leaders to stay true to the *laissez faire* faith, backed away.

Yet we should also attempt to understand the pressures on interest group leaders. A crucial characteristic of the American interest group system compared with those in most other advanced democracies[68] is fragmentation. Numerous groups compete for the support of potential members in each sector. Pluralist analyses of politics have generally assumed that no interest will obtain everything and others nothing. Yet such a theory, like all theories of bargaining, assumes that participants have some room for maneuver, for settling on a plan that may not be their first preference but that adequately accounts for their vital concerns. In an era when membership in interest groups—like so much in politics—

can be decided by sound bites, statesmanlike compromise is difficult. In sound bite politics it is much easier for the NFIB to criticize the Chamber of Commerce for compromise with the Washington establishment by accepting employer mandates than for the leaders of the Chamber of Commerce to explain why compromise was wise. Competition from the Association of American Physicians placed the AMA in a similar box. Analysts may advise this—or any future—administration to be more skillful in its interest group strategies in any future attempt to solve our health care problems. It is less easy to see how interest group leaders can obtain the freedom of maneuver necessary to play a more constructive role in policymaking.

Comments

Julie Kosterlitz: Graham Wilson has provided an interesting retrospective on the role of interest groups in the health care debate. His chapter helps explain why the Clinton administration—for all that it anticipated special interest opposition—was lulled—falsely, as it turned out—into thinking this opposition could be co-opted or outflanked.

It is striking, in retrospect, how tractable many of the major industry stakeholders in the health care debate seemed at its outset. Large employers, doctors, hospitals and large insurers all seemed willing to countenance government intrusions they once fought bitterly, because the dysfunctions of or changes in the marketplace were making life increasingly uncomfortable. Even the Health Insurance Association of America, despite representing the most change-averse small and midsized insurers, had abandoned its long-time opposition to employer mandates and embraced significant insurance reforms.

Wilson also provides useful insights into what caused interest group support for the Clinton plan to evaporate. The Clinton administration's tactical mistakes have already come in for a lot of attention. But other contributing factors have not—such as the "backwards lobbying" of interest groups by politicians, for example, and the game theory notion that shrillness and intransigence can be a useful marketing technique for interest groups in a competitive environment. He also makes a persuasive case that today's special interest politics stray from the Toquevillian ideal.

I wanted to respond briefly to two of Wilson's points before revisiting one of the more central questions he raises. First, I think he and others overestimate what genuine give-and-take with the Clinton administration might have accomplished. It's clear that the task force's go-it-alone strategy—leavened only slightly by token hearings—created an added level of mistrust and ill-will that came back to haunt it. But it's unlikely that the administration could have appeased the wide range of interest groups it confronted without eviscerating sweeping reform and abandoning its goals of universal coverage and strict spending limits. Whether it should have set such ambitious goals or made these nonnegotiable in early discussions with vested interests are other questions entirely.

Wilson may have also underrated in his analysis, as I think I did at the outset of the reform debate, how soft and how conditional was much of the original support or acquiescence by major interest groups to reform. Most of the major employer groups who supported a mandate, for example, supported it in mainly in the abstract, and then only if many other conditions were met. Moreover, I think Wilson overlooks that the hardening of some positions was not always because of ideological or institutional politics, but was based on a very rational cost-benefit analysis. In providing a simplified scorecard on where the players stood, I and many of my colleagues in the press often failed to attend sufficiently to the many contingent clauses in groups' broad statements of support for universal coverage. I wrote a profile on the Association of Private Pension and Welfare Plans, for example, as one of the last representatives of large employers to support the employer mandate, although the group had argued rather consistently that they were troubled by the Clinton plan's imposition of onerous conditions on large employers—who, they argued, were already doing the right thing by insuring their workers. Not too long after the profile, the group abandoned its support of mandates, having concluded that a host of surcharges, mandates, and limits on their freedom of maneuver would more than offset the gains from ending cost-shifting.

Moreover, the seeming support for reform by many interest groups for reform represented opportunism more than it did a genuine shift in their policy views. Not surprisingly, these groups seemed the most acquiescent when public sentiment for change seemed the strongest, and President Clinton was at his most popular. Appearing open-minded made political sense when the options seemed to be either cutting a deal with the administration or risking getting swept away in a tide of radical reform. But when public opinion began to shift against reform, so too did the groups' calculus of their self-interest.

I would have liked to hear more from Graham Wilson about his conclusions on the broad question he poses at the outset. "Was the failure of the Clinton plan just another, though particularly important, example" of special interests blocking meaningful reform?

The answer matters because, as others have noted, what observers take away from this debate will shape views on what can and should be done for years hence. And it matters because it can tell Americans how well their political system continues to serve them.

Having chronicled in some detail the massive girding up of interest groups for this fight, and watched these groups in action, I still find this question difficult to answer. Despite having been to the the press conferences, seen the ads and the polls unveiled, and interviewed the hired guns about how they gin up grass-roots support for their clients, I have not come up with a simple conclusion about how much difference they made in the outcome of this debate.

It seems clear to me that interest groups had an important role in undermining support for sweeping reform in a variety of ways. The influence of Harry and Louise, or of any single ad campaign in moving broad public opinion may be overstated. But the cumulative effect of the question raising (and sometimes outright fear-mongering) can't fail to have contributed to a generalized atmosphere of doubt. The sums spent on congressional campaign contributions, on the highest-caliber hired guns—many of them fresh from Capitol Hill—and on sophisticated grass-roots organizing by themselves leave no doubt that interest group activity played an important role.

Having lots of money to spend on an issue matters: interest groups had the time and expertise to analyze the legislation's likely impact on them, to poll and gauge public sensitivities, and to develop sophisticated and compelling—if often disingenuous arguments against elements of the reform. National organizations could selectively mobilize their local affiliates to lobby members on critical committees. And members do pay attention to who they hear from back home.

Indeed, strategic use of pressure by home-state interests appears to have been decisive in one critical skirmish over health care reform. The *Washington Post* chronicled in some detail the fight for the critical vote of Representative Jim Slattery, a centrist Democrat from Kansas on the Energy and Commerce Committee, then embroiled in a bid—unsuccessful it turned out—for the governorship.[69] Slattery came under great pressure from two home state industries—Hallmark and Pizza Hut—who vehemently opposed the employer mandate. In the end, despite heavy pressure from the powerful committee chairman, Slattery refused to support the bill. The sidelining of Dingell and the Energy and Commerce Committee may not have cost reform advocates the game, but it was undeniably a major setback.

But implicit in the accusation against interest groups—mainly by pro-reform advocates is that special interests were principally responsible for somehow frustrating public aspirations for sweeping reform—including universal coverage and cost controls. I think this is a more complicated proposition.

Although public opinion polls at the outset of the debate showed a public solidly in favor of sweeping reform, universal coverage, and cost controls, the public, as Daniel Yankelovich has persuasively argued, was far more ambivalent about comprehensive reform than the initial polls implied. If one accepts, as I do, that the public had yet to seriously grapple with the difficult trade-offs implicit in any plan that would guarantee universal coverage and clamp down on health care costs, then perhaps interest groups can be accused of inflaming opposition, but not of inventing it.

Did the interest groups foment fear and doubt by misleading the public? Clearly there was exaggeration and misinformation about what the plan would do. The National Federation of Independent Businesses' numbers on job loss, for example, were off the charts of any respectable economists. And when the HIAA's Harry and Louise fretted that the Clinton plan would create more government bureaucracy, or the possibility of rationing, they failed to point out that similar developments were already taking place in the private sector.

But some of the issues interest groups raised were legitimate—even if the groups had ulterior motives in raising them: the HIAA may have been trying to keep the world safe for cherry-picking by small-and-midsized insurance companies when it ran ads against expenditure targets with the tag line that asked, "So, what if the health plan runs out of money?" But the question got at justifiable public concerns about the implications of limiting national health care spending.

Such an ad is calculated more to inspire dread than the high-minded public deliberation Yankelovich would like to see. But by the same token the administration public relations campaign blithely dismissed these concerns and in the process resorted to some distortions in marketing its own plan. The assertion that government could clamp down drastically on the rate of growth in health care spending by cutting out only unnecessary care and other waste, fraud, and abuse was unproven at best.

If the interest groups hadn't raised the doubts and the spectre of sacrifice, would these doubts and fears have never surfaced? A good deal of the opposition was led by conservative organizations and politicians. Such groups as Citizens for a Sound Economy were probably able to amplify their message thanks to contributions from industry groups. But some of the most effective antireform campaigns were carried on by conservative talk-show radio hosts.

Blaming the interest groups who opposed reform also lets a lot of other players off the hook. Chief among them was the Clinton administration, whose ham-handedness in explaining and selling its own plan has been well-documented elsewhere. Even interest groups who nominally supported reform were often more concerned with advancing their narrow interests arguably at the expense of the public good as well. The unions and automakers wanted the public to bail out collectively bargained promises of early retirement health care benefits. Teaching hospitals fought for about $30 billion in no-strings-attached new subsidies over five years, mainly to train high-cost specialists already widely considered in excess supply.[70] Even community health centers, staffed by idealistic doctors deeply concerned about the plight of the uninsured, spent a good deal of their energy worrying about how to preserve their own institutions and jobs if reform provided private insurance and allowed the uninsured for the first time to choose other providers.

That leads me to a final, related point. As Jonathan Rauch has persuasively argued interest groups are no longer easily written off as representing only the elite and monied.[71] The astonishing proliferation of interest groups represented in Washington tells us that an increasing share of the citizenry is represented. The problem is that these people are not represented as ordinary citizens, but along narrower lines of perceived self-interest. Rauch argues that this "hyperpluralism" has led to both a dangerous expansion and paralysis of government. In the case of health reform, this representation-itis may have stymied government intervention—and not merely because Americans mistrust government. Although Americans supported the goals of reform in the abstract, once the plan became concrete, the emphasis shifted from what reform might do for the nation as a whole in the long run, to what it might do to me, now. People are insurance agents, hospital employees, medicare recipients, or kidney cancer patients first, and members of a commonwealth only second.

One can disagree with features of the Clinton plan and still argue that universal coverage and cost control might have been good for the nation as a whole—providing security, enhancing fairness, and freeing up resources for other pressing priorities. But the benefits of reform for most

Americans—who were already insured—were abstract and long term. Getting to universal coverage and cost containment would have invariably required a redistribution of resources, a dislocation, and sacrifices from specific individuals that were far more tangible and immediate.

I remember being on a call-in show with a San Francisco radio station in which a succession of callers argued that they would be hurt by the plan. A Silicon Valley entrepreneur, who had had a bad year, worried about what employer mandates would do to his small business. A self-proclaimed member of Generation X complained that community rating of insurance would unfairly raise premiums for the young . . . and on it went. The entrepreneur didn't seem able to imagine that a change in his circumstances might make the guarantee of insurance worthy of some sacrifice now, and the X-er didn't seem to imagine what it might be like to be a bad health risk who is laid off at age 55.

I leave you with no anwers, but rather a parting question. What precisely does it mean to blame special interests for the demise of health care reform if, as Rauch puts it—"Groups R Us?"[72]

Fred Grandy: The underlying assumption of policy conferences such as this one is that health care reform failed in the 103d Congress because the Health Security Act did not become law. That neither comprehensive nor incremental reform survived the health care wars of the last session leads to the easy conclusion by scholars and policymakers that the health care debate accomplished nothing substantive.

I do not share that view. This negative judgment does not consider the evolution of attitude by the American people as they watched the debate unfold. One can make a compelling case that their views were manipulated and exploited by special interests and, depending upon what side of the debate one was on, such manipulation is either a good or bad thing. But the conclusion that the more the American people learned about the Health Security Act the more *insecure* they felt is inescapable.

So the performance of the 103d Congress on health care should be evaluated more for the quality of the learning process than for the inability to produce a final product. By the November elections the majority of voters were not ready for the changes health care reform entailed, and Congress delivered just what the public was clamoring for. Nothing.

Ultimate failure on the health care issue will be more appropriately determined in the 104th Congress. Clearly, with a Republican majority in control, health care reform, if there is to be any, will be incremental. But as a former Republican member of the House (albeit an apostate in the eyes of some of my colleagues) and a casualty of the health care wars I would hate to see the knowledge and expertise acquired in the 103d Congress squandered or scorned in the 104th. The problems of cost, access, and quality persist, and with new issues emerging on both medicare and medicaid policy, the puzzle of providing affordable health care for all becomes even more difficult to solve. A successful solution depends on a new relationship between two major coconspirators in the last health care debate who, for some reason, Graham Wilson does *not* prominently feature—namely, congressional leaders and the American people.

In the last go-around the average American watching the health care debate was a conflicted consumer who sent a profoundly mixed message to his or her representative.

In September of 1993 after the president's "Health of the Union" address that message was loud and clear, "I don't know what I want and I want it now!" A year later that same constituent was just as firm in his or her conviction. Only now the message to Congress was, "Don't just do something, stand there!"

This complete flip-flop in attitude is either a triumph of electronic populism or a casualty of hyperdemocracy. But the national collapse in public confidence cannot be attributed solely to demagoguery. This is not just the cumulative handiwork of Harry and Louise, or Rush Limbaugh, or William Kristol, or even Jim McDermott and Paul Wellstone. Neither is it fair to say health care reform was sabotaged by an artful Republican conspiracy. Many Republicans, I among them, began the last Congress eager to cooperate in a major health care initiative only to find ourselves prematurely excluded from the early planning stages. The decision to discredit and destroy the Clinton plan grew partially from resentment at being shut out of the process by the administration and its allies on Capitol Hill.

My observation from the battlefield is that very early on Democratic House and Senate leaders made some decisions privately that ultimately derailed the Clinton plan publicly. Coupled with some events beyond the president's control, health care reform was terminally and irretrievably ill by January 1994. It took the rest of the year for the rituals of dying to be scrupulously performed. Health care died prematurely because any serious effort at a bipartisan compromise collapsed early in the House and eventually overwhelmed honest efforts in the Senate.

What follows is my chronology of critical events:

November–December 1992—Clinton is unwisely convinced by George Mitchell and Richard Gephardt that Democrats can pass health care reform without Republican support. The decision of Democrats to go-it-alone chilled a broad-based enthusiasm on the part of many Republicans to be part of a compromise solution. Long before Hillary Clinton's task force sequestered itself, Republicans in both the House and Senate felt excluded from serious discussions on reform.

This estrangement created the Managed Competition Act of 1993. The bill, also known as the Cooper-Grandy bill, was a refuge for Republicans and Democrats interested in changing health care but unwilling to swallow the Clinton program whole. As such it was always more defense than offense. The strategy was to build a strong bipartisan alternative that would pull President Clinton back to the center of the debate and win more GOP allies. This effort was more frustrating to centrist Democrats like Jim Cooper of Tennessee than to Republicans. Cooper endured hours of futile discussions with the White House only to have talks collapse in late 1993. In early 1994 Republicans started pulling off the bill.

In January and February 1993 the president suffered a severe tactical blow when his most important committee chairman and field general, Dan Rostenkowski, was indicted and forced to cede his power atop the Ways and Means Committee. Publicly, Rosty was a loyal Clinton lieutenant who had informed Republicans on Ways and Means that they should either accept almost all of the Clinton plan or forget about any amendments. Privately, Rosty knew the Clinton plan was in trouble and was looking for compromises the administration was not yet ready to make. We had begun to talk informally about Cooper-Grandy when the U.S. Attorney's office brought the indictment.

When Rosty was forced to step aside, power transferred not to the new chairman, Sam Gibbons, but to the long-time health care expert on the Democratic side of Ways and Means, Pete Stark. When Rosty went down, Clinton did not just lose a chairman. He lost a committee.

The power shift to Pete Stark was a major setback for the Clinton plan because Stark was no fan of the Health Security Act or its promoters. Indeed, first in subcommittee and then at the full committee level, he gutted large provisions of the bill and replaced them with his own creation, Medicare Part C, a brand new public health program for the poor. This strategy accomplished two ends. First, it essentially strangled the Clinton plan in its crib. By the time the bill left the full committee it had become the Gephardt bill. Clinton's imprimatur had been substantively and symbolically erased. Second, it unified Republicans in opposition to *any* Democratic initiative and made bipartisanship that much more difficult. Even though the Health Security Act was reported out of Ways and Means, it was little more than a specter that spent the rest of the session haunting Congress.

And this relative failure was President Clinton's most successful attempt at moving his health care ideas through the legislative process. The two other major panels through which health care had to pass—Education and Labor and Energy and Commerce—did not do as well by the president as Ways and Means. In Education and Labor the committee passed out not one bill but two, a version of the Clinton plan more expensive than the original and a single-payer option that the president opposed. In Energy and Commerce the votes could not be found to enact the key provision in the president's bill, the employer mandate. Chairman John Dingell concluded it was politically more prudent to do nothing than to risk rejection of the Clinton plan by his own cohorts.

The final blow came from the Congressional Budget Office. The Clinton plan had boasted that it would achieve universal coverage for all Americans while reducing the deficit. The Congressional Budget Office affirmed the former contention but contested the latter, and the president was stuck with a proposal that congressional accountants said actually raised the deficit over time. This ill-timed and unwanted rendezvous with reality magnified Clinton's biggest mistake throughout the health care debate, the attempt to beguile the American people into believing that universal health care coverage could be both comprehensive and cheap. Nobody ever believed that. And by the time Harry and Louise hit the airwaves, that suspicion did not need to be established, only reenforced.

From these actions a national mood of doubt was created and into this void rushed an army of special interests with a single agenda: finish off the wounded beast.

The battle that took place once the Clinton bill was seen to be in trouble was a series of skirmishes not a united campaign. But every glancing blow took its toll and at the end the Health Security Act did not even enjoy the dignity of falling on the floor of the House. It died in ignominy off stage.

Many narrowly focused special interest groups took part in the slow extermination of the Clinton bill, but three deserve particular mention here only because their activities were so stealthy that they have escaped notice in most of the analyses following the debate. Yet all were highly influential in shaping the final outcome.

The health care debate in the 103d Congress is a primer in how to foment fear. Very little has been written about the antiabortion groups in that process. They were formidable behind the scenes. Early on with the Clinton bill, the Republican alternative, and any variation on the theme, the pro-life groups said unequivocally that any provision dealing with reproductive health was de facto abortion on demand. Even the Cooper-Grandy bill, which tried to remain scrupulously silent on abortion, was condemned for the sin of omission. Because it did not specifically exclude reproductive services from the basic benefit package it was deemed to be underwriting abortions at taxpayer expense. This stance spread like wildfire through the 103d Congress and has consequences for the future. The current Republican majority talks periodically about health care reforms such as guaranteed portability of insurance, guaranteed issue regardless of pre-existing conditions, and assured renewability. These do not mean anything without some basic benefit concept, and once a basic benefit is postulated, abortion has to be left in or taken out. It's the same problem all over again.

The groups and associations of small insurers, although not as doctrinaire as the antiabortion advocates, were no less persuasive in their behind-the-scenes efforts to kill health care reform. Their strategy was to remain consistently inconsistent in their demands and their conditions for support. Their principal issue (or so we thought) was price controls. They raised the legitimate complaint, as did all representatives from the insurance industry, that they should not be singled out for price caps. Bill Gradison, president of the Health Insurance Association of America, argued persuasively that high-cost medicine and low-cost insurance cannot coexist in a free market. But once price controls were deleted in committee, the small-group guys moved the goal post. They quickly became sworn enemies of mandatory purchasing co-operatives, which were components of both the Clinton bill and Cooper-Grandy. Our argument had always been that without an employer mandate or price regulation, there had to be some compelling necessity to encourage small employers to join purchasing groups, and compulsory participation was the only way to insure universal access at low cost. The small-group folks activated a powerful grass-roots network and successfully vilified both the Clinton proposal and the Cooper-Grandy bill.

The final special interest players in the health care debate who successfully fulfilled their agenda behind the scenes were the chiropractors. For years chiropractic associations had been lobbying the hill for a level playing field with M.D.'s. In the health care debate they got a level playing field that tilted their way. Leery of managed care from the outset, near the end of the mark-up in Ways and Means, they advanced an amendment under the popular guise of physician choice that effectively gutted the Gephardt bill specifically and managed competition in general. This was the infamous any-willing-provider amendment, which succeeded in building temporary but nonetheless effective coalitions between single-payer advocates like Senator Paul Wellstone and antigovernment conservatives like Representative Bill Archer, now the chairman of the House Ways and Means Committee. Like small insurers, chiropractors have vast networks of grass-roots supporters, which they activated on this issue. The net result was to make first the Gephardt bill and eventually the entire health care reform effort totally unwieldy.

In combination, these rifle shots at the health care reform effort subtly but consistently made what one group or another regarded as perfect the enemy of the good. With so many special interests in the field a consensus strategy for passage was impossible.

But the special interests are not to blame for the downfall of health care reform in the last Congress. They were hyenas nibbling at a carcass that was already dying. The real demise of health care can be attributed to a very simple fact—nobody told the truth. Nobody leveled about the true costs and consequences of health care reform. We were all too consumed with hawking the benefits and the savings. And Americans, already fatigued by the posturing and doubletalk over the federal budget debate, were just not that easily duped this time.

Tip O'Neill is remembered for saying all politics is local. Health care goes him one better. It's personal. Each American tends to view the national health care debate through the prism of his or her own plan. Once Americans began to realize that their benefits could be affected by a national realignment, their potential loss of coverage was not offset by the knowledge that some people less fortunate than they might gain.

Near the beginning of the health care debate, former Surgeon General C. Everett Koop made an observation about the status of health care in the United States that was deeply insightful and probably too unsettling. He said the problem with health care delivery in America was not just that too many people had too little. It was that too many people had too much. Until we own up to that, the health care debate will continue to be ours to lose.

Notes

1. Robin Toner, "Health Impasse Souring Voters, New Poll Finds," *New York Times*, September 13, 1994, p. 1A.

2. Adam Clymer, "Hillary Clinton Says Administration Was Misunderstood on Health Care," *New York Times*, October 3, 1994, p. A12.

3. Neil A. Lewis, "Medical Industry Showers Congress with Lobby Money," *New York Times*, December 13, 1993, p. A1.

4. Julie Kosterlitz, "Hiring Spree," *National Journal*, September 4, 1993, pp. 2120–25.

5. Peter H. Stone, "An Industry in Pain," *National Journal*, October 23, 1993, pp. 2526–30.

6. Theodore R. Marmor provides an excellent analysis of the role of interest groups in the fight for and against medicare. Theodore R. Marmor, *The Politics of Medicare* (Aldine, 1973).

7. Theodore R. Marmor, *Political Analysis and American Medical Care: Essays* (Cambridge University Press, 1983), p. 140.

8. David S. Broder, "Health Plan's Chief Anticipated Criticism; Foes Would Label Effort Cumbersome, Aide Said," *Washington Post*, September 13, 1994, p. A10.

9. Graham K. Wilson, *Special Interests and Policymaking: Agricultural Policies and Politics in Britain and the United States of America, 1956–1970* (John Wiley and Sons, 1977).

10. Marmor, *The Politics of Medicare*.

11. David Vogel, "Why Businessmen Distrust Their State: The Political Consciousness of American Corporate Executives," *British Journal of Political Science*, vol. 8 (January 1978), pp. 45–78.

12. James Q. Wilson, *Political Organizations* (Basic Books, 1974).

13. Marmor, *Politics of Medicare*; and Marmor, *Political Analysis*.

14. Julie Kosterlitz, "Stress Fractures," *National Journal*, February 19, 1994, pp. 412–17.

15. Robert Pear, "A.M.A. and Insurers Clash Over Restrictions on Doctors," *New York Times*, May 24, 1994, p. A14.

16. Robert Pear "The Health Care Debate: The Doctors; Health Care Tug-of-War Puts A.M.A. under Strain," *New York Times*, August 5, 1994, p. A18.

17. Kosterlitz, "Stress Fractures"; and Pear, "The Health Care Debate."

18. Marmor, *Political Analysis*, p. 141.

19. Health costs for employers for Canadian hourly paid workers per year have been put at $3,200; the figure for American hourly paid workers is $7,600. Cathie Jo Martin, "Mandating Social Change: The Struggle within Corporate America Over National Health Reform," paper prepared for the 1994 annual meeting of the American Political Science Association, p. 13.

20. Robert Pear, "Health Costs Vary Greatly by Industry, a Survey Finds," *New York Times*, December 21, 1993, p. A20.

21. Ibid.

22. Joel C. Cantor and others, "Business Leaders' Views on American Health Care," *Health Affairs*, vol. 10 (Spring 1991), pp. 98–105, quotation on p. 100.

23. Cathie Jo Martin, "Mandating Social Change: The Struggle within Corporate America Over National Health Reform," paper prepared for the 1994 annual meeting of the American Political Science Association, p. 17.

24. Graham K. Wilson, *Interest Groups in the United States* (Oxford University Press, 1981), pp. 27, 22.

25. Kirk Victor, "Deal Us In," *National Journal,* April 3, 1993, pp. 807 and following.

26. Victor, "Deal Us In," p. 808.

27. Robert Pear, "Groups Laud Health-Care Reform in Theory, but Clash on Practice," *New York Times,* March 30, 1993, p. A1.

28. Steven Greenhouse, "Small Business Groups in No Mood to Relent on Opposition to Health Plan," *New York Times,* September 17, 1993, p. A20.

29. Victor, "Deal Us In."

30. Kosterlitz, "Stress Fractures."

31. Julie Kosterlitz, "Itching for a Fight?" *National Journal,* January 15, 1994, p. 106–10.

32. Peter T. Kilborn, "Unions Plan to Spend $10 Million to Promote Clinton Health Plan," *New York Times,* February 22, 1994, p. A14.

33. Kosterlitz, "Stress Fractures."

34. Sidney Wolfe, M.D., and Sara Nichols, letter to the editor, *New York Times,* November 7, 1993.

35. Clymer, "Hillary Clinton Says Administration Was Misunderstood."

36. Pear, "Groups Laud Health-Care Reform."

37. Toni Locy, "Settlement of Health Task Force Suit Rejected; Doctors Want Magaziner to Answer Charges He Lied About Members," *Washington Post,* August 16, 1994, p. A17.

38. David S. Broder, "Physicians Allege Conflicts on Health Care Task Force," *Washington Post,* March 24, 1994, p. A26.

39. Kosterlitz, "Itching for a Fight?"

40. Dana Priest, "Health Care Price Curbs Advocated; White House Pushes Idea of Short-Term, Voluntary Controls," *Washington Post,* May 1, 1993, p. A1 (emphasis added).

41. Dana Priest, "Hillary Clinton's Meetings of the Minds; On Hill and in Town Gyms First Lady Seeks Health Care Consensus," *Washington Post,* April 30, 1993, p. A1.

42. Dana Priest, "AMA Seeks Voice on Health Care Task Force; Doctors' Group Repeats Its Support for Attempt to Curb Rising Costs," *Washington Post,* March 4, 1993, p. A8.

43. Priest, "Health Care Price Curbs Advocated."

44. Adam Clymer, Robert Pear, and Robin Toner, "The Health Care Debate: What Went Wrong? How the Health Care Campaign Collapsed," *New York Times,* August 29, 1994, p. A1.

45. Abigail Trafford, "What Went Wrong; How Wonks and Pols and You Fumbled Universal Health Care," *Washington Post,* August 21, 1994, p. C1.

46. Paul Starr, "What Happened to Health Care Reform?" *American Prospect,* no. 20 (Winter 1995), p. 22.

47. Gwen Ifill, "Washington at Work; Clinton's 'Ms Fixit'; A Friendly Link to Black Interests and Big Business," *New York Times,* August 30, 1994, p. A16.

48. Martin, "Mandating Social Change," p. 27.

49. Elizabeth Drew, *On The Edge: The Clinton Presidency* (Simon and Schuster, 1994); and Bob Woodward, *The Agenda: Inside the Clinton White House* (Simon and Schuster, 1994), pp. 110, 147.

50. Kosterlitz, "Itching For a Fight?"

51. Martin, "Mandating Social Change," p. 28.

52. Interview with the author, January 1995.

53. Katherine Q. Seelye, "The Health Care Debate: The Lobbyists, *New York Times*, August 16, 1994, p. A1.

54. Ibid.

55. Dana Priest, "Health-Interest Donations to Campaigns Rise Sharply; Much Goes to Incumbents on Key Committees," *Washington Post*, July 18, 1994, p. A6.

56. Charles Lewis, "In Sickness and in Wealth; How a Swarm of Lobbyists Cornered the Debate on Health Care Reform," *Washington Post*, August 21, 1994, p. C2.

57. Raymond Augustine Bauer, Ithiel de Sola Pool, and Lewis Anthony Dexter, *American Business and Public Policy: The Politics of Foreign Trade* (Atherton Press, 1963).

58. *Campaigns and Elections* (Washington: ISF Reed, 1994).

59. Peter H. Stone, "Lost Cause," *National Journal*, September 17, 1994, pp. 2133–36.

60. Peter T. Kilborn, "Unions Plan to Spend $10 Million to Promote Clinton Health Plan," *New York Times*, February 22, 1994, p. A14.

61. David S. Broder and Spencer Rich, "Hope, Risks Run High in Health Plan Equation; The Politics: Route through Congress Is Strewn with Hazards," *Washington Post*, September 9, 1993, p. A1.

62. David S. Broder, "GOP Health Care Strategy Emerging; Despite Divergence of Alternatives, Republicans Hope to Shape Plan," *Washington Post*, October 11, 1993, p. A16.

63. Lydia Saad, "Public Has Cold Feet on Health Care Reform," *Gallup Monthly Poll*, August 1994, pp. 2–10.

64. For a summary of the normative arguments about interest groups, see Graham K. Wilson, *Interest Groups* (Basil Blackwell, 1990).

65. Robin Toner, "Following the Crowd on Health Care and Getting Lost," *New York Times*, March 20, 1994, sec. 4, p. 1.

66. Burt Solomon, "In Leaning on Congress, Clinton . . . Uses Carrots Instead of Sticks," cited in the *National Journal*, November 6, 1993, p. 2676.

67. Vogel, "Why American Businessmen Distrust Their State."

68. Wilson, *Interest Groups.*

69. Michael Weisskopf, "Delivering a Defeat for Total Coverage," *Washington Post*, July 19, 1994, p. A6.

70. Julie Kosterlitz, "The Spoils of Reform," *National Journal*, August 20, 1994, pp. 1970–74.

71. Jonathan Rauch, *Demosclerosis: The Silent Killer of American Government* (Times Books, 1994).

72. Ibid., p. 48.

PART TWO

How Can Information Be Improved?

CHAPTER SIX

Estimating the Effects of Reform

Linda Bilheimer and Robert Reischauer

As THE analytic capabilities of the social sciences have developed over the past several decades, participants in the public policy process have increasingly requested analyses and estimates of the likely costs, benefits, and other effects of legislative proposals. That information has become a critical input in policy formulation and the ensuing political debate. It has also become the standard fare of the congressional budget process. Estimates, many of which are highly uncertain, have come to play a central role in determining whether proposals are adopted, radically restructured, or abandoned altogether.

The recent effort to reform the nation's health care system had to surmount that less-than-perfect form of analytic scrutiny. In the end, it did not, and that inability contributed to the failure of the effort. Much of the focus in the health reform case was directed at the budgetary effects of the various proposals. One reason for that focus was that the effort to reform the health care system was launched when the nation was trying painfully to deal with its large, structural fiscal imbalance. To that end, Congress had established complicated rules, embodied in the Balanced Budget Act of 1985, the Budget Enforcement Act of 1990, and the budget resolutions for fiscal years 1994 and 1995. Those rules placed formidable procedural hurdles in the path of any initiative that would add to the deficit in the budget year or the budget year plus the ensuing four years. Ensuring that those constraints were met often shaped policy as much as did considerations of what made programmatic sense or was workable.

A second reason for the inordinate focus on budgetary impacts was that health reform was a primary policy response to the nation's long-run deficit problem. Budget projections indicated that the deficit would begin to rise in 1996, a rise entirely explainable by the continued rapid growth anticipated in medicare and medicaid spending. The belief was that if health reform could just slow the increase in spending for those programs, the need for further wrenching reconciliation efforts like those of 1990 and 1993 might be limited.

Because health reform had the potential to significantly transform an important service used by every member of society, restructure one-seventh of the economy, and affect employee compensation and taxpayer burdens, participants in the policy debate were also keenly interested in the likely nonbudgetary effects of the various health reform proposals. Analysts were expected to answer other questions. To what extent would reform increase insurance coverage? Would premiums rise or fall as a result of reform? How much choice would consumers have in a reformed system? How would the scope and depth of insurance compare with current coverage? Would the proposal affect employment? To what extent would reform slow the growth of aggregate health spending? The answers to those questions, of course, were inextricably entwined in the estimates of the budgetary effects of various proposals.

This chapter reviews how one agency, the Congressional Budget Office (CBO), went about answering those questions and developing estimates of the effects of the various health reform proposals considered by the 103d Congress.[1] The estimates that CBO provided to Congress were, for the most part, point estimates—single numbers—even though the agency recognized that significant uncertainty surrounded each number. Ranges would have more accurately reflected the state of analytic knowledge. But the enforcement procedures of the budget process require single numbers. Moreover, the information needed to estimate the widths of ranges—that is, the standard errors—was generally not available. That lack of information precluded providing ranges for such qualities as coverage that were not the focus of the budget process.

The Challenge

In designing and considering health reform proposals, analysts and policymakers required two sorts of information. First, they needed an accurate picture of the existing health care system—including its expenditures, coverage, and distribution of services—so that they could understand the underlying problem and the base on which a reformed system would be built. Second, they needed projections of the future health care system without health care reform, so that they could judge the need for reform, design the reform, and understand its likely effects. Unfortunately, current data and analytical methods were inadequate for meeting either of those information needs.

Information on the Current Health Care System

To construct a comprehensive picture of the health care system is impossible with today's databases. What is known must be pieced together from several inadequate or dated sources.

The March supplement to the Current Population Survey (CPS), an annual sample survey of some 57,000 households, can be used to estimate the number of people with and without insurance coverage, their demographic and socioeconomic characteristics, and the type of coverage (employment based, medicare or medicaid, for example) of those who have any. The March supplement also reports whether an employer paid none, some, or all of the premium for employment-based coverage.

This survey tells nothing, however, about the premiums that insured people pay, the types of health plans in which they are enrolled, or the generosity of those plans—in terms of either covered benefits or cost-sharing requirements. Nor can it be used to find out whether those people without insurance could have obtained insurance from an employer or another source but chose not to do so,[2] the fraction of the premium picked up by an employer, or—in the case of workers who reported having individual coverage only—whether an employer offered family as well as individual coverage. The CPS also provides no information on people's health status, their patterns of service use, or their health expenditures. The National Medical Expenditure Survey (NMES) provides answers to some of those questions, but the latest version of that survey is based on 1987 information.

Another source of data on the current health care system is the National Health Interview Survey (NHIS), an annual survey of about 50,000 households. It offers more information than the CPS about the types of insurance that people have and the reasons why some lack coverage. The NHIS can be used to link together health insurance coverage, health status, the use of health services, and socioeconomic variables. The survey lacks, however, the detailed information on income and employment found in the CPS. It also provides no data on premiums or cost-sharing requirements and nothing on the share of premiums paid by employers.

Because employers provide most of the insurance for nonelderly people, analysts also need to know the characteristics of companies and of the insurance they offer their workers. Unfortunately, little reliable information of that sort is available. An accurate picture even of the distribution of companies by size, payroll, and full-time-equivalent employment is difficult. County Business Patterns (CBP) data, which the Census Bureau compiles from a variety of sources, are the primary source of that type of information. But the CBP does not include data on full-time-equivalent employment—only on employment, full time and part time together. Moreover, the CBP data that are generally released relate to business establishments rather than to companies and cannot be used to analyze policies affecting companies.[3]

With a one-year lag, the Health Care Financing Administration (HCFA) estimates aggregate health care spending and spending for various medical services (for example, hospital services, physician services, dental services, prescription drugs, nursing homes, home health care, and so forth).[4] But that information is generally not available for states or substate regions, which were the market areas of most relevance in the health reforms debated in 1993 and 1994.

Projections of the Future Health Care System

To make matters worse, the health sector is evolving rapidly in ways that could not have been foreseen just a few years ago. Technology continues to unfold in unpredictable directions, offering new diagnostic tools and treatments and creating new demands from consumers and new types of providers. Institutional arrangements are changing swiftly. New forms of managed care have emerged. A wave of hospital consolidations has begun. The use of drug formularies has grown dramatically. And employers have become more aggressively cost conscious. The character of public programs is changing even without specific legislative impetus. States have tapped into medicaid's "disproportionate-share" provisions for fiscal relief.[5] The federal government has granted waivers that allow states to broaden the population covered by medicaid or to enroll medicaid beneficiaries in managed care programs. And medicare's reimbursement policies have underwritten an explosion in home health care and outpatient hospital services.

Given such rapid change, it is difficult to know what the future will look like if public policy is unchanged and, hence, what changes various proposals will cause. CBO develops projections of spending and coverage for a decade into the future, but those projections generally presuppose that recent trends will continue.[6] The HCFA makes spending projections using similar assumptions.[7] Those approaches are almost certainly wrong. Nevertheless, any other method would be little more than pure speculation and, more often than not, would generate estimates that were even less reliable.

It is against this backdrop of not knowing many important things about the current health care system and having little idea of how fast and in what directions the existing system might evolve over the next decade or two that CBO and administration analysts estimated the effects of reform proposals. That their results were uncertain and controversial is not surprising.

What Did the Estimators Need to Know?

Analysts needed to answer three basic questions to estimate the federal costs of a health care proposal and its effects on health insurance coverage, national health expenditures, and marginal tax rates. First, what premiums would different groups in the population face, initially and over time? Second, how many people in those groups would be covered and how many would remain uncovered? Third, what portion of people's premiums and other health care spending would be paid for out of pretax dollars, posttax dollars, or subsidies?

The answers to those questions were—and still are—interdependent and uncertain. How uncertain depends on the proposal: the more choice a proposal would allow individuals, families, and employers, the more uncertain would be their responses to policy changes. Those responses, in turn, would affect key variables—such as premiums—invoking further behavioral responses.

To develop answers, analysts need detailed information on the current distributions of health insurance coverage, insurance costs, health status, and health expenditures. Such information can be provided by national sample surveys that contain data on the income and employment characteristics of individuals and families, their health insurance coverage (type of plan, benefits, premiums, and employer payments), their health expenditures, and their health status. That information would also have to be linked to a survey of companies that collected data on the distribution of wages and fringe benefits within companies with different characteristics. Available national sample surveys do not come close to providing information of that sort.

Not only do estimators need reliable, up-to-date information about the current health care system, they also have to develop assumptions about how all the participants in that system would respond if it was fundamentally restructured. Although more research findings on such issues as employers' and families' responses to past changes in the relative price of health insurance would be helpful, such studies can credibly illuminate the effects only of marginal changes to the current environment. The large, systemic changes that major health care reform proposals would provoke lie far outside the boundaries of past changes. The behavioral responses of health care consumers and providers to markedly altered incentives would be difficult enough to predict in the next few years, let alone over the ten-year period that is the purview of the congressional budget process.

During the health care reform debate, the assumptions that analysts had to make about behavioral responses were, unavoidably, little more than informed guesses. But even with greatly expanded and targeted economic research, much of that uncertainty would probably remain. Current state experiments offer some hope. Some of them radically depart from current policy and may provide data for future research that could improve estimates of behavioral responses to fundamental reforms.[8]

Estimating Premiums

Premiums are the result of complex interactions between an array of supply and demand factors, many of which CBO could not take into account in its estimates. The most serious omissions were probably on the supply side. The task of modeling the effects of health care reform on providers and of estimating the consequences of providers' behavioral responses for the supply of health services was too complex to undertake in the time available. CBO assumed that the primary factors determining the level and growth of premiums were the nature of the covered benefits, the service-use patterns of the covered population (reflecting the health status of its members and their proclivities to use health services when covered by comprehensive insurance), and the effectiveness of policies to contain costs. The agency's confidence in its estimates of those factors varied considerably.

COVERED BENEFITS. Most of the proposals CBO estimated incorporated a standard benefit package but differed in the degree to which they actually specified covered benefits. With help from the Congressional Research Service, CBO made assumptions about how the benefit package of each plan would relate to the current average employment-based policy. For example, CBO judged the Clinton administration's plan to be 5 percent more costly than the current average policy; Congressman Gephardt's proposal, 3 percent more costly; and the plans proposed by the House Bipartisan group, the Senate Finance Committee, and Senator Mitchell, 3 percent less costly. CBO concluded that minor variations in benefits, which could be very important to the course of the political debate, had little impact on the premiums for a given population.

USE OF SERVICES. All the comprehensive reform proposals envisioned an insurance market with a community-rated pool for individual purchasers and small companies. Large companies were to be experience rated. The definition of "large" ranged from 5,000 or more workers in the administration's proposal to 100 or more workers in the Managed Competition Act and in the plans proposed by the House Bipartisan group, the Senate Finance Committee, Senator Robert Dole, and the Senate Mainstream group. The problem for cost estimators was to determine who would end up in the community-rated and experience-rated pools, and how much care each would use.

Even under proposals that included an employer mandate, those determinations were not straightforward since some two-worker families would be eligible for both pools and could choose coverage through either employer. Their choice would be affected not only by the premiums and the perceived quality of the plans available in them but also by the proportion of the premium paid by each spouse's employer. Given the lack of current information relating to the amounts firms now pay, it is virtually impossible to project which companies might pay more than the minimum required under the mandate.

The Clinton administration's proposal was particularly tricky for estimators, introducing added complexity and uncertainty because it gave large employers the option to participate in the community-rated pool if they met certain conditions. Moreover, large companies under the proposal faced disincentives to self-insure: those that chose to stay outside the community-rated pool would have had to pay a 1 percent payroll tax, forego subsidies, and subsidize their own low-wage employees. Little information is available on which to estimate the proportion of large companies that would choose to participate in the community-rated pool under those circumstances. More data on the relative health status of employees (and their families) in companies of different sizes and on the variation among large companies would have helped identify large companies whose employees could be better off financially if those companies joined the community-rated pool, but such data provide no insight into how many large companies would actually join the pool.[9]

In preparing its estimates of the administration's plan, CBO used data from the Current Population Survey to estimate, industry by industry, the average difference between a company's premium and the premium in the community-rated pool that would be necessary to offset the financial disadvantages of remaining experience rated. Those estimates varied according to assumptions about employers' discount rates and subsidies for their low-wage workers. To estimate the proportion of large companies that would choose experience rating, CBO then made assumptions about the distribution of premiums among large companies by industry group, the overhead costs of large companies, and how the attitudes of large companies toward participating in regional alliances and the community-rated pool might change over time. CBO concluded that costs of staying outside the community-rated pool were large enough that only about one-tenth of the eligible employees in large companies would be in corporate alliances—that is, experience rated—after 2001. Anecdotal evidence from large companies about their likely responses supported this conclusion.

Estimating who would end up in the community-rated pool and who in the experience-rated pool was considerably more complicated for those proposals that did not require people to obtain health insurance. The problem was simultaneous. Whether people would choose to purchase health insurance in the community-rated pool depended on the premium in that pool, their expected health expenditures, and their aversion to risk. But the premium itself depended on the characteristics of the population in the pool.

Neither the time nor the resources were available to conduct extensive iterations. Moreover, a complex iterative analysis could not be justified, given the limitations of the underlying data. Instead, CBO made simple assumptions about the participation rates of people who currently have private health insurance coverage or who would have their premiums fully subsidized under the proposal. To estimate who among the currently uninsured would choose to obtain coverage, CBO used the available research on price elasticities of demand for health insurance; it also used estimates from Lewin-VHI on the probability of purchasing individual insurance given the premium as a percentage of income.[10] Yet both approaches produce highly uncertain results. Using estimated price elasticities is particularly risky when the price changes are larger than those in the data used for estimating the elasticities and when the entire structure of the health care market is changing as well. Using the Lewin-VHI income-related probabilities implicitly assumes that the uninsured would behave the same way as those currently purchasing individual insurance—a tenuous assumption even in an unchanged marketplace.

For purposes of the cost estimates, CBO also assumed that once people were in the community-rated pool, they would not drop out. This was a heroic assumption because premiums could have spiraled if coverage was voluntary, if high-risk individuals were initially concentrated in the community-rated pool, and if healthier participants began to drop out of that pool because the premiums exceeded their expected benefit adjusted for their aversion to risk. CBO did not try to estimate such effects, but assumed that if, at the outset, people had opportunities to opt out of the community-rated pool and buy insurance through other groups (such as multiple-employer welfare associations) or to purchase catastrophic rather than standard policies, some would choose to do so. Without effective risk adjustment, premiums for standard coverage would be correspondingly higher. Since little is known about risk aversion, inertia, and other noneconomic factors that affect peoples' choice of policies, it was possible only to make an informed guess about the size of the premium adjustment.

Under either mandatory or voluntary approaches, the community-rated pool would include population groups—medicaid beneficiaries and the currently uninsured—whose potential patterns of service use when given standard health coverage are highly uncertain.[11] More research on that issue would be extremely beneficial. As states enroll increasing numbers of medicaid beneficiaries in private managed care plans, analysts should be able to gather more information about whether such groups, if guaranteed access to well-managed care, have health expenditures that are higher, lower, or the same as comparable privately insured people.

CBO generally assumed that medicaid beneficiaries would be more costly to insure than people who had employment-based coverage, but how much more depended on their eligibility category. For example, medicaid beneficiaries who receive aid to families with dependent children would be less costly to insure than beneficiaries receiving supplemental security income (SSI). An issue of particular importance when determining premiums was whether SSI beneficiaries, who typically have large health expenditures, should be included in the community-rated pool. Because of the adverse effects on community-rated premiums of including SSI beneficiaries, most of the voluntary proposals established separate premiums for them.

Compared with medicaid beneficiaries, the uninsured population poses even more of a conundrum for estimators because it comprises several disparate groups: people who have been denied coverage because of pre-existing conditions; those who would like to be insured but cannot afford the premiums available to them through their employer or the individual market; and those who could afford coverage but have other priorities, including healthy young adults who assume that they have little need for insurance. All of those groups would be insured under mandatory proposals, and their members would be split between the community-rated and experience-rated pools. In a voluntary world, those with poor health status would be the most likely to participate.

To gain a better understanding of the potential effects that the uninsured could have on the premiums in the two pools, analysts need improved information about the relative sizes of the three different groups that make up the uninsured population and the employment status and health risks of the members of each group. At present, analysts know only how the average health care use of uninsured people compares with that of demographically similar people with health insurance. Based on data from the National Medical Expenditure Survey, CBO assumed that spending by uninsured people would increase, on average, by 57 percent if they were covered by a comprehensive policy with standard cost-sharing requirements.

EFFECTIVENESS OF POLICIES TO CONTAIN COSTS. The effectiveness of a proposal's policies to contain costs would affect the rate of growth of premiums. Some proposals—such as those advanced by Senator Dole, the Senate Mainstream group, and the House Bipartisan group—included no substantial cost containment provisions. Other proposals relied on enhanced market forces, regulations, or both to slow growth of health care costs. The effectiveness assigned to those mechanisms could only be an educated guess. That those judgments would be highly controversial was also unavoidable, both because so much could ride on them and because they went to the heart of people's underlying beliefs about how consumers, providers, institutions, and political forces respond to incentives and restraints in the health care system.

Some analysts have argued that experiences in competitive markets in the United States or in such programs as the California Public Employees

Retirement System (CalPERS) or the Minnesota State Employee Insurance Program (SEIP) indicate that competitive forces will drastically slow the growth of health spending nationwide. Although those programs offer useful insights, the inferences that one can draw from them are limited. None of these programs is more than a few years old. It is impossible, therefore, to know whether any slowdown in spending growth is temporary or enduring. Furthermore, these programs are operating in an environment that differs substantially from the markets that would be created by the restructured health care systems of the various proposals.

Lacking an alternative, CBO developed effectiveness ratings based largely on informed judgment for competitive proposals. CBO concluded that eight features were essential for the effective functioning of a health care system based on managed competition: (1) regional health insurance purchasing cooperatives would oversee a restructured insurance market, in which health plans competed on the basis of price and quality; (2) access to health insurance would be universal and on an essentially equal basis, accomplished by open-enrollment periods, community-rated premiums, and limited restrictions on coverage; (3) insurance coverage would be universal; (4) all health plans would offer a standard benefit package; (5) purchasing cooperatives would provide comparable information on both price and quality of care for each health plan; (6) health plans would have substantially nonoverlapping networks of affiliated providers; (7) payments to health plans would be adjusted for the risks of their enrollees; and (8) the amount of a health insurance premium that could be sheltered from tax would be limited to the level of the least expensive plan offered through the purchasing cooperative.[12] CBO evaluated the competitive proposals according to how well they met those eight criteria and made corresponding judgments about how much they would reduce the growth of spending, and hence premiums, below the baseline rate.

The Managed Competition Act came closest to meeting all eight criteria fully; it did not assure universal coverage, but it contained part or all of the other seven features.[13] CBO assumed that the proposal would restrain the growth of health care costs in two ways. First, the incentives created by managed competition would accelerate the shift in insurance enrollment to effectively managed plans. That shift would slow the growth of acute care spending on covered benefits by 0.6 percentage point for each of the first five years. Second, competitive pressures fostered by the proposal would cause all insurers to intensify their efforts to control costs. Those efforts would dampen the growth of costs by a gradually increasing amount that would reach 1 percentage point after ten years. Other plans with competitive aspects were accorded fractions of those effects. The proposals put forward by the Senate Finance Committee and Senator Mitchell, for example, were judged to have only one-quarter of the cost containment punch of the Managed Competition Act.

CBO's approach to proposals that relied on regulatory approaches to cost containment was similarly judgmental. CBO judged the effectiveness of each plan's cost containment mechanisms on the basis of the clarity, specificity, automaticity, and enforceability of the regulatory provisions. The experience with medicare's cost containment efforts informed those judgments.

CBO was criticized for concluding that the regulatory cost containment provisions of the administration's plan would be fully effective. That conclusion was reached only after CBO had extensively examined the detailed legislative language that was so tightly constructed that it offered little or no room for administrative flexibility. New legislation would have been needed to relax the cost control limits, and that legislation would have been scored with associated costs. CBO's judgment was not a statement that the limits on cost were politically achievable.

The assessment of the effectiveness of the cost containment provisions in Congressman Gephardt's proposal, the other plan that relied heavily on regulation to contain costs, was far less favorable. CBO judged that the mechanisms for containing costs in the private sector would be ineffective from 2001 through 2003 and only one-quarter effective in 2004. By contrast, it assumed that the limits on medicare spending would ultimately prove to be 75 percent effective.

Coverage

Premiums and coverage are inextricably linked. To estimate premiums, one has to know the number and types of people who would be covered under a restructured health care system; to estimate coverage in nonuniversal systems, one has to know the premiums that participants would be charged. The proposals put forward by the administration, the Ways and Means Committee, Congressman Gephardt, and Senator Mitchell (one variant) contained employer and individual mandates that CBO assumed would produce universal coverage. Yet that assumption was debatable. As Eugene Steuerle of the Urban Institute has pointed out, a mandate is only as effective as its enforcement mechanisms, and enforcement in the case of health care could be difficult.[14]

Estimates of the coverage resulting from the various voluntary proposals were politically sensitive and much more problematic. All advocates of reform expressed concern over the plight of the 39 million Americans—15 percent of the population—who lacked health insurance. The president emphasized that everyone would have coverage under his plan. When mandates came to be regarded as poison, some advocates of reform tried to relax the meaning of the term universal as it related to health insurance. Senator Moynihan pointed out that even so-called universal programs such as social security had participation rates of around 95 percent to 97 percent; he then concluded that an acceptable level of coverage might be in the 92 percent to 95 percent range.

Not surprisingly, estimates of coverage assumed a mystique of their own. Estimates of the fraction of the population that would be covered became a crucial dimension on which the competing plans were compared. Some sponsors went through programmatic contortions to achieve the coverage they believed minimally acceptable. The proposal introduced by Senator Mitchell represented the extreme case. Under that plan, the failure to reach 95 percent coverage voluntarily by 2000 would trigger mandates on employers and individuals. In an effort to attain that threshold, the plan extended subsidies for children and pregnant women to those with incomes up to three times the poverty level, provided special subsidies for the temporarily unemployed, and permitted families eligible for more than one type of subsidy to combine their subsidies to purchase coverage for all or some family members. In addition, the plan allowed those who were eligible for full subsidies to sign up for health insurance with health care providers whenever they sought services. Those "presumptively eligible" people, who may not in fact have been enrolled at the time, were to be counted in determining the fraction of the population that was covered. Through those devices, which were added one at a time as the legislation was crafted, Senator Mitchell's plan was able to claw and scrape its way to the promised land of 95 percent coverage. Given the unavoidable crudeness and uncertainty inherent in CBO's estimates, such fine-tuning was ludicrous and reflected the manner in which the numbers drove policy. Few cared about the administrative nightmares and consumer confusion that the myriad subsidy mechanisms would create.

Sources of Payment

Under most of the health care proposals, individuals and families would pay their health insurance premiums out of pretax dollars (in the form of contributions from employers), posttax dollars, or some combination of the two—as they do today. Those payments would be reduced by subsidies for low-income individuals and families and, in some plans, for employers. Out-of-pocket health expenditures for cost sharing and noncovered services would generally be paid out of posttax dollars, with some proposals also subsidizing cost-sharing amounts for low-income families. Some proposals would also have permitted people to buy catastrophic health coverage supplemented with a medical savings account. Those accounts would let people use pretax dollars to pay for out-of-pocket health expenditures.

Determining the distribution of payments for premiums and cost sharing among these sources was critically important for the cost estimates and for assessing the effects of proposals on labor markets. Changes in both spending and revenues would affect the federal budget; larger subsidies would result in greater direct spending for the federal government, and more pretax spending for premiums would mean lower federal revenues. Subsidies would also influence the supply and demand for low-wage workers—whether to work at all (because of the effects of subsidies on marginal tax rates) and whether to work for an employer offering health insurance coverage.

CONTRIBUTIONS BY EMPLOYERS. Even under proposals with mandates on employers, contributions by employers are difficult to estimate because some employers may pay for more than the mandate requires. Such estimates are critical in determining the costs of subsidies and the tax expenditures associated with employment-based health insurance. Although most of the proposals introduced in the 103d Congress specified the minimum percentage of a benchmark premium that employers had to pay,[15] none prohibited employers from paying more than that amount, either for coverage under the standard benefit package or for supplemental coverage. Moreover, some proposals would have allowed the employer's entire contribution to be tax exempt, as under current law.

One cannot assume that all employers would pay only the minimum amount required. Employers who were currently offering more generous benefits would have no particular reason to cut them, unless the standard benefit package under reform cost more than their more generous benefit package,[16] or unless the additional contributions were no longer tax exempt. Developing assumptions about how employers would behave in those circumstances is extremely difficult, however, because so little is known about what employers currently pay, the percentage of the premium that that payment represents, and the generosity of the benefit packages that they now offer relative to the standard benefits called for in a restructured health care system.[17] Those are important areas in which more survey research is needed, although collecting such information from self-insured companies is difficult.

Given the expanded choice that workers—especially those in the community-rated pool—would have under most of the proposals, some employees would choose plans that were more or less expensive than the average or benchmark plan. The difference between the full premium and the portion paid by the employer would generally be paid with posttax dollars. But existing databases and research do not provide much help in determining the cost of plans people would choose.

The problems in estimating employers' payments under voluntary proposals are compounded by the possibility that some employers who currently offer coverage might choose not to do so in a restructured market, while others might start offering insurance. Some companies might drop coverage for people who were eligible for subsidies. Others might drop coverage for all of their workers if their premiums rose significantly—a possible outcome for some small employers with young, healthy workers who were required to buy coverage through the community-rated pool. Market reforms, of course, could lower premiums for some companies that currently do not pay for coverage for their employees and entice some into the market. No data or research exist that could be used to estimate those opposing impacts. Consequently, CBO did not take the potential effects of changes in premiums into account when estimating the proportion of employers who would offer coverage under the new system.

SUBSIDIES FOR PREMIUMS. To determine the costs of subsidies, analysts must estimate the rates of participation in subsidy programs by individuals, families, and companies. Most of the subsidy regimes proposed would have operated on a sliding-scale basis, and—at least in the voluntary world—participation rates would vary with the subsidy.

Under proposals that imposed mandates on employers and individuals, CBO assumed that all of those eligible for subsidies would claim them. Nonetheless, determining the subsidy amounts was not an easy matter. Estimating subsidies for companies was particularly difficult, since those subsidies depended both on the characteristics of the companies themselves (size and average payroll) and on premiums, which would vary according to the family types of employees. Because data are not collected jointly for companies and employees, CBO could not classify companies by size, payroll, and characteristics of workers. Further data collection in that area is badly needed if future reform proposals are going to maintain a system of employment-based insurance. Yet, even with such information, a good deal of uncertainty will exist as long as there is little consensus about the elasticities of labor supply.

Estimating subsidies for employers was further complicated by the incentives those subsidies would create for low-wage workers to sort themselves into subsidized firms in order to minimize their premium liability.[18] Employers who were not eligible for subsidies would also have incentives to contract for low-wage work with subsidized firms rather than hire their own low-wage workers. CBO based its estimates of the potential magnitude of those responses on average payroll alone. Basing them on the distribution of wages and fringe benefits within companies of different sizes would have been more appropriate.

Most of the proposals that were voluntary provided subsidies for individuals and families but not for employers. The uncertainty that surrounded CBO's estimates of the costs of those premium subsidies arose primarily from a limited knowledge of participation rates. Research on what affects people's decisions to buy insurance is sparse, in part because researchers have no knowledge of the prices that uninsured people face.[19]

Yet participation rates were uncertain even for people who under the proposals would receive subsidies covering their entire premium. Medicaid data suggest that only 75 percent of eligible people participate in that program, and CBO used that rate in developing assumptions about participation. At issue, however, is how the nominal participation rate for the medicaid program should be interpreted. Do that program's provisions for year-round, open enrollment with no exclusions for preexisting conditions make the concept of a participation rate—in the sense of the proportion of the eligible population that is formally enrolled in the program—meaningless? Some people who meet all of the program's eligibility criteria but whose proclivities to use health care services are low may not be enrolled in the program. They could, nonetheless, obtain coverage if they needed it. Others may not enroll because they have private coverage or because they can get services from public or nonprofit providers. Still others may not enroll because of a dislike of government programs or because they lack information about the program. Further investigation into why people who appear to be eligible for medicaid are not enrolled in the program would be extremely useful.

More problematic yet for CBO's estimates were the participation rates of individuals and families who would be eligible for partial subsidies of their premiums. CBO based its calculations on the Lewin-VHI analysis of the individual insurance market mentioned previously. As with people eligible for full subsidies, however, analysts need a better understanding of how various market reforms—such as open enrollment and prohibitions on excluding pre-existing conditions—would affect participation of those individuals eligible for partial subsidies.

Also important for estimating subsidies in the voluntary world are the behavioral responses of employers and employees. Employers would have incentives to drop coverage for low-wage workers who were eligible for subsidies. Those incentives would be shared by employees, too, if the savings realized by employers that stopped providing coverage translated into higher wages. For the same reason, workers eligible for subsidies would have incentives to seek employment in companies that did not offer insurance.

Although some health reform proposals included provisions to limit such responses, it is unclear how effective they would have been. Existing research sheds little light on the magnitude of the responses, and CBO's estimating assumptions were inevitably somewhat tenuous. Much more research needs to be done in that area because the potential effects on subsidy costs are large. CBO estimated, for example, that the reallocation of low-wage workers among firms would account for about $11 billion (7 percent) of the costs of premium subsidies in 2004 under the Bipartisan proposal, about $13 billion (8 percent) under the Senate Finance Committee's proposal, and about $14 billion (7 percent) under Senator Mitchell's proposal without the mandate in effect.

SUBSIDIES FOR COST SHARING. Besides subsidies for premiums, many of the proposals would also have provided low-income people with subsidies for cost-sharing amounts. Some proposals would have restricted such subsidies to situations in which low-cost-sharing plans were not available at a reasonable premium; others would have subsidized cost-sharing expenditures, even if low-cost-sharing plans were available. CBO used the findings from the Rand Health Insurance Experiment to estimate the probable increase in use of health services that would result if low-income people effectively had first-dollar coverage.[20] These data are of high quality but are old, having been generated between 1974 and 1981, and may not correctly characterize current behavior. That estimate was important—not only for the estimates of subsidies but also for the feedback effect on premiums. The more people with access to cost-sharing subsidies, the higher would be the premiums.

Information Needs for Implementation

The estimates that CBO prepared of the various comprehensive health care proposals assumed that the proposals could be implemented as the sponsors intended. Anyone considering the magnitude of the changes envisioned by those plans, however, would have to question the feasibility of implementing many components of those proposals within the foreseeable future. Yet CBO had no reasonable way to factor those concerns explicitly into its estimates. Instead, it chose to discuss them extensively without quantifying their effects on already highly uncertain estimates.

Most of the reform plans called for creating complex new entities, such as geographically based insurance purchasing cooperatives, that would have had substantial responsibilities that no existing institution now performs. State governments and federal agencies also would have been assigned major new tasks. No research evidence exists to support estimates of how long it might take to bring off such institutional changes or to determine just what the limits of the administrative capabilities of those entities might be.

In addition to new institutions, most of the plans would have required huge amounts of new information to operate effectively. The data needs and reporting requirements to develop an effective mechanism for adjusting risks among health plans would have been extensive. New information and evaluations would have been needed to help consumers choose rationally among health plans. Information would have had to be collected and analyzed to monitor the quality of care.

Besides such plan-level data, some proposals required the collection and processing of demographic, income, employment, and health expenditure data at the state and substate levels to support administering subsidies and for monitoring and regulating health spending. Administering subsidies would have also required extensive cooperation among the purchasing cooperatives or states to track the income, family status, and program participation of low-income individuals when they moved among states. Databases and information systems with those capabilities do not exist, and many analysts are skeptical that they could have been developed within the few years envisioned by the proposals.

The competitive health care markets that are being developed in some of the states and the experimentation going on under the medicaid waivers call for some of the information and institution building that would have been required on a massive scale by the reform proposals. Tracking the success of those efforts as they try to develop appropriate data systems and administrative structures should inform those who will be charged with estimating the effects of future fundamental health reform proposals.

Conclusion

CBO's estimates of the effects of the major health proposals played an important role in the deliberations of the 103d Congress over the desirability of the alternative methods of health care reform. Unfortunately, those estimates were quite uncertain and therefore controversial. If a sustained effort had been mounted in the late 1980s to collect more complete and up-to-date information and to conduct the economic research on the responses of consumers, providers, and businesses to various changes in incentives, the uncertainty surrounding some of those estimates could have been reduced substantially. Nevertheless, huge residual uncertainty is inescapable whenever legislative proposals call for systemic change. When proposals fundamentally restructure the health care system and change the incentives and relative prices faced by all participants, the best data from the existing system and the most sophisticated research will only be able to provide partial insights into what that brave new world will look like.

Comments

John F. Sheils: Linda Bilheimer and Robert Reischauer do an excellent job of summarizing the limitations in the data available for estimating the cost of major health reform initiatives. Moreover, the Congressional Budget Office (CBO) should be congratulated for its contributions to the policy process last year. As at CBO, we at Lewin-VHI developed financial analyses of the costs of several major health reform initiatives ranging from mandates to voluntary programs. We too are intimately familiar with the limitations of the available data. However, we seem to differ over the nature of these data deficiencies.

As the authors explain, estimating the cost of major health reform initiatives involves two steps. First, the analyst develops a "base case" projection of health care coverage and costs under the current health care system for the year in which the health reform plan would be implemented. Second, the analyst estimates coverage and costs under proposed reforms in that same year. The difference between costs under the reform plan and costs under the base case represents the net cost of the health reform plan. The more detailed simulation models also show the net cost of the plan to employers by company size and industry; state, local, and federal governments; and households by income level and other family characteristics.

What makes health reform modeling so difficult is the surprising lack of data available on current health expenditures. Even the national health accounts data are based upon fragmentary information from disparate sources that potentially suffer from underreporting, misclassification, and double counting. Moreover, these data provide little information on the distribution of health spending across various demographic and employment status groups. Such details must be estimated from other data sources such as the National Health Interview Survey (NHIS) or the 1987 National Medical Expenditure Survey (NMES) data. Thus in many cases the net cost of reform for a particular group of payers is estimated by taking the difference between simulated costs for these groups under reform and a base case spending estimate for these groups that is itself the product of a simulation.

Cost estimating is further complicated by the fact that many health reform plans would rely upon delivery system reforms that never before have been attempted on a broad scale in the United States. For example, some health reform plans would rely on market forces to control costs by altering incentives for consumers, providers, and insurers. One can try to estimate the effects of such a program by extrapolating from cost data for managed care plans, provided that the effects of managed care plans can be isolated from selection effects and other factors that are correlated with health plan costs. However, as the authors point out, it is unclear whether the cost performance of managed care plans is representative of what costs would be under the unique incentive structures created by these reforms.

Our experience indicates that the lack of data on employers is more serious than the authors suggest. Both the administration and CBO used the County Business Patterns (CBP) data to develop estimates of employer premium subsidies for low-wage companies under President Clinton's health reform plan. The CBP data provide comprehensive data on wages and employment for private employers but do not provide information on the age and family status characteristics of individuals within these companies. This deficiency is serious because low-wage workers are about twice as likely to be single and without dependents as are higher-wage workers.[21] This correlation tends to reduce employer premium payments for dependent coverage in low-wage companies, which in turn reduces employer subsidy payments to these companies under President Clinton's plan. In fact, our analyses suggest that because of these data deficiencies, both the administration and CBO substantially overestimated the cost of these subsidies for a given level of premiums.

In our analysis we used a survey of employers conducted by the Health Insurance Association of America (HIAA). Although these data suffer from nonresponse problems, they provide information on employment within individual companies by age, wage level, part-time/full-time status, and family/single coverage. These data enabled Lewin-VHI to control for the correlation between wage levels and family size and resulted in substantially lower estimates for low-wage companies than CBO estimated. In fact, we found that controlling for these correlations reduced our estimates of employer premium subsidies under President Clinton's plan by about $11.0 billion a year. However, much improved employer data are required to adequately capture these relationships.

As the authors point out, the cost impacts of health reform are driven by the health service utilization characteristics of individuals who would find themselves in various community-rated pools under these reforms. For example, several health reform proposals would pool families in small companies with families where there is no worker (excluding medicare recipients). This feature is important because compared with workers, the nonworking population uses about twice as much hospital care, and individuals are about three times as likely to report themselves to be in poor health.[22] Consequently, pooling small employers with nonworkers can result in an increase in small employer premiums of up to 30 percent while reducing premiums for nonworkers by as much as 50 percent. This correlation also tends to reduce federal premium subsidy payments because most nonworkers are in low-income groups that qualify for these subsidies.

We found that these effects were largely unexpected by the authors of the various bills. For example, some bills would have pooled the relatively costly medicaid population with individuals and employers in the community-rated pool. This policy tends to reduce federal costs for the medicaid population because the community rate would be less than their actual costs under the current medicaid program.[23] However, it would increase premiums for small employers by pooling workers in these companies with higher-cost populations. Although this policy reduces federal costs, it also has the largely unintended effect of shifting costs from public programs to small employers through the community rate. Although the NMES and the NHIS data are useful for quantifying these effects, more reliable data on the relative differences in utilization across various demographic and employment status groups are required.

Another area of great uncertainty is the likely cost of covering the current medicaid population under private insurance plans. Some health reform proposals would shift many medicaid recipients into subsidized private insurance plans. This shift represents such a major change in the delivery system that it is difficult to estimate the costs under the reform. In some instances, costs would increase because provider payments under private insurance plans can be up to three times higher than medicaid payment rates for the same service. However, managed care plans employ management techniques that reduce use of hospital inpatient and emergency room care. In fact, anecdotal evidence suggests that existing medicaid managed care programs have dramatically reduced hospital utilization for these groups. More research is required to understand the cost implications of these reforms.

The authors might have devoted more attention to their assumptions in scoring programs with health expenditure limits. Like CBO, we too assumed that the spending controls in President Clinton's proposal would be fully effective.[24] After all, if Congress were to enact a cost control program as draconian as that proposed by President Clinton, it hardly would be appropriate for private estimators to assume that Congress does not mean to see it enforced. The problem is that it is highly unlikely that Congress would have the sustained political will to enforce a major reduction in the growth in health spending well into the next century. If congressional will weakened, the result would be higher program costs over time. The policy process might be better served in future cost analyses by providing a range of estimates under alternative scenarios for cost growth regardless of the demand for point estimates in the budgeting process.

Despite these many data deficiencies, those of us who estimate health reform program costs have perfected our craft to the point where we can "hit the broad side of a barn." Although point estimates are sure to be wrong, our models are capable of identifying the relative costs of alternative health reform plans. But budgetary effects cannot be estimated with certainty. Policymakers should recognize that any major health reform initiative will require continued refinements in program design and financing over time.

Len M. Nichols: Robert Reischauer and Linda Bilheimer have written a predictably first-rate description of some major estimation issues in the health reform debate of 1993–94. I could add others,[25] but I have no substantive disagreements with their chapter. My agreement should not surprise anyone, as everyone involved in the developing of cost estimates grappled with the same questions and imperfect data for two years. We often tried to help each other sort out the implications of proposals and meet relentless deadlines. I will add a general perspective on the role of quantitative estimates in the policy debate and a brief discussion of ways to address the data and research shortcomings that persist.

How Serious Was the Lack of Information?

Why do we need quantitative information, or more broadly, what is the responsibility of quantitative analysts in social policy debates? I believe that we have three responsibilities: to inform public policy choices, so that decision-makers and the public know the implications of the choices; to protect the treasury from financial ruin by alerting policymakers to rosy scenarios; and to enable policy reform to have a chance by highlighting areas of analytical agreement and carefully delimiting areas of remaining uncertainty. Such information is essential for the public deliberation Daniel Yankelovich describes. Uncertainty is certainly large in health system reform estimates, but it should not be overstated. Since the enemies of reform and activist presidencies always exaggerate uncertainty for their own ends, it is essential that serious analysts define the contours of agreement and remaining uncertainty precisely.

Overall, in 1993 and 1994 quantitative health reform analysts informed and protected but did not enable. Analysts made clear to decisionmakers the broad consequences of choices. They fashioned fail-safe mechanisms that all serious bills contained and developed the reasonable

Congressional Budget Office cost estimates to protect the federal treasury. The CBO estimates minimized the risk of disastrous future consequences from tightly binding constraints. However, early disputes about deficit reduction created an exaggerated impression of great uncertainty and risk that was never removed and that colored the future debate.

My basic point is simple. The Health Security Act (HSA) may have had flaws, and the Clinton administration's political strategy made comprehensive health reform a hard sell, as others have said. But it is possible to construct a health plan based on reformed private insurance markets and employer mandates that will deliver universal coverage and at least rough deficit neutrality even without a broad-based tax increase.

The administration surely thought so when it released its official estimates in November 1993. The independent consulting firm Lewin-VHI reached the same conclusion in December 1993.[26] Had CBO confirmed this basic judgment of the HSA in its February 1994 report, a major body blow to the president's credibility in the entire health care debate would have been averted, and the political dynamic in early 1994 would surely have been different.

If the administration had been able to work with CBO, as major committees and the leadership routinely do, the HSA could have been altered slightly to hit a modest deficit reduction target. I do not want to apportion blame for the fact that CBO and the administration and its allies in Congress failed to work together in this way. From what I know about the administration's policy development processes, it is not clear that the administration would or even could have supplied CBO with sufficiently detailed legislative language within the time constraints. What is clear is that an opportunity was lost for serious and credible analysts to reach a reasonable consensus on the technical feasibility of the administration's goals as embodied in the Health Security Act, and that losing this opportunity was costly.

In any event, quantitative information of adequate quality was eventually produced, but it was very unevenly disseminated. Robert Reischauer eloquently defined "adequate" during testimony about CBO estimates of the HSA. When asked by Representative Barbara B. Kennelly, "Are you sure you're [your estimates] in the ballpark?" he replied, "We're in the town the ballpark is in."[27]

I understand all too well that human nature and the policy process require point estimates. I would submit, however, that ten-year point estimates of major reforms should be rounded to the nearest $100 billion (1994 dollars). If both the administration and CBO estimates were rounded in this way, they would have easily fallen into the same range. All comprehensive reform bills had subsidy cost estimates for 1996 to 2005 in the $1 trillion ballpark. Plus or minus $100 billion is equivalent to plus or minus 10 percent. Given the inherent estimation difficulties, plus or minus $100 billion over ten years, or $10 billion each year, should be good enough for major social reforms in a $7 trillion economy and with a $1.5 trillion dollar annual federal budget. Original social security and medicare predictions were nowhere near this close, and whatever their current problems, those programs must surely be counted among our greater political and social successes. Current budget rules hold major social reforms to a standard that is often impossible to reach.

Accurate quantitative information is unevenly distributed. I focus on the problems of three groups: the press, the public, and Congress. Complex and ambiguous quantitative information does not fit the preferred format of the press, and most press coverage of "numbers" issues focused on adversarial quotations and reporting conclusions without reflection or analysis. "He said, she said" in quantitative matters leads the public to believe that "no one knows." The oft-repeated belief that "no one knows" can kill any proposal, good or bad.

By "the public" I mean both interest groups and individuals. Interest groups reduce their general credibility by acknowledging or releasing data only if it supports their current positions. Graham Wilson's account in this volume reports that interest groups found it hard to decide what to be *for*. Perhaps. But I can assure you, most powerful interest groups showed little doubt about what to be *against*. This dichotomy may have contributed to the general focus on the negative during the legislative struggle of 1994.

Most individuals do not know what amount they are paying for health insurance now through their employers, and little effort was devoted to this educational prerequisite for a serious public discussion about reform options. Given this unfortunate fact, the exaggerated uncertainties during the debate, and the complicated redistributions implicit in any comprehensive reform proposal, it is not surprising that few believed rhetorical claims that "everyone's a winner." In the end the lack of faith in reform and in reformers is what killed health reform in Congress.

Members of Congress, like the press, are heterogenous. Some are brilliant and exceptionally well informed about health care matters. Some are neither. This heterogeneity forces officials to provide a "lowest common denominator" type of briefing. This approach can be effective in the short run, but it leaves any estimate vulnerable to interest group coun-

Figure 6-1. *Existing Data on Health Care Delivery and Financing*

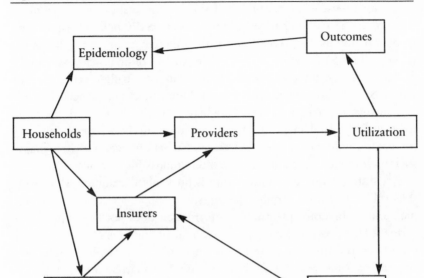

terassertion, because the methods and rationale behind the numbers never get explained.

Many members prefer credible cover to detailed analysis. Most really only want to know, "What will CBO say?" which gives enormous power to CBO. Given the capable stewardship of past CBO directors, this abdication of personal responsibility has been, on balance, a good social bargain for the United States. But it would be better for the republic and Congress itself if representatives and senators were more demanding and willing to accept the sometimes bad news of cold, hard analysis that CBO was created to deliver.

And What Can Be Done About It?

Some important technical issues have not yet been mentioned today but deserve attention.

Figure 6-1 is a schematic diagram of data on our health delivery and financing systems. Start with household demographics at the far left-hand side, and move horizontally through providers to utilization. Everything on this line and above it, with the notable exception of medical outcomes, is quite well captured in national probability surveys, usually annually, by at least one in the set of National Health Care Surveys[28] conducted by the National Center for Health Statistics. The nation has extremely good annual information linking household demographics and utilization.

Now return to that same first horizontal line linking households and utilization, and this time think about it plus everything below it. The National Medical Expenditure Survey (NMES) of the Agency for Health Care Policy Research provides many of these data. This survey is the nation's primary source of information about the distribution of household health expenditures and financing sources: households themselves, employers, insurers, governments, and providers. Unfortunately, the NMES is conducted only once a decade, the last time in 1987. So the only nationally representative data on the distribution of expenditures by demographic subgroup—data that were crucial for premium estimation und:r the myriad alternative risk pools in the health reform proposals of 1993–94—were seven years old. But the health delivery system of 1987 was quite different from today's. The allocation of data collection resources is out of balance when expenditure data are collected once a decade, while utilization data, which does not vary nearly as much, is collected annually.

As Bilheimer and Reischauer point out, the two biggest estimation issues affecting cost estimates concerned the level and growth of premiums. The triangle in the lower left-hand corner—household demographics, employers, and insurers—represents key linkages. The truth is that analysts know embarrassingly little about insurance markets. We have good information about the type of coverage the public has, but we know little about how people came to make those choices. We need much improved surveys on the choices employers face and make, on the contingent choices households then make, and on how the local insurance market conditions affect these offers and choices. The CBO, the administration, and Lewin-VHI did creditable jobs of estimating the long-run equilibrium premiums for the Health Security Act, but each assumed effectively enforced mandates, complete insurance reforms,[29] community rating, and perfect risk adjustment believed by all bidding insurers. Basic research is needed on the quantitative significance of relaxing any of these assumptions to support analyses of proposals centered on voluntary approaches with incomplete insurance reforms.

Additional research should focus on the trapezoid formed by insurers, providers, utilization, and expenditures (figure 6-1). What strategies might actually reduce cost growth? The premium caps in the Health

Security Act were little more than assertions of will in the face of what some analysts thought was possible. Since overall health spending may not be slowing down without reform as much as some may have hoped,[30] interest in caps on spending growth may revive. Although developments in the private sector currently hold some promise of slowing spending growth, research should accompany the experimentation so that systematically successful strategies spread as rapidly as possible, and so that the effects of successful strategies on technology and quality are clearly understood. For this reason, it is important to pay attention to the outcomes emanating from the trapezoid.

Finally, two new surveys would greatly improve health reform cost estimation. Information on the wage distribution within companies would support improved predictions on how various premium subsidies (including medicaid expansions) and income tax changes targeted to low-income households might affect the decisions of employers to sponsor coverage. Serious thought should also be given to reorganizing and co-ordinating the multiple data-gathering efforts of the National Center of Health Statistics (NCHS) and the Agency for Health Care Policy Research, perhaps finally combining the efforts into a single household panel survey that traces interactions among employers, insurers, and providers, all the way to expenditures and outcomes. Properly designed with appropriate supplements, this panel should be capable of generating data on insurance, utilization, and expenditures much more often than once a decade, without sacrificing the ongoing monitoring of the evolving health delivery system that the NHCS does now.

Kenneth Thorpe: I commend Linda Bilheimer and Robert Reischauer for providing an excellent summary of the data issues raised during the recent national health reform debate. Their chapter nicely summarizes the major issues facing those seeking to estimate the effects of major state or national health care reform proposals. My reflections will simply extend their observations.

Those estimating the impact of health reform proposals face several obstacles. Such estimates generally start with a microsimulation model that necessarily simplified greatly the complex interactions in the health care sector. These models require detailed data on individuals, their employers, and their health insurance. Answering the series of "what if" questions also requires modelers to incorporate several assumptions about the behavior of individuals, employers, and health care providers under various health reform options. As Bilheimer and Reischauer note, the data currently collected by the federal government are not sufficient for these tasks. Moreover, the results from the health services research community do not provide a sufficient basis for solid behavioral assumptions that must be incorporated within models used to simulate the effects of health care reform. Both shortcomings increase dramatically the uncertainty of reform estimates. They also guarantee that point estimates of reform impacts will differ across agencies. These differences confuse users of these estimates and provide opportunities for opponents of legislative initiatives to selectively pick estimates to advance their agendas.

Although we will never completely eliminate differences among estimates of various agencies on effects of large-scale health reform proposals, it is possible to improve data and thereby narrow the range of disagreement and to focus on differences driven by behavioral assumptions. Improving the quality of these estimates is critical, I believe, given their central role in policy formation both within the administration and Congress.

I briefly illustrate how the lack of data limits the ability of planners to produce reform estimates and why estimates will ultimately differ across models. I believe the quality of estimates can be improved by collecting more complete and timely data for simulation models. Moreover, health services research could assume an important role in providing more guidance on key behavioral assumptions used in microsimulation models.

Within the administration, financial estimates of the costs and savings of the president's plan served as important inputs into the final formulation of the Health Security Act. Estimates of the federal costs of the plan served to inform the size of federal budget savings needed to pay for the program and to contribute to deficit reduction. Estimates of federal costs and savings proceeded in several interconnected steps. A critical step concerned the insurance costs (premiums) associated with the benefits outlined in the president's plan. The Department of Health and Human Services spent several weeks refining estimates of these costs. Our approach relied both on econometric estimates of the "premiums" and on more conventional actuarial estimates. These estimates were complicated since the president's proposal extended private health insurance to the currently uninsured as well as to medicaid beneficiaries, populations about which the private insurance industry knows little.

To mitigate the financial impact on small companies and low-income individuals, the president's plan provided premium discounts that varied by company size and average company payroll and by family income. We applied this subsidy schedule to our premium estimates to estimate the federal costs of the premium discounts.

Estimates of the insurance premiums and their growth over time were critical for calculating revenue impacts as well. By convention, financial estimates generally assume that workers "pay" for mandated health benefits through lower wages. Conversely, slower growth in health insurance premiums generated through efforts to slow the growth in costs results in higher wages. Since employer-financed health insurance is not included in income subject to the individual income tax or payroll taxes, these assumptions influence the growth of taxable income and, hence, of government revenues. Holding other factors constant, higher estimates of health insurance premiums result in slower growth in tax receipts over time. These "indirect" effects of health reform are often overlooked in the public debate, but on occasion served as important points of departure between the administration estimates and those provided by the Congressional Budget Office (CBO).

We also produced several other analyses that focused on total health care spending, as well as the distribution of spending among employers, individuals, and governments. These analyses allowed us to understand the financial effect of the Health Security Act on households by income, companies by company size and industry, and for each of the states. On their own merit, such estimates are complicated, requiring simulations of individual and company behavior in newly constructed insurance markets not previously observed. Such estimates are also complicated by two other issues. First, the data underlying the estimates are woefully inadequate and out of date, forcing analysts to improvise. Second, such estimates require several assumptions about company and individual behavior. In many cases, these assumptions are educated, though debatable, guesses. Finally, analysts produce single, point estimates that cannot, by nature, convey the underlying uncertainty.

Data Requirements

The data requirements underlying these estimates are daunting. The data should include timely information linking individual income and insurance status (both whether individuals are insured and the nature of the coverage) to characteristics of the company the individual works for and the type of health insurance the employer offers. Bilheimer and Reischauer lucidly outline these data requirements and current shortcomings. For instance, the primary source of data, the National Medical Expenditure Survey (NMES), collects data once a decade. Though it is a rich source of data, it does not provide financial detail on households or state-level data required for most health care reform proposals. These deficiencies could and should be corrected.

Since there is no timely, comprehensive source of health care data, microsimulation modelers must link several data sets. The administration and CBO used slightly different data to construct their simulation models and included different assumptions about today's spending on health care. One example of these differences concerns current spending on private health insurance. The CBO estimates of baseline spending on private health insurance were higher than those estimated by the actuaries at the Department of Health and Human Services. Such differences are, of course, completely understandable given the dearth of information on health insurance premiums.

These differences contributed, in part, to the higher premiums estimated by CBO under the Health Security Act (CBO's premium estimates were approximately 15 percent higher than those produced by the administration).

Use of Point Estimates

Point estimates of the cost of program initiatives are required for budget estimates, but such estimates do not reveal uncertainty. For instance, using data from the Rand Health Insurance Experiment (HIE), estimators can estimate the cost of covering the uninsured.[31] To be complete, these estimates should also include a standard error used to create a confidence interval. These ranges are not provided. Neither the administration nor the Congressional Budget Office provides such ranges. Point estimates provide a false sense of confidence in the results. Moreover, when the uncertainty is genuine, producing a single number also guarantees that different analysts will generate different estimates, though not necessarily ones that are statistically different. As a result, opponents of legislative initiatives may then use statistically insignificant differences among point estimates as an argument against action and to challenge the veracity of supporters. The recent debate over health reform illustrates this dynamic. The administration and CBO produced similar estimates of the costs of the administration program. Estimates of medicare savings, revenues from the tobacco tax, and the impact on national health spending were remarkably close. They differed on the distribution of effects of health reform among the federal government, state and local governments, and the private sector. CBO estimated higher federal costs and substantially higher savings to state and local governments than the administration did. Opponents of reform used these differences, particularly the impact on the federal budget, to undermine the credibility of the administration estimates and the plan in general. Given the uncertainty underlying the analyses, it is unlikely that the estimates were statistically different.

Behavioral Assumptions

Various estimators made different assumptions about the behavior of companies and individuals. Two brief examples illustrate the importance of these assumptions. The first concerns the behavior of employers and employees with generous health insurance benefits. The second concerns the treatment of cafeteria plans. In the HSA, higher federal income and payroll tax receipts resulting from the proposal's cost containment provisions constituted a major source of revenue included in both the CBO and administration budget estimates. The notion here is that slower growth in health insurance premiums leads to faster growth of (relative to current policy) wages and therefore to additional tax receipts. The magnitude of these additional revenues was substantial and represented a critical source of finance in many health reform proposals. These indirect tax effects represented the largest source of revenue—$125 billion between fiscal year 1996 and 2004—in the HSA according to CBO.[32] The next largest was the tobacco tax at $94 billion.

Underlying these estimates is the fact that many employers currently provide benefits more generous than those found in the HSA and the assumption that some would reduce their benefits to the mandated package. To the extent that this assumption is correct, the savings would result in higher wages and therefore additional tax receipts. This issue is clearly interesting and important, but little health services research is available to guide estimates. Consequently, differences among assumptions with important implications for estimates of the indirect tax effects of reform are likely and, with current information, unresolvable.

A second example concerns changes in the tax treatment of cafeteria plans envisioned under the HSA. Under this proposal, workers could not use cafeteria plans to purchase health insurance with pretax dollars. At issue is whether workers would accept a reduction in cash wages in return for their employer's payment of health insurance with pretax dollars. If this occurred, income and payroll tax receipts would be lower than expected, resulting in "higher" costs of the proposal. The extent of such strategic bargaining among employees and employers has a large effect on estimated "indirect" tax receipts. Again, reasonable analysts can and do disagree on this issue, and their disagreements have a large impact on the "cost" of such proposals.

In sum, estimates underlying large-scale health reform involve substantial uncertainty. Inadequate data, combined with often unspecified underlying behavioral assumptions, complicate comparisons among estimates. With respect to the former, government can and must collect more timely data. This step will involve substantial changes in current data collection methods. Providing more accurate, timely, and extensive data will enable improved estimates that vary less across modelers. Moreover, health services research can assume a major role in shaping the behavioral assumptions underlying simulation estimates. Several interesting areas of research are suggested by our recent health reform experience.

Notes

1. See, for example, Congressional Budget Office, *An Analysis of the Administration's Health Proposal* (Washington, February 1994); and Congressional Budget Office, *An Analysis of the Managed Competition Act* (Washington, 1994).

2. The April supplement to the Current Population Survey provides a limited amount of information on this issue. Unfortunately, it is conducted only every five years. At the time CBO was preparing its estimates of the health proposals, the latest available data from the April supplement were for 1988.

3. CBO was extremely fortunate to be able to work with the Census Bureau to conduct analyses using the bureau's firm-level data file. With the assistance of Census Bureau staff, CBO supplemented the file with data from other sources to analyze the effects of the administration's health proposal.

4. Katherine R. Levit and others, "National Health Spending Trends, 1960–1993," *Health Affairs*, vol. 13 (Winter 1994), pp. 14–31.

5. Medicaid's disproportionate share provisions provide special payments to hospitals serving disproportionate numbers of low-income persons. Before the payments were capped in 1993, some states used provider tax and donation schemes and intergovernmental transfers to increase their disproportionate share payments and provide state fiscal relief.

6. Congressional Budget Office, *Projections of National Health Expenditures: 1993 Update* (Washington, 1993).

7. Sally T. Burner and others, "National Health Expenditures Projections through 2030," *Health Care Financing Review*, vol. 14 (Fall 1992), pp. 1–29.

8. Under medicaid statewide waivers, Florida, Hawaii, Ohio, Oregon, Rhode Island, South Carolina, and Tennessee are beginning substantial initiatives to cover low-income people. Delaware, Illinois, Louisiana, Massachusetts, Missouri, and New Hampshire have applied to the Health Care Financing Administration for waivers; several other states are considering applying.

9. Some large firms that, in a narrow sense, would have been financially better off by self-insuring might have chosen to participate in the community-rated pool to reduce administrative burdens and remove health insurance from the list of potential labor-management problems.

10. Congressional Budget Office, *Behavioral Assumptions for Estimating the Effects of Health Care Proposals*, prepared by Sandra Christensen (Washington, 1993); and Lewin-VHI, Inc., "Expanding Insurance Coverage without a Mandate," draft report for the Health Care Leadership Council, Fairfax, Va., May 1994.

11. Not all currently uninsured people who would gain coverage under a proposal would end up in the community-rated pool. Some people working for large firms would be in the experience-rated pool.

12. Congressional Budget Office, *Managed Competition and Its Potential to Reduce Health Spending* (Washington, 1993).

13. Congressional Budget Office, *An Analysis of the Managed Competition Act.*

14. C. Eugene Steuerle, "Implementing Employer and Individual Mandates," *Health Affairs*, vol. 13 (Spring II 1994), pp. 54–68.

15. The benchmark premium might be the lowest available premium in the area, an average of the premiums in the area, an average adjusted for cost controls, or the firm's premium in the case of experience-rated firms.

16. Such a situation might be the case for some of the employers forced into the community-rated pool who had a low-risk group of employees.

17. Workers report on the Current Population Survey when their employer pays their entire premium, but nothing is known of the dollar amount or the covered benefits.

18. Only the plans proposed by the administration, the Ways and Means Committee, and Congressman Gephardt provided subsidies for employers. Family subsidies would, however, provide the same kind of incentives to sort.

19. Congressional Budget Office, *Behavioral Assumptions for Estimating the Effects of Health Care Proposals.*

20. Willard G. Manning and others, "Health Insurance and the Demand for Medical Care: Evidence from a Randomized Experiment," *American Economic Review*, vol. 77 (June 1987), pp. 251–77.

21. Lewin-VHI, Inc., analysis of Bureau of the Census, Current Population Survey (Department of Commerce, March 1994). Data available from author.

22. Lewin-VHI, Inc., "Permitting Voluntary Enrollment in Regional Alliances under the Health Security Act: The Impact on Spending for Employers and the Federal Government," final report prepared for the Henry J. Kaiser Family Foundation, Fairfax, Va., April 21, 1994.

23. John F. Sheils and others, "Health Insurance Coverage under Alternative

Health Reform Proposals," prepared for the Henry J. Kaiser Family Foundation, Lewin-VHI, Inc., Fairfax, Va., November 1994.

24. Unlike CBO estimates, the Lewin-VHI estimates included an adjustment for the aging of the non-medicare population, which appears to have been permitted under the president's plan.

25. For an alternative survey of this list, see L. Nichols and L. Blumberg, "Federal Budget Effects of Alternative Health Reform Proposals," paper presented to Allied Social Science Association, January 1995.

26. Lewin-VHI, "The Financial Impact of the Health Security Act," Fairfax, Va., December 1993.

27. Dana Priest, Spencer Rich, and staff writers, "Health Plan Will Swell Deficit," *Washington Post*, February 9, 1994, p. A1.

28. These surveys are the National Ambulatory Medical Care Survey, the National Hospital Ambulatory Medical Care Survey, the National Hospital Discharge Survey, the National Survey of Ambulatory Surgery, the National Nursing Home Survey, and the National Home and Hospice Care Survey. When coupled with the National Health Interview Survey, the items above the horizontal are covered very well, save for managed care providers and outcomes.

29. Standard benefit package; guaranteed issue, renewability, and portability; and limits on pre-existing condition restrictions.

30. Haiden A. Huskamp and Joseph P. Newhouse, "Is Health Spending Slowing Down?" *Health Affairs*, vol. 13 (Winter 1994), pp. 32–38.

31. Data were collected from 1974 to 1982. For a summary of the HIE, see Joseph P. Newhouse and the Insurance Experiment Group, *Free for All? Lessons Learned from the RAND Health Insurance Experiment* (Harvard University Press, 1993).

32. Congressional Budget Office, *An Analysis of the Administration's Health Proposal.*

PART THREE

What Does the Future Hold?

Market-Based Reform:
What to Regulate and by Whom?

Alain C. Enthoven and Sara J. Singer

B EYOND producing efficiency in the allocation of resources, market forces have several other important positive features. They motivate innovation in products, services, technology, quality improvement, and cost reduction. Market-based systems are flexible and motivate continuous adaptation to changes in technology and tastes. As Charles Schultze wrote, "Market-like arrangements not only minimize the need for coercion . . .; they also reduce the need for compassion, patriotism, brotherly love, and cultural solidarity as motivating forces behind social improvement. . . .The market . . . reduces the need for hard-to-get information. . . . Efficiency-creating changes are not seriously impeded . . . [because] those who may suffer losses are not usually able to stand in the way of change.[1]

Indeed, in health care now—at least in competitive markets such as California's—market forces are motivating large innovations in cost reduction and customer service improvement. Government programs, however, are often associated with waste, pork barrel, complexity, rigidity, and coercion.[2] For example, although the federal medicare program has achieved much by ensuring health care for our elderly, it is complex and rigid, and its hundreds of pages of laws provide rich opportunities to create particularized benefits that can be used to reward political supporters. A revolution has occurred in health care financing in the private sector over the past fifteen years with the introduction of preferred provider insurance (PPI) and rapid growth of membership in health maintenance organizations (HMOs). Medicare has not kept pace. It needs to be modernized to offer beneficiaries an annual choice among competing health plans. Very large gains in efficiency would ensue.

Thus important advantages can be gained by leaving resource allocation to the private market. But market forces in health care if left un-
checked also produce undesirable results or block the ability to produce
good results. Therefore, collective action at some level (private sector,
local, state, or federal government) is often needed to correct these problems. In some cases, there is no alternative to government intervention;
in others, with appropriate rules and incentives, collective action in the
private sector may produce desired results. The practical problems with
health insurance markets can be characterized as supply-side or demand-
side problems.

Supply-Side Problems

Supply-side problems are those related to health plans, doctors, hospitals,
and other providers.

Variation in Expected Medical Costs

Medical expenses are distributed very unevenly. In 1993 about 80
percent of total health care spending was spent on the 15 percent of the
population with the highest costs.[3] To survive in an unregulated market
and to protect those who buy insurance from escalating costs, an insurer
must seek to cover "good risks," who are unlikely to need much care,
and to avoid "bad risks," who are likely to need care. And if an insurer
cannot avoid covering bad risks, the insurer must charge them high
premiums proportionate to the expected costs of providing the health
care services that they will require. In the individual and small group
market, this incentive has motivated development of strategies to cover
the healthy and avoid the sick. In the large group market, carriers typically price to a group according to the cost of the group's prior experience
(experience rating) or adjust an average rate for an entire community
according to prior use (utilization-adjusted community rating). In both
cases, the large covered group serves, in effect, as its own insurer.

Strategies to avoid insuring high-risk or ill individuals (risk-avoidance
strategies) have led to high transactions costs in the individual and small
group markets, noncoverage of high-risk people, or coverage of them
only at prohibitively expensive premiums. Universal access to coverage

is a compelling goal because it is not morally acceptable to allow sick or injured people to suffer, die, or be disabled for lack of medical care because they cannot pay. So people who are not covered and cannot pay get care at the expense of providers and those who are covered and do pay for care. If everyone is to have access to coverage at a reasonable premium, we need to create rules that counter the behavior motivated by free market incentives, rules such as guaranteed issue and renewal to require health plans to contract with anyone who desires and can pay for coverage; limits on exclusions of coverage for pre-existing medical conditions, used by health plans as protection against free riding; and some limitations on the price of premiums charged high-risk people. Of course, for individuals with low incomes, direct government subsidization is also required.

Yet there is an inherent tension between ensuring access via guaranteed issue and deterring free riding through limitations on pre-existing condition exclusions. If anyone could step up anytime and buy coverage without such exclusions, people would have an incentive to wait to buy coverage until they became sick, thus driving premiums up to unafford-able levels. Reforms typically characterized as incremental, such as un-restricted guaranteed issue and complete prohibitions of pre-existing condition exclusions, have the potential to destroy a market without universal coverage because they would encourage free riding. We need a balance of rules and incentives that produces a high level of coverage, while holding down the amount of free riding. In the absence of universal coverage or at least adequate subsidies for low-income individuals, some limits on guaranteed issue are necessary. Proposals that would limit guaranteed issue include a one-time unlimited guaranteed issue period followed by limitations on pre-existing condition exclusions or waiting periods for people without prior, continuous coverage; (2) guaranteed issue only during an annual open enrollment period during which everyone chooses among plans being offered; limiting pre-existing condition exclusions to a fixed time period; and limited guaranteed issue with different prices for different age categories to encourage young, healthy individuals to enroll.

However, the question arises of whether even unlimited "guaranteed issue" by itself can really guarantee issue, or whether some neutral institution must exist to enforce guaranteed issue, through which the would-be insurance purchaser can enroll. Great ingenuity has been exercised in the effort to encourage good risks to enroll and to discourage bad risks.

Government-Created Supply-Side Market Failures

Some major governmental policies drive the market away from an efficient outcome. They include excess hospital capacity, excess specialists, the free-choice, fee-for-service insurance model, and provider protectionism.

—Excess hospital capacity. After World War II, the federal government decided that more hospitals were needed. Congress enacted the Hill-Burton hospital construction program with a goal of 4.5 acute beds per 1,000 population.[4] That will soon be at least three or four times the beds really needed. The hospital building boom was fueled by the medicare program, which reimburses capital expenditures on the basis of costs and generous treatment of capital under medicare's Prospective Payment System. Short-sighted public policy contributed to the problem, and private employers and insurers were forced to contribute by paying the resulting prices.

Excess hospitals and bed capacity lead to strategies to fill beds and lead to excess costs. For-profit hospitals will close when their owners project continuing losses. Assets will be re-deployed into more productive uses. Nonprofit hospital boards do not have such an incentive, and nonprofit hospitals are in excess supply and are proving extremely difficult to close.

It is probably true that there is no better answer than to leave this problem to market forces. But thought should be given to possible development of a public policy that would facilitate market exit by nonprofit hospitals in communities where they are in excess supply.

—Excess specialists. We are clearly heading toward an excess supply of physician specialists as managed care expands and makes more efficient use of them.[5] Too many specialists are bad in terms of cost and in terms of health. Specialists may do too few procedures per doctor and therefore lack proficiency, or they may do too many per capita and therefore provide inappropriate services. Again, the main force creating this situation is public policy, especially federal policies that subsidize hospital residency programs.

Subsidizing an excess supply of specialists has many negative consequences. For one, valuable government funds are spent that could be directed toward other worthy purposes. For another, unemployed specialists and specialists who fear the personal consequences of managed care have become a political force against it.

As Uwe Reinhardt has recently recommended, the federal government should phase out subsidies to residency programs.[6] One place to start would be to limit subsidies to no more than three years of residency, the average time it takes to complete primary care training. And the government should invest in the development and provision of information to medical students about current and projected supply and demand in different specialties.

—The "free choice" fee-for-service model. The private market has been moving away quite rapidly from traditional health care coverage with free choice of doctor and fee-for-service reimbursement of doctors, hospitals, and other providers, especially in competitive states like California and Massachusetts where HMOs and PPI are well developed. Indeed, the traditional model usually has not survived in competition on a level playing field because it prices itself out of business. But medicare and medicaid favor the traditional model, and they remain very inflationary programs.

States should be given greater flexibility to contract with managed care for medicaid instead of having to navigate through the current complex waiver process. And medicare should be converted to a truly competitive model.[7] Health plans would compete on quality and price in providing a medicare benefit package and supplemental packages. The current fee-for-service medicare program would also continue to be available, but government would no longer pay its extra cost. Such a model would provide beneficiaries not only with choice of physician but also choice of health plan. Competition could substantially reduce the growth in medicare outlays. The existing model, based on inflationary fee-for-service reimbursement, offers little hope of that result despite efforts to continue to shift costs to other sectors of the health care market.

The Civilian Health and Medical Program of the Uniformed Services, which provides health care services to the military, also relies on the traditional fee-for-service model and should be exposed to market forces and individual choice. Currently, CHAMPUS contracts with one carrier in an area, threatening to require everyone to change health plans when contracts are renewed.

—Provider protectionism. Laws proposed at the national level, and in some cases enacted by states, are designed to protect providers from market forces and block the cost-reducing effects of competition. Such laws include the following:

—"Any-willing-provider" laws that require HMOs to make contracts agreed to with one type of provider available equally to any other willing provider of that type. This, of course, destroys the ability of managed care organizations to negotiate selectively, to drive hard bargains, to select for quality and cost-effective practices, and to match numbers of doctors to members' needs.

—"Due process for doctors" who must be given written explanations for why they are not selected or why they are being dropped. This rule is a radical departure from the normal business principle of contract at will and an invitation to a great deal of costly litigation.

—A point-of-service requirement that every managed care plan must allow any enrollee to see any doctor outside the plan's network with cost-sharing comparable to that for fee-for-service coverage. This requirement would, in effect, transform every HMO into a fee-for-service insurance plan, a defective concept that caused the current cost explosion.

—Various proposed exemptions from antitrust laws established to protect against anticompetitive practices.

—A requirement to allow women to see an ob-gyn without obtaining a referral from their primary care doctor. If this requirement were to pass, a long line of other specialists would demand similar "gatekeeper bypass" provisions, again grievously undermining managed care.

—Requirements that managed care plans contract with academic medical centers and "essential community providers," narrower versions of any-willing-provider rules.

—Requirements that health plans cover the services of certain providers that could be performed by other clinicians.[8]

Approximately 56 million Americans have already chosen HMOs, but these laws eliminate the opportunity to choose a tightly managed and coordinated network that seeks to maintain the health of the population it serves at minimum cost.[9]

State treatment of these provisions varies considerably. To allow the market to function efficiently, if the states cannot or will not eliminate these provider protections, federal legislation should preempt their ability to enact them.

Natural Monopolies

Thinly populated areas and remote small communities, where market forces fail to provide quality products at affordable prices, are frequently mentioned as natural monopolies. People therefore suggest that these areas are candidates for price controls that would fix rates or limit rate increases for services.[10] There is no assurance, however, that this type of public utility regulation would lower prices below monopoly levels. And it would be difficult to draw lines separating "competitive areas" where price controls are inappropriate from "noncompetitive areas" where price controls might be appropriate.

Alternative strategies exist for bringing cost-effective medical care to such communities.[11] Competition *for* the field where there cannot be competition *in* the field would involve aggregating purchasing power and using it to contract with a health care delivery system to staff and operate outposts in the desired area. Contract prices might be keyed to prices in competitive areas. Discounting fee-for-service contracts and moving gradually toward capitation (that is, fixed payments per person per month) could also introduce rural providers to managed care. Some strategies suggest increasing price elasticity of demand by developing substitutes. For example, the monopoly hospital might face competition from transportation of patients to metropolitan areas at one end of the severity spectrum or increased use of outpatient procedures at the other. Hub and spoke strategies envision rural care delivered by satellites of metropolitan systems.

To date, the biggest problem in remote areas and small communities has usually been paying enough to attract providers to practice there, not holding down their pay.

Demand-Side Problems

Demand-side problems are those related to purchasers.

Special Moral Quality

Access to health care has a special moral quality: we want people to have it. It is not morally tolerable to allow people to suffer and die for lack of care because they cannot pay for it. So our government has constructed a safety net made up of local public providers, medicaid for the categorically needy, medicare for the elderly, various subsidies and special programs, and rules for hospitals against dumping patients. Market forces will not produce universal coverage because some people cannot reasonably afford coverage, and others are motivated to take a "free ride" and do not buy coverage. Free riders are deterred from buying coverage by their low risk of illness, the high cost of coverage, the availability of the safety net, and the easy access to coverage when they get sick if there is "guaranteed issue" without exclusion of coverage for pre-existing conditions or waiting periods. Thus to produce universal coverage, the market needs to be supported by a system of incentives, subsidies, or possibly compulsion (mandates or taxes).

Pooling Expected Medical Expenses

Health insurance requires "pooling" of coverage of a large number of people to spread their health expenses and to achieve economies of scale in administration. Pooling is done both by insurers (including HMOs), especially in the individual and small group markets, and by employers when they self-insure, especially in large groups. Pooling entails spreading variations in expected medical expenses among people to make coverage affordable to people with high expected expenses and spreading over time the variations in each person's expenses.

Market forces attack pooling of expected medical expenses. The comparatively low-risk members of any pool have an incentive to escape the pool and get a lower price that reflects their lower expected medical costs. Carriers can profitably sell to them at a lower premium. This phenomenon besets all voluntary pooling arrangements. Even the California Public Employees Retirement System (CalPERS), a nearly one million member purchasing group in which participation by public agencies is voluntary, is periodically threatened by depooling despite its tremendous economies of scale.

Theoretically, if market forces were completely unrestrained—if we had a free market at the individual level and insurers did not form pools—then each person's premium would reflect his or her expected medical costs plus administrative costs. We need some social institution that motivates pooling and holds pools together in the face of heterogeneous risks to ensure that insurance remains affordable to high-cost people.

Two major institutions make it possible for insurers and large employers to pool groups with heterogeneous risks in society today. First, government legislation excludes employer contributions for employees' health benefits from the taxable incomes of the employees. Thus employees have a powerful incentive to take a part of their compensation in the form of employer-paid health care coverage and buy through their employment group rather than take cash and buy coverage themselves. Second, regulations require health plans to offer the same price to purchasers in a designated market (that is, community rating), by "class" such as age class (for example, individual adults under age 35), or "rate bands" that limit the extent to which a premium can deviate from the carrier's average. Such regulations have been enacted by states and the federal government for certain portions of the market. For example, the state of New York requires community rating by all carriers in the small group market up to groups of fifty employees.[12] The federal government requires federally qualified HMOs to apply community rating, community rating by class, or community rating within a 10 percent band for employment groups with one hundred or fewer employees.

One way to reduce high costs for high-risk individuals would be to require all plans to community rate all their groups and individuals and to participate in the small group and individual markets. This step would bring into the risk pools those large groups that still pay much of the premium and would keep their lower-risk people in the risk pool to lower the average cost. However, unless done by the federal government or accompanied by Employee Retirement Income Security Act (ERISA) waivers for the states, this requirement would be limited to insured health plans and would create added incentives for self-insurance by low-risk groups. Employers currently have the ability to escape the risk pool by self-insuring, taking advantage of the ERISA preemption of state regulation of employee benefits by the federal government. Although ERISA is important to large multistate employers' ability to apply uniform policies across the country, many small employers with better-than-average risks simply use ERISA to escape the risk pool. This prevents the broadening of risk pools. The availability of reinsurance with very low deductibles that allows self-insured employers to protect against unexpected costs and hospital and physician networks that can be rented by self-insuring employers enhances the feasibility of this option.

Moreover, areawide community rating deprives individual groups of the reward of a lower price for bargaining hard or for creating cost-conscious employee choice among health plans. And it allows groups that do not do so to "free ride" on the hard-won gains of other groups. This result would argue for community rating or community rating by class within sponsored groups large enough to spread risk, but not among groups.

Another way for good risks to escape the pool is through health plan design. Take, for example, two products: one with first-dollar coverage and one with a high deductible, say $3,000. If people have a choice, the good risks will pick the high deductible and get a low premium. The poor risks will prefer first-dollar coverage. Even if they do not have choice of plan, the healthy will pay less than the chronically ill for care and coverage. So pooling requires some standards for plan design as well as premium-setting rules.

The pursuit of the pooling objective must be balanced against the pursuit of other objectives. For example, by mandating full community rating in a voluntary market for all groups up to fifty, the state of New York may have inadvertently increased the number of uninsured by increasing the premiums for groups of young people.[13]

Small employers (at least those with under fifty employees) are too small to spread risks, too small to achieve economies of scale in administration (especially of multiple plans), too small to manage competition, and usually too small to offer multiple choices of plans. All of these problems can be corrected by health plan purchasing cooperatives (HPPCs), which pool purchasing for individuals and groups, offer wide choice of health plans, and manage the competition among plans. Such HPPCs may be voluntary if precautions are taken to ensure protection against adverse selection.[14]

In the individual market, adverse selection results from healthy individuals' choosing to forego coverage, leaving increasingly high-risk people in the pool and driving up costs. The problem is acute in the market of those newly unemployed who were previously insured. That is because those who expect not to use their coverage are more likely to drop it. In the absence of generalized community rating over a wide population, the excess burden of cost from adverse selection in the individual market must be allocated to someone. How to do this fairly is a problem yet to be solved.

Adverse selection is not inevitable. This problem would be solved by universal coverage. It would be possible to ameliorate the problem by subsidizing the individual purchase of health care. The more incentive for healthy people to keep their coverage, the less adverse selection.

An alternative mechanism for pooling expected medical expenses is government programs such as medicare or a single-payer system in which the federal government would pay for all health services for all Americans. However, this approach is subject to the infirmities of government mentioned at the outset.

Public Goods

In the United States we have traditionally regarded both basic scientific research and education as public goods that benefit all of society. We also realize they would be underproduced in a free market unless collective action were undertaken to correct the loss. Government financial support for basic scientific research has served America well in terms of economic development, international balance of trade, and access to advanced medical technologies. Education produces social benefits beyond what can be recaptured in the private market by the beneficiaries. Support by government of basic scientific research and education should continue, although such support should not completely shelter academic medical centers from market forces. Where not explicit, as in medicare, medicaid, graduate medical education, and disproportionate share hospital payments, government support should be explicit and directed for maximum efficiency.

Price-Inelastic Demand

Many features of the market for health insurance contribute to making demand price inelastic, in which case market forces do not work to motivate reduction of prices and costs. They include complexity and ambiguity of contracts; market segmentation; lack of choice among competing plans; no side-by-side comparison; lack of information about quality; employer contribution policies reinforced by government tax policies; and risk selection. Preferable would be a market with price-elastic demand, in which customers were willing and able to switch to lower-priced health plans.

—Complexity and ambiguity of contracts. Health insurance contracts are extremely complex, ambiguous, and hard to understand. Very few people read and understand their coverage contracts. If they do— typically after they become ill and need treatment—they find hidden exclusions (air pockets) and ambiguous language. What does "medically necessary" mean? This phrase causes a great deal of litigation. All this difficulty makes for high transaction costs and inelastic demand, as people fear changing plans once they have found one with which they are comfortable.

Standardization can simplify comparisons and reduce the costs of contract administration. If all the choices offer the same contract, people will be less afraid of changing plans because of fear of air pockets. Standardization has been very helpful for CalPERS, Stanford University, and other employers. An important area in need of standardization is technology assessment and a coordinated approach to coverage of expensive emerging technologies such as autologous bone marrow transplants, a treatment being used to treat an advanced form of breast cancer. An individual health plan that covers one of these technologies could experience adverse selection if others do not follow suit. However, health plans that do not cover new technologies risk costly law suits, a very expensive process that produces uneven results. Development of one or more authoritative bodies to provide external review of new technologies could help.

—Segmentation. The health coverage market is extremely easy to segment by plan design because there are so many different health conditions and so many different possible coverage options. An individual with bad eyes, for example, is likely to choose a plan with good vision care coverage even if it costs slightly more.

The most common form of segmentation occurs on the basis of differences in cost-sharing requirements of enrollees in different plans. This type of segmentation discriminates against the sick who choose plans with low deductibles or comprehensive HMOs, the prices of which increase because of adverse selection. Segmentation is also increased, in the case of managed care plans, by differences in location of facilities and systems and styles of care. These circumstances contribute to the inelasticity of demand. Standardizing the coverage contracts of all competitors within a sponsored group is an important tool for reducing segmentation and increasing price elasticity of demand.

—Lack of choice among plans. Price-elastic demand will not occur in a market in which consumers cannot make choices among health plans. In the current environment this is often true. Some large employers believe they can negotiate a better deal with a single carrier. Small employers are too small to offer choice of health plans to individual subscribers. If an HMO wants to be offered as a choice in a small group, the traditional indemnity insurer will usually decline to participate, arguing (with some accuracy) that offering a lower-cost choice would split the group, raise administrative costs, and leave the insurer with the poor risks.

In a world of managed care, in which there are contractual links between carriers and doctors, changing health plans may mean changing doctors. To persuade a whole group of people to switch from one health plan to another, a high level of agreement is required. This requirement can make it very difficult for a managed care plan seeking to serve the group to win the business, even if it offers a substantial price reduction. Thus demand for health plans in this market is quite inelastic with respect to price. A company's sole carrier can raise prices substantially before management is willing to take on the burden of making employees change plans, which attenuates or destroys the incentive to reduce price normally created by competition.

This problem can be ameliorated by sponsors' deliberately expanding the range of choices, by rules requiring them to do so, and by grouping individuals and small groups into HPPCs that can offer multiple choices of plans. Requiring large employers to offer competing choices may be attacked as interfering with employers' freedom to act as they wish, but individual choice of plan is important, not only as a means of fostering elastic demand and public acceptance of managed care, but also as a value in itself.

—No side-by-side comparison. An efficient market does not happen naturally. Would-be purchasers of coverage on an individual basis who would like to shop for coverage must visit different agents and brokers, try to understand different contract terms, deal with different premium pricing categories (rating classes), and possibly with different renewal dates. In health insurance, as with insurance generally, especially in the individual and small group market, it is costly to get a side-by-side comparison of the price and quality of the same coverage from different carriers at the same time, although brokers provide available information. Price elasticity of demand would be increased if institutions existed that would create efficient markets by enabling purchasers to review all the health plans on offer during an annual open enrollment period when the plans would be presented side-by-side, preferably with standard coverage terms and information on prices and quality. Then individuals could make independent decisions.

—Lack of information about quality. Some people will be more reluctant to switch from familiar plan A to unfamiliar plan B to save $20 a month premium if they lack information to assure them the change will not be bad for their health. Thus the availability of reliable information on quality is important for elastic demand. Without such information, competition will proceed on the basis of incomplete information, and quality may suffer.

—Employer contribution policies reinforced by government tax policies. Another cause of price-inelastic demand is the health plan contribution policies of employers. Many employers subsidize more expensive policies against cost-effective managed care arrangements. A frequent pattern is to pay 100 percent of the premium of whichever plan an employee chooses, which makes demand perfectly inelastic up to the price of the high-priced (typically fee-for-service) plan. Almost as bad is to pay 90 percent or 80 percent, in which case the employee is personally responsible for only 10 percent or 20 percent of premium differences.

Employers got into this pattern in the 1950s, 1960s, and 1970s when health care costs were much lower and HMOs were rare, and therefore choice of plan was rare. Employers became used to the idea that they would pay the full premium of plans offering fee-for-service reimbursement for hospitals and physicians and free choice of doctor for enrollees, and employees came to regard this policy as an entitlement. Adopting a contribution policy that requires an employee to pay the full difference for a more expensive plan is regarded as a take-away. These decisions were reinforced by unions, which demanded "employer-pay-all" as a trade-off for smaller wage increases and the Internal Revenue Code, which did not tax employer-paid health care benefits. A collective action problem can arise: one employer, acting alone to convert to defined contributions set at or below the price of the low-priced plan, risks antagonizing employees by taking away the entitlement but does not benefit from a cost-effective health care delivery system in return. For that to happen, a critical mass of employers in the area must make the change. When Stanford adopted a "defined contribution policy" (that is, Stanford pays 90 percent of the low-cost plan regardless of the plan an employee chooses), we got a large organized employee protest. That is one reason why many employers, particularly those with union employees, choose to stay with "employer-pay-all" or similar policies.

Some employers have switched to defined contributions to create premium-price sensitive employees. For example, Stanford and Harvard Universities and the University of California have made the change with very positive results.[15]

The open-ended tax exclusion of employer-paid health benefits has further weakened sensitivity to premium price and made demand inelastic. That employer-paid health benefits are tax free to the employee without limit has encouraged "employer-pay-all" and similar policies that subsidize more expensive health care plans and destroy premium price sensitivity; encouraged employees to spend more money on health care than if they were fully responsible for differences in costs despite the best efforts of some employers to instill cost consciousness; and weakened the incentive for health plans to lower their price as a means of competing for new customers. The result has been the continued escalation of health care costs.

The need to motivate responsible, price-conscious choice of health plans by individuals and the need to limit the revenue loss to the federal budget have led many to recommend either a limit on employer contributions that are tax free to the employee (tax cap) or the abolition of the tax break and its replacement by a refundable tax credit for individuals for the purchase of health insurance.[16] Both could fix the current government-created market failure of price-inelastic demand by encouraging employers to enact contribution policies that create full sensitivity by consumers to premium price and encourage competition among health care plans.

Choosing between cap and credit is important and complex. On the plus side for the credit, it gives individuals portability from one job to the next; gives the same amount to low-income people as to high-income people and could be structured to give more; and can be readily characterized as giving something to people as opposed to a tax cap that is taking something away.

But the tax credit carries a danger that is not inherent in a tax cap. The employment-related tax exclusion is an important part of the "glue" that holds employment groups together as risk pools for purchasing health care benefits. In today's market, a low-risk employee who would prefer to take his or her employer-paid health benefit in cash and buy cheaper insurance priced according to expected costs or prior experience in the individual market is inhibited from doing so by the following factors: the tax break is applicable only to employer-paid coverage; the employer has scale and ability to develop or hire expertise to use in purchasing, thus getting better deals and lower transaction costs; and the employer may refuse the request, preferring to use the employer contribution to hold together the risk pool of the employment group and thereby to hold down average costs.

A tax cap would limit the amount that could be excluded from an employee's income but would still be applicable only to employer-paid coverage. If tax subsidies made directly to individuals are used, we weaken the glue and risk unraveling the employment-based system. A market based on underwriting at the individual level would exhibit many or all of the pathologies observed today in that market. However, the credit could be structured so that it would not dismantle the employment-based system. For example, only health care purchased through an employer (or HPPC for those not employed) could be made eligible for the credit. Once the tax break is capped or converted to a credit, several viewpoints have been advanced on the question of how to resolve the employee contribution issue. One would leave the employer contribution policy to employment groups to decide (in the belief that employers and employees will find it in their own best interest for employees to be price sensitive). Or tax breaks on contributions could be made dependent on employers' making employees responsible for premium differences. Capping employers' deduction of health care expenses to accelerate the process of change toward price-conscious contribution policies may also be necessary. Finally, cost shifting from cost-conscious to cost-unconscious employers will force the latter to adopt the policies of the former, so the market will take care of the problem without help.

—Risk selection. With or without deliberate efforts by different carriers to select good risks, health risks may fall unevenly among health plans. If plan A gets the good risks, plan B the bad ones, then plan B's ability to compete with plan A is impaired, and plan A is likely to experience less elastic demand than it would if it got the same risk mix as plan B. Moreover, the competitive disadvantage experienced by plan B gives it a disincentive to develop excellent programs in areas that attract high-cost patients. This problem can be corrected by a system known as "risk adjustment of premiums," whereby the health risks of the populations enrolled in the different plans are measured and payments are made to compensate plans experiencing unfavorable selection.[17] This could be done at the large employer level or at the state level for individuals and small groups as in New York.

Who Should Ensure the Efficient Functioning of the Health Care Market?

Any of several institutions could take many of the collective actions necessary to correct the flaws associated with unrestricted market forces: government, employers, HPPCs, or others. Which institution should perform which functions, and why?

Government must perform some of these functions because they rely on the taxing powers or other coercive powers of government or because they are a correction of defects in existing government programs. Subsidizing access for those who cannot afford or obtain coverage, including medicaid, state and local government direct-provider programs, and antidumping laws that require insured people who are insured to pay for care of the uninsured through premiums is best done by government. Subsidizing research and education, correcting the effects of the unlimited exclusion of employer-provided health care benefits in the internal revenue code, correcting the structures of medicare, medicaid, and CHAMPUS that block those programs from adopting competitive managed care belong to government. Preempting anticompetitive, antimanaged care legislation and changing ERISA to allow states to require small employers (up to fifty or one hundred employees) to participate in large risk pools also fall under government purview. Alternatively, states could restrict the accessibility to reinsurance to relatively high deductibles ($10,000 or more per claim) to make self-insurance a less attractive option for very small companies. But much could continue to be done, probably more effectively, by private purchasers or public purchasers acting as private purchasers of coverage for their employees (such as FEHBP and CalPERS).

Some functions could be performed by government or by the private sector. For example, insurance rules may be enacted at the federal, state, or sponsored group level. In the private sector, health plans serving Stanford employees guarantee issue and renewal, have no pre-existing condition exclusions, and spread the health risks of the Stanford community enrolled in their plans because the university as sponsor requires them to do so. Spreading of risk may be done by some carriers voluntarily (for example, some HMOs charge all small employers a community rate or community rate by class of age, sex, industry, and so on, and phase in rates adjusted for expected utilization for larger employers). But generally, if spreading of expected costs is not done by a sponsor, it should be done by government.

Similarly, the need for standardization of benefits does not necessarily mean there must be one national uniform benefit package. For purposes mentioned here, there could be a different one for each large sponsored group. The standardization function may be carried out better in the private sector. Because the members of the sponsored group bear the financial consequences for the coverage decisions they make, they thus have some incentive (though attenuated by the tax code) to choose value for money. In contrast, a government-designed benefit package has the potential to become a great pork barrel for provider interest groups. Legislators can give away many favors without having to vote explicitly for higher taxes.

Production of standard quality-related information that can serve as the basis for risk-adjusted measures of health care outcomes is a public good whose production may, but does not necessarily have to, be done by government. Indeed, government is often hobbled by providers who use their political power to block collection of such information. In some communities—notably Cleveland and Cincinnati—employers have successfully demanded cooperative efforts to produce quality-related information. But this is likely to work only where there are a few dominant purchasers with the market power to enforce their demand. HPPCs could also serve this role, but they are not yet available to much of the population. The problems of costs and free riders are likely to overwhelm the data collection effort. Public action may be required to compel production of systematic performance information on all providers in the same way that it took enactment of the securities laws to achieve uniformly available financial information on companies that are sold to the public.

Competing Visions for the Future

At least two competing visions of the structure of the future competitive market exist. Both envisage informed, cost-conscious consumer choice among a variety of health care financing and delivery plans as the fundamental driving force in the market. The likely outcome will be a blend of the two. Perhaps the greatest challenge is devising a set of rules under which the two can coexist.

One vision—call it the "sponsored group model"—would build on the successes of the present employment-based system, correct its defects in incremental steps, and extend it to people who are now outside it. Everybody would be covered through one or another sponsored group, each of which offers price-conscious multiple choice of plan and cost savings through economies of scale: large employers, medium-sized employers pooled in HPPCs or other employer coalitions, small employers pooled through HPPCs, freestanding individuals who are not members of employment groups (that is, early retirees, unemployed, self-employed) pooled through HPPCs or permitted to buy through a public sponsor agency, medicare beneficiaries through their own competitive system, and low-income subsidized beneficiaries through a public sponsor agency.

Each sponsored group would be held together by some incentive or subsidy. Each sponsor would carry out the following functions by contracts with health plans and covered beneficiaries: guarantee issue and renewal within limits; limit or abolish pre-existing condition exclusions; determine the health plan premium rating rules; create a market with annual open enrollment (and changes of enrollment with changing circumstances), side-by-side comparison, and individual (household) choice; standardize coverage contracts (usually one or a few standard benefit packages; adjust premiums for risk; make or require employer contributions that make employees responsible for differences in health plan prices; survey beneficiaries about their experience with their health plans and acquire or produce quality-related information; and innovate in ways that improve the efficiency of the market and the suppliers. In short, sponsors would act as makers of competitive markets of health plans on behalf of their sponsored populations.

To prevent adverse selection among sponsors in the individual and small group markets, rules related to limited guaranteed issue and renewal, exclusions of pre-existing conditions and rating practices must be applied in a consistent manner across sponsored groups and so must be established at the state level. And unless and until everyone is in a large sponsored group, risk adjustment must be performed across the entire market at the community level to avoid selection against HPPCs.

The alternative vision is a market made up of individual purchasers who "own" their own individual health insurance policies. These people would have complete portability, with no job link or job lock, and their choice of insurance coverage would be completely independent of where they work. Most important, the regulatory functions needed to make this market work would have to be established and performed by some institution—almost certainly the state or federal government. Such a policy carries certain risks. Experience with the individual market to date does not inspire confidence that it would work well, even with a great deal of detailed government regulation. This model would be a radical change with a very uncertain outcome. Provider interests in this model would dominate because they have much lower costs than consumers to aggregate the resources needed to lobby. The system is likely to suffer rigidity, inflexibility, and costly uniformity.

The sponsored group model has some important additional advantages. For one, the market-perfecting functions are decentralized, pluralistic, and to some extent competitive and therefore oriented toward consumers' satisfaction. The market-makers are close to the beneficiaries and acting on their behalf. They are responsible to employers and employees. Sponsors are purchasers. Employers, for example, compete for employees by offering attractive benefits, and they profit by buying them at a good price. As purchasers, they institutionalize consumers' interest and can do so with expertise and resources. Different sponsors might use different rules (for example, different coverage standards) to suit their different constituencies. This model is far more conducive to innovation on the purchasing side; each sponsor can innovate without first obtaining the approval of state government and providers. Thus adaptation to changing conditions would be reasonably quick.

Another important advantage to this strategy is that it represents incremental change—the safety of relatively small steps with fairly predictable outcomes. It does not risk tearing down an existing, relatively successful institution (that is, employment-based health care purchasing) that works tolerably well and whose defects might be corrected. For most non-aged, nonpoor individuals, private employers and other purchasing groups already create and enforce the necessary rules to manage competition (albeit imperfectly) within the group through private contracts with health plans.

Finally, many of the deficiencies of the employment-based system associated with the nonemployed, the newly unemployed, and new employment (that is, new application of exclusions of pre-existing conditions and waiting periods for coverage) can be ameliorated. For example, today people who belong to a federally qualified HMO through employment can keep membership, without limit of time at a community rate, upon leaving their employment group. That rule might be generalized. Employment-based HPPCs might be structured to permit former employees to continue membership in the plan of their choice through the HPPC and to participate in the annual open enrollment, much as the Consolidated Omnibus Budget Reconciliation Act (COBRA) enables people recently unemployed to maintain existing coverage (though for a limited period) today. Although a burden of excess risk would still exist because of the tendency for newly unemployed, healthy people to drop coverage, this risk would fall on the prior employment group. This would reduce, but not eliminate, the burden of adverse selection in the individual market. Insurance reforms would help to ensure continuity of coverage for people changing jobs. People who transfer to a large employer that offers fewer plans than the HPPC might be required to change plans. However, if the new employer offers a broad choice, chances are that employees could keep their primary care doctor. At least, they will have some choice of plans. If every state had HPPCs for small businesses, like California and Florida, inter-HPPC transfer arrangements for individuals who are moving might be created.

For freestanding individuals who never were part of an employment group, institutions must be created in the private or public sectors to create and enforce the necessary rules. This is likely to require some public action, such as mandating the creation of HPPCs for individuals and small employment groups, as envisioned in the Managed Competition Acts of 1992 and 1993.[18] Or government could create incentives for their formation by linking favorable tax treatment to plans purchased through a qualified HPPC. People purchasing outside a sponsored group forego multiple choice of plan and the customer-oriented service and economies of scale offered by HPPCs. However, so long as rules regulating the market are applied consistently, coexistence is possible.

Notes

1. Charles L. Schultze, *The Public Use of Private Interest* (Brookings, 1977), pp. 17–20.

2. According to Vice President Al Gore in the 1993 National Performance Review, "We have spent too much money for programs that don't work. . . . In the name of controlling waste, we have created paralyzing inefficiency. . . . The Federal government seems unable to abandon the obsolete . . . the federal government is not simply broke; it is broken. . . . In Washington's highly politicized world, the greatest risk is not that a program will perform poorly, but that a scandal will erupt. Scandals are front-page news, while routine failure is ignored." See National Performance Review, *From Red Tape to Results: Creating a Government That Works Better and Costs Less: Report of the National Performance Review* (Washington: Government Printing Office, 1993).

3. Alan Monheit, Agency of Health Care Policy and Research, based on 1987 National Medical Expenditure Survey data.

4. Judith R. Lave and Lester B. Lave, *The Hospital Construction Act: An Evaluation of the Hill-Burton Program, 1948–1973* (Washington: American Enterprise Institute for Public Policy Research, 1974), p. 9.

5. Jonathan P. Weiner, "Forecasting the Effects of Health Reform on U.S. Physician Workforce Requirement," *Journal of the American Medical Association*, vol. 272 (July 1994), pp. 222–30.

6. Uwe E. Reinhardt, "Planning the Nation's Health Workforce: Let the Market In," *Inquiry*, vol. 31 (Fall 1994), pp. 250–63.

7. See, for example, the Medicare Choice Act of 1994. Senator Dave Durenberger and others, *S.1996: Medicare Choice Act of 1994;* and Paul M. Ellwood and Alain C. Enthoven, "Responsible Choices: The Jackson Hole Plan," *Health Affairs* (Summer 1995), pp. 24–39.

8. Health Security Act, HR 3600, October 27, 1993, as reported by the House Committee on Ways and Means, July 14, 1994; and Health Security Act as reported by the Senate Finance Committee, S1757, August 4, 1994.

9. GHAA, *HMO Magazine*, July–August 1995.

10. Richard Kronick and others, "The Marketplace in Health Care Reform: The Demographic Limitations of Managed Competition," *New England Journal of Medicine*, vol. 328 (January 14, 1993), pp. 148–52.

11. See, for example, "Rural Health Care: Improvements through Managed Competition/Cooperation" (Jackson Hole, Wyo.: The Jackson Hole Group, July 1993).

12. "Rules to Assure an Orderly Implementation and Ongoing Operation of Open Enrollment and Community Rating of Individual and Small Group Health

Insurance," Regulation 145, 11NYCRR 360, New York, Insurance Department of the State of New York, December 22, 1992.

13. Robert Pear, "Pooling Risks and Sharing Costs in Effort to Gain Stable Insurance Rates," *New York Times,* May 22, 1994, p. 22. The New York commissioner later testified in defense of the New York community rating rule, claiming that it did not adversely affect coverage.

14. For a discussion of the precautions necessary for implementing effective voluntary HPPCs, see the Jackson Hole Group HPPC manual. Tom Glassberg, Michael Moore, and Charles Buck, *Governors' Guide to Forming and Implementing Health Plan Purchasing Cooperatives* (Jackson Hole, Wyo.: Jackson Hole Group, December 1993).

15. Stanford University's weighted average premiums for 1995 were 6.2 percent below those of 1994; the University of California's were 7.8 percent lower; Harvard University's were 10.5 percent lower. See also Thomas C. Buchmueller and Paul Feldstein, "The Effect of Price on Switching Among Health Plans," *Health Affairs*, forthcoming, which reports that the response of University of California employees suggests that 26 percent of health plan enrollees will switch to a cheaper plan when the monthly premium for their own plan rises by $10.

16. Alain C. Enthoven, "A New Proposal to Reform the Tax Treatment of Health Insurance," *Health Affairs*, vol. 3 (Spring 1984), pp. 21–39.

17. Richard Scheffler and Louis Rossiter, eds., *Advances in Health Economics and Health Services Research,* vols. 6, 10, and 12 (Greenwich, Conn.: JAI Press Inc., 1985, 1989, 1991).

18. Congressmen Jim Cooper, Fred Grandy, and others, *H.R. 3222: The Managed Competition Act of 1993*; and Senators John Breaux, David Durenberger, and others, *S.1579: The Managed Competition Act of 1993.*

CHAPTER EIGHT

How Does Antitrust Enforcement Fit In?

Steven C. Sunshine

T HERE is little doubt that the United States is experiencing dramatic changes in health care delivery. Approximately one hundred hospitals close or merge each year. At the same time, the growth of managed care is a nationwide phenomenon, with penetration exceeding 90 percent of private-pay patients in some markets. New forms of multiprovider networks, combining providers of competing and complementary services, are emerging in markets across the country. And continuous advances in technology change the nature of the services offered to and demanded by patients.

Although it would be difficult to explain all of the forces behind this process, it is nonetheless safe to say that at bottom these changes are driven by market forces. As total health care expenditures approximate one-seventh of the nation's domestic national product, increasing cries for cost containment are heard. Employers have looked for ways to lower the cost of insuring their employees. Payers have devised innovative new systems to spread risk and monitor use. In response to competitive pressures, hospitals have sought to capture efficiencies and eliminate duplication. These efforts have resulted in decreased use, particularly of in-patient hospitalization, exacerbating the problem of excess capacity.

Changes in technology have fundamentally affected market demand. New procedures allow patients to be treated with higher quality and in a less intrusive fashion than in the past. Many of these improvements have increased use of out-patient procedures and obviated the need for hospital admissions. New equipment, often highly capital intensive, offers improved treatment or diagnosis. Not all providers, however, can afford to invest in such equipment.

These market forces have spawned widespread efforts to rationalize and eliminate excess capacity. Antitrust enforcers are called on to review many of these efforts, including mergers among competitors, vertical mergers, partnerships and joint ventures, and a host of contractual arrangements, all designed to secure for the participants a place in the changing market.

The Role of Antitrust Policy

What is the role of antitrust review in this dynamic market? Before answering that question, let us begin with a basic assumption—competition works in the health care industry. It works best when knowledgeable purchasers can base purchasing decisions on adequate information and purchasers have the financial incentives to select the services that offer the best combination of price and quality. But, of course, competition works only when purchasers have choices.

The Virtues of Competition

To date, managed care is the best available instrument of competition and cost containment. The success of managed care rests on its ability to assemble information, provide financial incentives, and to shift demand to preferred providers. Many analysts have shown its effectiveness. For example, in California where managed care has achieved high levels of penetration, the average bed days per thousand patients and hospital prices and price increases are significantly lower than the national average.

Competition produces more than static benefits. Competition is also the best way to insure innovation, and innovation allows markets to evolve into more efficient delivery systems. Since 1993, the Department of Justice has emphasized the importance of innovation. For the first time ever, the department has challenged a merger on the grounds that it would lessen competition in an innovation market. That case, *United States* v. *General Motors Corp.*, involved a heavy-duty truck transmission market, but its principles are just as apt in health care.

Innovation in health care has promoted efficiency. Many physicians now assume risk for their patients' use of services, encouraging physicians to contain costs and to reduce unnecessary treatment. Managed care providers are innovating point-of-service plans. Competitive conditions have spurred hospitals to work with their managed care customers to reduce use and improve care. Hospitals are participating in networks and are teaming with other providers and insurers to offer innovative new services.

The role of antitrust in health care is to promote consumer welfare primarily through competition in free and open markets. Open markets promote price and quality competition, increased information, and, perhaps most important, innovation. As an antitrust prosecutor, however, the department does not view itself as a regulator of these markets. Generally speaking, the market ought to be left to market forces—with antitrust enforcement stepping in only when noncompetitive market structures or restraints imposed by private parties threaten competition.

Antitrust, of course, is not blind to efficiencies. Efficiencies may be achieved through cooperation among parties in mergers and joint ventures and through contractual arrangements. The department typically balances the procompetitive effects of the likely efficiency gains of a proposed arrangement against its likely harm to competition.

Antitrust polices markets in two principal ways. First, antitrust enforcement prevents noncompetitive market structures, typically through merger policy. Second, antitrust enforcement prevents and removes private restraints that can lead to excessive prices, entry barriers, foreclosure and denial of access, or other competition-limiting practices.

The Department of Justice and Federal Trade Commission's Statements of Enforcement Policy reaffirmed the vitality of antitrust enforcement in health care. The statements were issued first in September 1993, and then expanded in September 1994. The statements describe antitrust enforcement policy and provide clear guidance to the health care community on how enforcement affects nine major practices. With clear guidance, the health care community can plan and carry out innovative business arrangements without fear of antitrust challenge. For those types of practices that are close questions, the parties can secure an expedited business review letter from the department.

The importance of competition and antitrust does not mean that other social problems may not possibly require other solutions. There may be issues of risk selection, universality, uncompensated care, and cost shifting that cannot always be adequately solved through competition. But the existence of these issues does not diminish the belief that competition is a principal avenue for cost containment and innovation in the health care industry.

As in any other industry, mergers may promote efficiency or enhance market power. The department uses the 1992 Horizontal Merger Guidelines to gauge a merger's likely competitive effects and efficiencies and to determine whether the transaction is likely to lead to higher prices, reduced output, or lessened innovation. The merger guidelines are flexible and general enough to subsume many specific health care issues. For example, the department takes account of the effect of insurance on incentives; the effect of regulatory constraints on price and availability of new services; the role of the physician in the physician-patient relationship; the nonprofit status of some market participants; and the implications of an individual's lack of information.

Although the department reviews many health care mergers, its enforcement actions to date have been limited to hospital mergers. Health maintenance organizations typically compete with other HMOs and often face competition from other insurance plans. Physician groups typically face competition from many other physician groups. To date, proposed HMO and physician group mergers have not raised competitive concerns, although this situation may change. Increasing HMO penetration and consolidation may lead to situations in which an HMO merger could create or enhance market power. As physician groups in many local markets grow, the point may be reached where additional mergers—whether horizontal or vertical—raise concerns.

In 1994 the department challenged two hospital mergers. In the *United States* v. *Morton Plant Health System, Inc.*, the department challenged the merger of two hospitals with a combined share of 60 percent of the Clearwater, Florida, market. Approximately two months after filing that case, the department reached a settlement with the hospitals. The second hospital merger challenge was *United States* v. *Mercy Health Systems*. In that case, the department sought to prevent the merger of the only two hospitals in the Dubuque, Iowa, market.

The department's analysis of hospital mergers is in principle no different from its general merger analysis. The department examines the likely anticompetitive effects and possible efficiency gains to determine whether the transaction's net effect will harm consumers. In hospital merger analysis, the department typically focuses on in-patient services. It usually concludes that the merger will not harm out-patient services, either because there are non-acute-care hospital providers of these services in the market or entry into those services would be easy. In hospital mergers, two key issues are almost always local market definition and efficiencies.

Merging parties often claim that the transaction is needed to balance the hospital's power against the growing power of managed care. The department does not credit arguments of countervailing power. It is skeptical that monopsony power wielded by managed care providers is likely to have serious welfare effects since demand for in-patient service may be quite inelastic. Without a clear view of a welfare loss, the department would not be inclined to intervene when the alleged "harm" is lower prices.

The department puts great importance on analysis of efficiencies. In 1994 several mergers were allowed to proceed on the basis of likely efficiency gains even though the mergers exceeded structural guidelines for presumptive anticompetitive effects.

Four general criteria guide the department's analysis. First, it evaluates the likely size of the claimed efficiencies. Next, it asks whether the efficiencies will be realized, especially in light of the desires of the relevant medical staffs and the local community. Third, the department asks whether the efficiencies are merger specific. For instance, claims of efficiencies through improved "best practices" are viewed with great skepticism since best practices can be and usually are achieved without merger. Finally, the department asks if the benefits from the merger are likely to be passed on to consumers directly or indirectly through lower prices and costs.

As a general matter, merger efficiency analysis is complicated by the fact that the parties are not starting from a blank slate; each has significant sunk costs. For instance, analyzing the efficiency gains if two 200-bed hospitals come under common ownership may be a far different question from determining the efficiency of one 400-bed hospital compared with two 200-bed hospitals.

Typically, few efficiencies arise from the mere unification of economic ownership. The department is most likely to credit maximum efficiencies if a hospital merger results in a consolidation of campuses. However, hospital merger partners rarely propose consolidation of campuses, perhaps because of a number of factors: because existing hospitals represent large sunk costs, it may be less costly to keep two hospitals open then to shut one down and expand capacity at the other; the medical staffs at the two hospitals may make consolidation difficult; and the community may object to the loss of the convenience of two campuses.

Merging hospitals typically propose consolidation of clinical services as part of their strategic planning. This consolidation may provide both operating and capital savings. However, the savings may be small if both hospitals fully use their minimum staffing requirements, so that additional staffing is a variable cost.

The most extreme situation concerning efficiencies arises when the parties seek to justify a merger to monopoly on the grounds of efficiencies. Of course, the analysis must weigh the anticompetitive effects of the monopoly against the expected efficiencies. But the Justice Department starts with the presumption that the anticompetitive effects of monopoly are severe. A move to monopoly means a loss of price competition and, in fact, regulation is often imposed to prevent natural monopolies from setting price significantly above marginal cost. Regulation is usually not workable in the hospital context, and certainly not one the Justice Department would initiate.

Monopoly may also lessen innovation, either by the monopolist itself or because the monopolist refuses to accommodate the innovative efforts of others. In today's dynamic health care market, the possible efficiency losses are large.

The Justice Department also questions whether proposed efficiencies will be achieved over the long run in the absence of competition. Monopolists usually have strong incentives to lower costs, but a hospital's incentives, especially those of nonprofits, may get distorted by other interests. The interests of the medical staff or community may override a hospital's interest in certain cost-saving measures. In addition, many nonprofit hospitals are part of a larger nonprofit organization, and revenue from hospital services may be used to cross-subsidize other causes.

For all these reasons, the department remains skeptical of approving natural monopoly on the basis of efficiency gains.

One transaction in which the Department of Justice was able to promote efficiency gains was in its settlement of *United States* v. *Morton Plant Health Systems, Inc.* That suit challenged the proposed merger of the two largest hospitals in Clearwater, Florida. The Florida state attorney general joined that challenge.

Two months into the litigation, Justice Department officials met with the merging hospitals and explored ways to accomplish most of the parties' proposed efficiencies without a full-scale merger. After days of intensive negotiation, the negotiators agreed on an innovative solution that made business sense to the parties and promoted rather than lessened competition.

The settlement had two parts. First, the merger was prohibited, and the two hospitals agreed to remain independent providers of in-patient acute care services. Both hospitals agreed to continue to contract separately with managed care. Second, the hospitals could capture efficiencies through a production joint venture. The services that could be performed by the joint venture fell into three categories: certain tertiary services; out-patient care; and ancillary services.

Competition for the services contributed to the joint venture was protected in two important ways. First, the services in the joint venture would face competition from many other sources either because the markets (for tertiary care, for example) were broader geographically than the general in-patient services market or because organizations other than the acute-care hospitals were participants or likely entrants. If the market for these tertiary services extended just to the Tampa Bay area, many other hospitals provide comparable services. The department found that out-patient services were provided by urgent care facilities, doctors' offices, and clinics. Last, ancillary services such as laundry, billing, management information services, and purchasing were all provided in a much larger market than just the Clearwater, Florida, area.

The second protection is that the venture is limited to production only. Although the venture can jointly produce the services, it must sell them back to each parent hospital at cost. Each hospital will separately market those services to managed care plans and others, often in competition with one another.

The joint venture has been in operation now for about four months. The hospitals have reported that the joint venture is likely to save $8 million in its first year. Interestingly, the hospital administrators said that the consolidation of clinical services is far more difficult than they first imagined. They have scaled back their plans but are still planning some future clinical consolidations.

Antitrust enforcement has an important role to play in the market-driven reform of the health care industry. Free and open markets usually lead to innovative and efficient solutions. Antitrust enforcement, to the maximum extent possible, keeps those markets free and open.

Comments on Chapters 7 and 8

William L. Roper: The various observations of Alain C. Enthoven and Sara J. Singer combine to make one major point: that there are appropriate roles for both the private and the public sectors. I share this view and want to develop it further.

The elections in November indicated a clear change of public attitude. A growing distrust of government at all levels, especially the federal government, is clearly visible. Enthoven and Singer provide an excellent overview of the appropriate application of regulation, and I would like to emphasize its relevance to the marketplace today and to The Prudential Health Care System.

As one of the largest managed health care companies and as a concerned corporate citizen, Prudential wants to maintain the integrity of the competitive marketplace without burdensome, unnecessary government regulation. In the health care arena, Prudential is responding to the marketplace because of the competitive process and because employers like Xerox are demanding that we be quality leaders. Employers, in short, are demanding accountability.

There is much to criticize about the various private sector efforts to date. But the major employer purchasers of health care and the leaders in organized health care delivery systems have been working to increase quality and efficiency of health care delivery.

Level Playing Field

To build on this work and not undermine progress, the government should ensure a level playing field, with fee-for-service and managed health care organizations regulated consistently. This nation's health care system can earn and maintain consumer confidence only if regulations are consistent and promote fair competition. For example, changing current ERISA law to allow each state to design and implement its own system would significantly increase regulation—and costs.

Prudential has long been an advocate of competition. However, no special rules should exist for certain health delivery systems, such as provider/hospital organizations (PHOs), academic medical centers, or Federally Qualified Health Centers. In the end, favoritism does not protect the ultimate purchaser of health care—the consumer.

For example, PHOs are large and growing fast, with 500 to 700 in operation nationwide, up from 200 in only three years, and another 900 to 1200 in the developmental stages.[1] Most PHOs compete directly with health insurers and managed care plans. PHOs may perform virtually all the same functions as health insurers and health maintenance organizations—develop procedures for efficient delivery of care, create new health care coverage products, market directly to employers, collect premiums, and determine covered benefits.

Although PHOs have an awesome responsibility for health care delivery and manage millions of dollars in premiums, only two states, Minnesota and Iowa, regulate them. PHOs have the potential to increase competition and efficiency to the health care marketplace, but their capitalization, financial soundness, and fair market practices should be regulated in the same ways as other health plans.

Public Sector Programs

Concerns about the cost and quality of health care in medicare and medicaid have led to greater regulatory oversight of these programs. Programs such as the professional review organizations (PROs) have attempted to provide proper oversight of providers in the medicare marketplace.

While I was administrator at the Health Care Financing Administration I set the goal of improving the quality of medicare-financed care as one of the top priorities. To be clear, quality improvement was already under way at the HCFA—but I chose to push it to the top of the agenda. We made a virtue of necessity and decided to pursue vigorously the general issue of quality—through the refinement of hospital mortality information, activities of PROs, publication of nursing home standards, and providing information about nursing home quality.

In the mid-1980s, we were also pushing the policy notion of "medicare's private health plan option"—managed health care in medicare. With 37 million medicare enrollees, 8 percent in managed care, and 33 million medicaid enrollees, 15 percent in managed care, the United States should vigorously pursue the private health plan option and remove the cumbersome statutory and regulatory impediments to greater use of managed care in medicare and medicaid.[2] These programs should also incorporate real outcomes measurement and carefully managed oversight. Remember, regulation of these programs is an activity designed to protect public beneficiaries, but medicare and medicaid should be allowed to benefit from private sector innovations.

The Role of Private Sector

The government does some things very well. It is good at getting people's attention, bringing together interested parties, and setting an agenda. However, the private sector enjoys significant competitive advantages over the public sector. Although private companies cannot regulate and compel with the force of law, they are much more flexible and more integrated with the medical community. The private sector, in many respects, regulates itself through competition over price and, especially, quality, the pursuit of which has become the driving competitive force in the marketplace.

Prudential has a targeted, multifaceted program, "Quality Beyond Words," to help it deliver quality health care and to compete in this marketplace. The Prudential Center for Health Care Research is a key element of this program. Leading scientists develop information and methods to improve quality and enhance effectiveness in Prudential's health care systems and in managed care in general.

The National Committee for Quality Assurance (NCQA) is an independent, nonprofit organization that reviews and accredits managed health care plans. Its findings are unbiased and objective. Prudential was the first national health care company to invite the NCQA to scrutinize every one of its health plans. Every aspect of the plan is evaluated; the physicians, plan management, and monitoring of communication with members and physicians and the role of physicians in decisionmaking.

When the NCQA published its results in mid-1994, more Prudential plans were accredited, by far, than any other company's. The NCQA continues to improve these processes, and the standards are becoming even more demanding, but Prudential is committed to this accountability. Right now, 88 percent of Prudential plans are NCQA accredited, with the remainder in the process of or waiting for review.

Prudential published report cards on all its health plans, based on the measures of the Health Plan and Employer Data Information Set in September 1994, the first national health care company to do so. These report cards focus on evaluation in five areas—membership, stability, utilization of services, quality of care, access to care, and member satisfaction. Prudential is committed to continuing the process annually.

These activities comprise a real world example of the innovation the marketplace is delivering.

The Risk of "Anti-Managed Care" Actions

Government legislation to protect health care providers from market forces and to block the cost-reducing effects of competition could stifle marketplace innovation. Enthoven and Singer list them. They include "any-willing-provider" laws, exemptions for providers from antitrust laws, "due process" for doctors, mandatory point-of-service requirements, and forced contracting.

State regulations on these provisions vary considerably. To allow the market to function efficiently, states must eliminate inappropriate provider protections, or federal legislation must preempt the ability of states to enact such measures.

In short, there is an appropriate regulatory role for government. But it is the private sector marketplace that is transforming itself and reforming health care in America. We seek to continue to do just that, and we ask to be held accountable for our performance.

Helen Darling: This was a hard assignment because I agreed with virtually everything in the two chapters—Alain C. Enthoven and Sara J. Singer's as well as Steven C. Sunshine's—and it is usually easier to disagree or raise new issues than to just agree. Along with the authors, we at Xerox believe that the market works. We also agree that protections are needed to forestall possible problems in the health care market.

But, all other things being equal, we would rely more on market forces and incentives and less on government actions, because we believe that the market will encourage innovation and demand efficiency. In contrast, governments and large bureaucratic businesses that are shielded from market forces have poor records in innovation, efficiency, quality of care, and customer service.

One of the reasons Xerox supports the positions Enthoven and Singer take is that the Xerox strategy includes virtually all of the design elements they recommend. Some unsolved problems remain, including ones Enthoven and Singer describe. We know we need to work on them and are seeking help from policy analysts and researchers to find solutions. Meanwhile, our contracts with health plans protect our employees. Almost everything that we do for our employees can be done for any large-enough group. Indeed, many employers need only a concentration in a particular geographic area to have leverage with health plans and to benefit from economies of scale.

Public Policy Agreement

Xerox's experience confirms the Enthoven-Singer contention that large purchasing groups can ensure that health plans compete on quality, service, and access, and that they do not distort coverage or hide behind plan design or interpretation of medical necessity to get out of providing medically necessary and appropriate services.

We also believe with Enthoven and Singer that standardized plans are desirable, although small and well-publicized differences may be permitted as long as they are clear and understandable to the consumer and are linked to small price differences.

Since any kind of tax cap or methods of taxing benefits will be seen as a takeaway and would hurt many families in the short term, we would rather see a type of fixed annual health care benefits allowance that each person or head of family would have, which could then be applied to any one of a number of options that are priced to the individual based on the relative efficiency or costliness of each plan. Within states, small employers or companies may be able to join purchasing groups. There should be more than one depending on the size of the state, but the purchasing groups should not be able to compete by attracting healthy people or discouraging enrollment of people with problems.

All employers, sponsoring groups, and other purchasers should get data based on the Health Plan and Employer Data Information Set—HEDIS 2.0 and its later versions. HEDIS 2.0 is a standardized data set developed by heath plans and corporate purchasers to be used by plans in their reporting to purchasers. HEDIS was developed under the auspices of the National Committee for Quality Assurance. Data should be audited, but the necessary auditing techniques have yet to be designed. Consumers should receive at least annually plan performance reports that cover key organizational and performance measures, including number of members, percentage of eligibles enrolled, rates of growth and disenrollment, medical loss rations, number of care locations and services at each site, top four admitting hospitals, availability of centers of excellence by type of procedures, physician turnover, profit or nonprofit status, and other relevant information.

Xerox strongly supports the idea that everyone needs easily available health care coverage through employers, purchasing pools, or government programs. We must start with a reasonable, affordable package of coverage and build universal coverage in incremental steps, using purchasing pools, medicaid, Consolidated Omnibus Budget Reconciliation Act of 1995 (COBRA), medical support orders, and all of the existing tools to bring people into a system in which no one need fear, and therefore price against, abnormal adverse selection.[3] This way may not be ideal, but we can make enormous progress if we take sensible incremental steps.

Antitrust Policy

It is gratifying to hear from the antitrust division that it is willing to be—indeed has already been—flexible regarding hospital mergers and acquisitions and that the Justice Department recognizes the power of organized systems of care to maintain a competitive environment. In numerous cases markets change dramatically when new health plans, health maintenance organizations (HMOs), move into a market previously lacking managed care. It is also gratifying to hear that the Department of Justice recognizes the roles of managed care and competition among managed care organizations in driving down cost increases and improving the quality and appropriateness of care. Xerox has experienced such effects. If set up correctly, managed care can bring considerable "value-added" to the health system and not be just another layer as some of the most skeptical believe.

The Xerox Story

The good news from Xerox is that its method of purchasing health care is working remarkably well for its employees given the complexities in the health system and the difficulty in changing habits developed over more than thirty years and fueled by generous third-party payments of demanding ever more medical care and any new technology. About 73 percent of our employees have already chosen HMOs. Xerox continues to offer everyone a fee-for-service indemnity plan. Xerox encourages its employees, through a fixed benefit allowance (keyed to the lowest-cost HMO in that service area for that calendar year) to understand value and to choose the plan that best balances services and cost. Employees who choose a more costly plan pay the difference.

Xerox recognizes that it is also benefiting from efforts made by other employers and purchasers to change the dynamics in the health care delivery and financing system. Purchasers and consumers are beginning to understand that health care benefits are—as economists remind us—foregone wages. They are becoming aware that if they want the best mix of cash compensation, health care, and other fringe benefits, they must become knowledgeable and discerning consumers in order to get the best package with their money.

Our system is not perfect, and we seek continuously to improve. But we are convinced that we have an increasingly consumer-friendly, accessible system. More than half of our health care plans are now accredited by the National Committee for Quality Assurance (NCQA). These plans are willing to report standardized data on plan performance and are committed to research on outcomes and effectiveness of care.

Important Research and Demonstrations Needed

If Xerox is to continue to move forward, research and operational evaluations are essential. If managed care in its various forms is to become the dominant mode of health care delivery and organization in the country, then the managed care industry needs to improve its benefits, eligibility determinations, and even treatment methods for the mentally ill and those with chemical dependency problems. Right now, some HMOs and other managed care companies control use by benefit design and very narrow eligibility determinations. Managed care should not dispense open-ended benefits for life transition and adjustment problems, as many indemnity plans did throughout the 1970s and 1980s (including Xerox, much to its financial harm). Nor should HMOs be paying for treatment of behavioral problems, personality problems, or learning problems just because plans used to pay for them because the problems were "medicalized" and were given diagnostic codes.

But there can be value in medically necessary care that helps to restore mentally ill people to functional levels. HMOs like the Harvard Community Health Plan, Group Health Cooperative of Puget Sound, and Kaiser Permanente are generally much more willing to authorize medically necessary treatments than some other HMOs.

The HMO industry needs to be sure that all HMOs are covering psychiatric problems and that patients are getting their fair share of appropriate treatment for these conditions. At the same time, we need more research on the effectiveness of brief therapy and of alternatives to inpatient care. As more and more Americans receive their medical care in HMOs and other managed care settings, it will be harder to avoid dealing with the complicated problems associated with mental illness and chemical dependency patients.

Another major challenge is to develop and test appropriate reliable methods of risk adjustment for premiums. Health plans that provide necessary quality care to people with complex, chronic, and sometimes very expensive problems should not be financially penalized for insuring such patients. High-quality organized delivery systems can provide the best setting and the best people for dealing with the many coordination and integration problems that seriously or chronically ill patients face. But the reimbursement for that care must be adequate to protect plans from financial ruin if they ensure that patients are properly cared for and protected.

Finally, the nation needs to have clear procedures for deciding when new technologies are worth what they cost, when they are not, and for deciding which classes of patients fall in which category. Unfortunately, many Americans fear that an insurance company, employer, or managed care company may deny them beneficial diagnosis or treatment in order to save money. Only objective criteria, open and verifiable procedures, and fair-minded policies based on empirical evidence can lay those fears to rest. David Lawrence put the point directly, "NCQA and other groups [should] expand their reviews to include the ethics of decisionmaking related to benefits and care decisions—who makes the decisions and by what process and ethical standards.[4]

ERISA Is Not the Problem

Xerox is a corporate purchaser that believes that significant positive changes are occurring because of the drive and commitment of employers to change the health care delivery system and the nature of the health care product being purchased. Accordingly, we are dismayed to hear assertions that the Employee Retirement Income Security Act of 1974 (ERISA) gets in the way of state health care reform.

ERISA is not the problem. ERISA protects from state regulation the very successful, self-insured, large, multistate plans that have been leading the way in innovation, health information system design, plan performance reports, required accreditation for quality, and report cards to consumers. During the same time period, states, who are often the largest health care purchasers through their provision of insurance for their employees, families, and retirees, and program beneficiaries typically have done little or nothing to change the delivery system and what they are buying. It is ironic that the purchasers lagging in innovation and sophisticated purchasing strategies would work to dismantle the employers' plans that are revolutionizing health care organizations in the United States.

If the main interest is to ensure a reasonable minimal standard of services, benefits, and consumer protections, and Congress agrees that such requirements are needed, then Congress can enact such standards and protections under ERISA. If some small employers have used ERISA to duck their responsibilities for helping their employees, then Congress can establish standards under ERISA. The choice would be the individual employer's, no matter what size. Included in this would be the requirement that any employer who meets federal standards does not have to meet state standards as well. There is serious danger that federal standards would become the floor and states just another level, as happened with the Family and Medical Leave Act.

In short, state and federal regulation of taxation of self-insured plans threatens to dampen or extinguish current incentives for them or so regulate them that reform would be impossible. If they will just be patient, we believe two good things will happen. First companies such as Xerox can help revolutionize the health care system through the power of informed purchasers. If they forebear they will discover ways to provide better care and better value than in the past for their employees and beneficiaries of state programs.

Notes

1. Interview with the executive director of the American Association of Physician-Hospital Organizations, Glen Allen, Va., December 1994.

2. For medicare see Group Health Association of America, *Medicare at 30: An Opportunity for all Americans* (Washington, July 1995). For medicaid see General Accounting Office, *Medicaid: Spending Pressures Drive States toward Program Reinvention* (Washington, 1995).

3. Medical support orders are court orders used to require noncustodial parents to provide medical coverage for their children. Under federal law, employers must honor the support order, even if the parent does not voluntarily cover the child for benefits. Also, the employer must cover the child for health care benefits, even if the employer has a requirement that the child must live with the employee to be an eligible dependent.

4. John K. Iglehardt, "Changing Course in Turbulent Times: An Interview with HMO Executive David Lawrence," *Health Affairs*, vol. 13 (Winter 1994), pp. 65–77.

PART FOUR

Incremental Reform

CHAPTER NINE

Steps toward Universal Coverage

Judith Feder and Larry Levitt

T HE health care reform debate of 1993–94 revealed widespread recognition that our nation's health care system has significant problems. These problems did not end with the debate's end in the 103d Congress. New efforts to address these problems will reflect not only values and policy judgments but also political lessons from our recent experience.

The goal of universal coverage can be pursued in steps. But these steps must be chosen to build public support for and confidence in policy initiatives. Further, policymakers must be sensitive to the risks of unintended consequences and invest in public education about costs and benefits.

Where Are We Going?

For reasons of policy and values, the Clinton administration remains firmly committed to guaranteeing affordable health insurance for all Americans. This commitment to universal coverage reflects both human and economic concerns.

Clearly, health care reform should aim to ensure access to appropriate health care. Although evidence tying insurance to specific health outcomes is limited, ample evidence shows that insurance makes a difference in the timing, type, and, in some cases, quality and outcomes of health care.[1] Universal coverage is therefore a necessary if not sufficient condition for everyone's getting health care when they need it.

Universal coverage is just as crucial to achieving equitable health care financing and efficient delivery of health care services. In particular it is important to control costs by improving efficiency, not by shifting costs from one payer to another or by reducing access to necessary care. Minimizing uncompensated care by expanding coverage is critical to the success of promoting competition as a means of cost containment.

We feel that it is important to be clear about the health care security we believe Americans ought to have (and seem to want).[2] Equally important, setting down concrete goals can prevent policymakers and stakeholders from claiming victory prematurely. And while the goals of universal coverage and cost containment leave ample room for differences of opinion—for example, defining operationally what it means for coverage to be affordable—it enables us to distinguish proposals that move us forward from those that would actually move us backward.

Experience in the 103d Congress indicates that health reform can be achieved only in steps. Clarifying why this is so can help point to strategies that are both desirable and viable from a political perspective.

Health care reform arose as a major political issue because the majority of Americans, most of whom have insurance, became concerned that their coverage would not be there when they needed it.[3] However, fears about the current system in no way precluded fears about reform. The inability to enact comprehensive reform legislation is attributable, at least in part, to the fact that people became more worried about their prospects under reform than under the status quo.[4] The policy debate suggests that the risks of disruption are easier to communicate than are the benefits of secure coverage. For a variety of reasons, (rightly or wrongly) the public came to see reform as riskier than the status quo.

This experience teaches two lessons applicable to a step-by-step approach to reform: (1) Minimize disruption. Particularly in the short term, it is necessary to build public comfort and confidence in taking action. (2) Make sure the targets of reform are clear. Each step must be understood as providing more security of coverage and better affordability than does the status quo.

Incremental reform may also have incremental advantages. It may be easier to communicate the value of each step than the net value of a more comprehensive and complicated proposal. But incremental reform poses its own political and policy risks. Indeed, the pursuit of comprehensive reform by the Clinton administration reflected not only the basic values and goals outlined earlier, but also a desire to avoid certain unintended consequences associated with partial change.

Insurance reforms, for example, present a greater risk of disruption under incremental reform than under comprehensive reform with universal coverage. Without universal coverage, increasing access would raise overall premiums because sicker people, who have been excluded from the system, would now be able to obtain coverage. Younger and healthier people (and the businesses that employ them) may tend not to purchase coverage as the cost of being covered rises. In a universal system, in which both the sick and the healthy are covered, such "adverse selection" cannot occur.

Also, compressing premiums—that is, limiting the ability of insurers to charge the sick or elderly substantially more than they charge the healthy or young—means that while older and sicker people will pay less than under the status quo, younger and healthier people will pay more. Although universal coverage cannot eliminate this disruption, it can cushion it by reducing uncompensated care and associated cost shifting, which in turn should reduce premiums. An effective cost containment strategy—which many believe is aided by universal coverage—can further cushion the effects of premium compression.

The risks of disruption from incremental reform can be neither ignored nor eliminated. In moving forward, however, several precautions can be taken. First, policy can and should be designed to mitigate the risk of disruption. Second, leaders should not overpromise. They should acknowledge the risks as well as the benefits of policy initiatives and monitor their effects over time, as they try to build the public confidence needed for broader reform.

What Next?

There are many possible paths to the objective of secure, affordable coverage. We highlight three of them as initial steps: insurance reforms, expanded coverage for working families (especially children in working families), and support for long-term care.

Insurance Reforms

The current system is unfair. People who are sick—and, arguably, have the greatest need for health coverage—can be charged premiums that are prohibitively high, and in some cases are denied coverage altogether. Furthermore, the current insurance marketplace works against efficient competition.

Two types of reforms would address these problems. The first would require insurers to guarantee access to coverage regardless of health status. This guarantee would include assured issuance and renewal of coverage, limits on pre-existing condition exclusions for persons newly purchasing coverage, and elimination of pre-existing condition exclusions for persons changing insurers (for example, when changing jobs). Outright elimination of pre-existing condition exclusions would be desirable but is possible only under universal coverage because people with the option to be uninsured would be tempted to wait until they were sick to buy coverage. However, eliminating exclusions for people changing insurers would address an important concern about the current system. Every major health or insurance reform bill introduced in the 103d Congress (by both Democrats and Republicans) included such reforms.

The second type of reform would limit or prohibit rating practices that permit insurers to charge some people (such as those who are sick) grossly more than they charge others. Some type of rating reform is necessary to make the promise of guaranteed access to coverage real. Otherwise, insurers could simply charge unaffordably high premiums to persons who are sick, effectively denying them access to care.

The issue at the heart of insurance rating reforms is who should be pooled with whom. To make insurance accessible and provide the rudiments of competitive pressure, the sick should be pooled with the healthy. That is, insurers should be prohibited from charging higher premiums to those who become ill. Pure community rating would go further in limiting the rating factors that an insurer could use, generally to standard family size and geography categories. In other words, the old would be pooled with the young, blue-collar workers with white-collar workers, and so on. The more factors that are eliminated, the more risks are shared and the more current practices are disrupted.

To eliminate the most discriminatory of current insurance rating practices and to make access to coverage real, we recommend that experience rating be eliminated or phased out quickly. Maintaining age-based premium variations is necessary to mitigate disruption created by compressing premiums and to avoid the chance that younger persons would drop coverage in the face of higher rates. Such variations could, however, be limited—for example, insurers could be permitted to charge an older person no more than two or three times more than they charge a younger person.

Insurance reforms are often touted as issues on which everybody agrees. But that perception reflects the limited policy debate these issues have received (relative to employer mandates, for example) rather than a genuine consensus. In fact, the specifics of insurance reform are highly controversial. Most (if not all) parties to the debate support insurance reforms that provide nominally greater access to coverage. But without limits on insurers' rating practices, the promise of increased access is largely an illusion, and there is hardly any consensus on how to accomplish this type of reform.

Perhaps even more controversial than the reforms themselves is the decision about the population to whom they should apply. Here perhaps are the most profound conflicts over the distribution of health care costs and who should share risk and costs with whom. An obvious issue is the business size to which the reform would apply. Two of the less obvious but equally significant of these distributional issues are the treatment of self-insurance and trade associations and the handling of individually purchased insurance.

SELF-INSURANCE AND TRADE ASSOCIATIONS. Support is widespread for permitting small businesses to self-insure or to purchase coverage through a self-insured or experience-rated trade association. In either case, if small companies employing healthier workers are permitted to avoid being pooled with small companies employing sicker workers, the benefits of any rating reforms will be attenuated.

INDIVIDUALLY PURCHASED INSURANCE. If insurance reforms were applied to individual purchasers of insurance (for example, the self-employed), premiums likely would rise significantly because of adverse selection. The difficult distributional question is, who should bear this higher cost? Is it the individual purchasers themselves (for example, by creating separate risk pools for individuals and employers)? This approach would likely make insurance prohibitively expensive for individual purchasers. Is it individuals and small businesses (for example, by creating a single risk pool for individuals and small businesses)? This would raise costs for small businesses—which may be unfair and politically difficult. Finally, is it individuals and all businesses (for example, by creating a risk pool for individuals and small businesses and by requiring larger businesses to pay an assessment to cover a portion of these costs)? This approach was advocated by Senate Majority Leader George J. Mitchell in the 103d Congress. It may be the fairest approach, but it obviously is politically difficult. As with most distributional questions, this one has no easy answers. However, avoiding the question by leaving individual purchasers out of insurance reform also is not appealing.

Finally, these issues cannot be fully addressed without reconsidering how the states and the federal government share responsibility for regulating insurance. Although states have generally enacted certain insurance reforms for small businesses, federal policy is required to address many of the more difficult distributional issues. The Employee Retirement Income Security Act (ERISA), for example, largely prevents states from prohibiting individual firms from self-insuring or from assessing large employers to cover a portion of the cost of individually purchased insurance.

There should be no illusion that insurance reform will be politically easy. Some risks may be acceptable in light of the attendant benefits, while others may need to be mitigated before reforms are enacted. Regulating insurers' rating practices creates two major risks. First, there will inevitably be some losers. But even the losers will gain the security of knowing that their premiums cannot be raised in the future if they become ill. Although the benefits of security may be harder to convey than the costs of immediately higher rates, they are nevertheless real.

Second, there is the risk of adverse selection. A selection spiral is a collective problem that brings little or no compensating benefit. Compressing premiums for small businesses too much, for example, could reduce pooling if larger firms escape the community risk pool through self-insurance or trade associations.[5] Indeed, states now have authority under ERISA to regulate associations of small employers that self-insure. Legislation that undermines this authority could worsen insurance pools instead of improving them.

Efforts to mitigate risks to specific policy proposals should not be viewed as obstructionist. Rather, they are critical to achieving positive policy change.

Expanded Coverage

Insurance reform alone is insufficient to achieve universal coverage. Proposed legislation in the 103d Congress by both Democrats and Republicans recognized that many people cannot afford insurance coverage even if it is available, and that financial assistance should be provided to help them buy insurance. A key question for step-wise reform is where to focus resources at the outset.

With an eye toward legislative agreement it is important to target resources based not only on need but also on the ability to generate political support. Need suggests targeting based on means testing and on beneficiaries who lack access to some other form of coverage. Generating political support suggests targeting primarily children in middle-income working families. Under current law, medicaid is phasing in coverage for all children in families with incomes below poverty. An expansion could cover children in middle-income families who now lack insurance.

Medicaid's expansions in the past decade indicate political support for targeting aid to children, as do recent initiatives in several of the states. Expanding that coverage also is consistent not only with assuring continued protection of children but also with improving the incentive to leave welfare for work. Further, such an initiative could build on a number of state programs that involve private insurers in covering children.[6]

As with insurance reforms, expanding coverage for children will pose risk and controversy. However, here the risk is not so much disruption or harm to people, but rather that some portion of the new financing allocated to expanding coverage might in fact substitute for existing public or private funding sources. For example, states that have expanded medicaid beyond the mandated levels for children or created state-only programs for providing coverage to children would be likely to drop coverage if a new program were available (unless, of course, there were a maintenance-of-effort requirement, which carries its own controversy).

Similarly, if not for the existence of the new public subsidy, some children eligible for the new program might have received an employer contribution toward coverage. This substitution could be reduced, for example, by making ineligible children who have some threshold employer contribution available.

These issues will be raised and should be debated. But they should not be allowed to stymie action. Without mandating employer contributions toward health care coverage—which seems quite unlikely in the near future—some substitution is inevitable with any subsidy program. In addition, substitution is not necessarily bad. Substitution for current state spending provides fiscal relief to states. Also, working families who substitute publicly subsidized coverage for employer-financed coverage for their children should see an increase in wages.

In pursuing this step of reform, it is important to pursue policies that do more than replace current coverage. But the fact that some funds will go to the already insured—that is, that we are unable to target with perfect efficiency—should not become an obstacle to moving forward.

Long-term Care

If secure and affordable protection against the costs of illness is an objective of reform, long-term care cannot be ignored. The financial and emotional burdens of addressing the nonmedical costs associated with chronic illness are at least as compelling as lack of protection for acute care services.

Republicans and Democrats alike have advocated changes in the tax treatment of long-term care insurance as an element in addressing long-term care needs. Clarifying that tax preferences for health insurance and medical care apply to long-term care as well may strengthen the demand for these policies. That action also has value as a consumer protection if it is accompanied by standards that ensure consumer information and prohibit abusive marketing practices prevalent in the long-term care insurance market.[7]

Improving value for the dollar in private long-term care insurance, however, is at best a long-term strategy for reducing the financial burdens of long-term care. Such insurance is in the early stages of development, too expensive for many seniors, and generally not available to persons who are already impaired.[8] To address current long-term care needs, it is necessary to do more. We recommend addressing what is now the most glaring gap in our system of long-term care financing: support for home- and community-based care.

Although states have expanded their provision of these services under medicaid, the availability of support varies greatly across the country. Matching grants to states, with more substantial federal participation than medicaid now provides, would enable all states to develop home- and community-based services. A new program could establish certain minimum federal eligibility and service requirements but allow states broad flexibility to tailor support to the varying needs of individuals. Such flexibility also would recognize differences in the way communities are providing services, for example, some relying more on agencies, others on individual providers for care.

Concern about existing, let alone new, entitlement programs has hindered expansion of public financing for long-term care. This approach would address that concern by capping the federal funds available for the program, with amounts made available to each state based on its share of the nation's disabled population. States, not individuals, would have entitlement to funds.

Designing a home- and community-based care program, like other steps in health care reform, poses risk. As with children's coverage, there are issues of substitution of new federal funds for existing state dollars. Decisions would be required about how to relate existing medicaid coverage to new programs so as to balance the desire for expanded service with states' interest in fiscal relief. Controversy would exist over how limited funds should be targeted. Means-tested programs efficiently target support but enjoy limited political support. Furthermore, the disabled population is made up of various subpopulations—children with disabilities and chronic illnesses, persons with mental illness, persons with developmental disabilities, other working-age adults with disabilities, and the disabled elderly—with stakes in resource allocation. Here too any action will be controversial. But progress can be made.

Pitfalls in Incremental Reform

Two general risks attend a step-by-step approach to reform of health care financing.

The first is the possibility of cutbacks in benefits masquerading as expansions. In the 103d Congress, for example, some reform bills included caps on funding (generally called entitlement caps or fail-safe mechanisms), which generally reduced eligibility for subsidies if costs exceeded the authorized funds. Some of these bills included current beneficiaries (for example, persons receiving medicaid) under these caps. Capping new programs may be appropriate. But such caps should not be permitted to jeopardize coverage under existing programs. Existing coverage would be particularly at risk if a new program's funding is tightly constrained or its costs are uncertain or unstable.

The second risk is unabashed cutbacks in public programs that provide valued protection—medicare and medicaid in particular. Medicare now provides universal coverage for the nation's senior citizens and many persons with disabilities. Cuts that destroy this basic mission of medicare, or that undermine its capacity to achieve it, clearly would be a step backward. Similarly, although there is considerable interest in medicaid reform, medicaid must be recognized as an important safety net for poor children, the elderly, and persons with disabilities. Indeed, without the recently legislated expansions in medicaid the number of uninsured Americans would have increased even faster than it has, given the decline in employer-based coverage.[9]

Conclusion

The last round of health care reform made clear that proponents must pursue their goals a step at a time. The individual steps should be framed with an eye toward the ultimate objectives: providing secure and afford-able coverage for all Americans.

Certain initial steps are consistent with any number of paths toward secure and affordable coverage. Reforming the insurance market—with a focus on the most discriminatory of current practices that erect barriers to access—provides a foundation for broader coverage and more efficient service delivery. Some people lack insurance because they cannot afford it, and addressing this problem by beginning with children in working families may generate broad support. Finally, some movement to address long-term care problems is an important substantive and political element of any incremental step taken.

Reformers should be aware of the disruption that each incremental step can cause and try to mitigate the risks and ensure that risks are balanced with benefits. Moving step by step offers an opportunity for public education as reform proceeds. But a step-by-step approach to reform should not become an excuse for action that would reduce, rather than improve, health care coverage. Cutbacks are not reforms.

Notes

1. U.S. Congress, Office of Technology Assessment, *Does Health Insurance Make a Difference?*, OTA-BP-H-99 (Washington, September 1992).

2. CBS/*New York Times* poll, cited in "CBS/NYT: Clinton and Congress Share Health Care Blame," *Healthline*, September 13, 1994; and Princeton Survey Research Association survey, cited in "Newsweek: Health Debate Makes More People Unsure," *Hotline*, August 8, 1994.

3. R. J. Blendon and J. N. Edwards, "Caring for the Uninsured: Choices for Reform," *Journal of the American Medical Association*, vol. 265 (May 15, 1991), pp. 2563–65.

4. A *Washington Post* survey, cited in "Washington Post: Assesses Impact of Delay," *Healthline*, July 7, 1993.

5. Similarly, if we enacted tax-preferred medical savings accounts, we could further segregate the sick (who would tend to choose plans with little cost sharing) from the healthy (who would tend to choose plans with high cost sharing).

6. Patricia Butler, Robert L. Mollica, and Trish Riley, "Children's Health Plans," National Academy for State Health Policy, Portland, Maine, July 1993.

7. The Health Insurance Association of America testified before the Ways and Means Subcommittee on Health that consumer confidence in these products

will be increased if tax clarification is accompanied by "reasonable Federal standards." See Health Insurance Association of America, *Tax Incentives for Long-Term Care Insurance as Part of the Senior Citizens Equity Act*, hearings before the Subcommittee on Health of the House Ways and Means Committee, 104 Cong. 1 sess. (Government Printing Office, 1995). See also General Accounting Office, *Long-Term Care Insurance: High Percentage of Policyholders Drop Policies*, GAO-HRD-93-129 (Washington, August 1993); and General Accounting Office, *Long-Term Care Insurance: Risks to Consumers Should Be Reduced*, GAO-HRD-92-14 (Washington, 1991).

8. Joshua M. Wiener, Laurel Hixon Illston, and Raymond J. Hanley, *Sharing the Burden: Strategies for Public and Private Long-Term Care Insurance* (Brookings, 1994).

9. John Holahan, Colin Winterbottom, and Shruti Rajan, *The Changing Composition of Health Insurance Coverage in the United States* (Washington: Urban Institute Press, 1995).

CHAPTER TEN

The Conservative Agenda

Stuart M. Butler

INCREMENTAL reforms of the U.S. health care system should be offered only within the context of steps toward larger reform goals, so that the American people can evaluate the final destination as well as the individual steps. Preferably, these specific reforms should be discussed as part of a sorely needed national debate about the basic features of the system, which Congress should construct in stages. Indeed, public understanding of the merits of rival proposals is hardly possible without such an open debate on the fundamentals. Whatever structural reforms Americans achieve should not be the haphazard result of disconnected incremental actions, nor should they be the undisclosed objectives of step-by-step reforms.

Most incremental reforms under discussion would move the health care system in one of three broad directions. The first group of reforms would expand on the current system of employment-based coverage, with varying degrees of new government regulation and subsidy. In the second group of reforms, government would determine the level and allocation of health care services for each person and the cost of those services to each family. The third group of reforms would move toward a "consumer-based" system in which individuals and families would own their own plans and determine the components of coverage. The government's role in this latter system would be limited to subsidizing lower-income families and establishing minimal rules to permit the health care market to function efficiently. I focus here on the third structural reform, which, I believe, is most in tune with the instincts of the American people.

Aims of a Consumer-Based Health System

Proposals to achieve a consumer-based health care system are based on the premise that today's employment-based system is failing because the normal producer-consumer relationship in the health care market has been undermined by the employer's role as a quasi-consumer, and on the idea that this unnatural role continues only because of perverse features of the tax code. Employed Americans enjoy a huge tax break for health care, valued at some $90 billion in federal and state tax relief in 1994 (or an average of $1,012 per family).[1] But there is one crucial requirement: employees must cede ownership and control of their health insurance to their employer and allow the employer to determine each worker's coverage, paid for with funds that otherwise would be part of each worker's cash compensation.

A consumer-based health care system would create a new economic relationship, in which households would own their own health plans and determine how much of their compensation would be devoted to coverage and what that coverage would include. The market for health care would thus become much like those for other services; that is, consumers would own their coverage and control the dollars. This situation would represent a more normal relationship between consumers and providers of health services than now exists. Health insurers would have to compete by satisfying the health care consumer, not the employer, regarding quality and price. This restructuring, reinforced with the tax reform discussed below, would introduce the normal pressures for efficient cost control in a consumer-driven market.

Another result of individual ownership would be security—the issue well understood by President Bill Clinton as the most potent in the politics of health care. The structure of benefits would no longer depend on decisions made by an employer, and employment changes would have no direct impact on the family plan. "Job lock" related to health care would cease. Although the primary objective is to create this new economic relationship for working Americans, the aim also is to make the same basic change in medicare and perhaps medicaid. I return to this point later.

The legislative key to the consumer-choice approach is tax reform to encourage people to own their own coverage and to make economic choices between insurance and direct payments. The ultimate aim is to amend the tax code so that it treats purchases of insurance and direct expenditures in exactly the same way and treats insurance the same way whether purchased directly or indirectly through an employer or another organization, such as a union or a church.

In principle, two broad methods exist to achieve tax neutrality. One is to eliminate the existing exclusion from taxable household income of company-sponsored health plans. The other is to replace the exclusion with a new tax break for households that would apply equally to household purchases of insurance and direct expenditures on health care (including funds in an earmarked savings account).

This latter tax reform is the core of the structural health care reform proposal developed by the Heritage Foundation and the legislation introduced in 1994 (S. 1743, H.R. 3698) by Senator Don Nickles and Representative Cliff Stearns.[2] The refundable tax credit in the Heritage plan and the Nickles-Stearns bill also provides a subsidy to lower-income families. The bill includes language to reform insurance underwriting rules to make it easier for families to retain affordable coverage or switch plans even if their health were to deteriorate. Other than the draft legislation offered late in 1994 by Senator Robert Dole, intended as a political *coup de grace* to President Clinton's initiative rather than as a serious bill, the Nickles-Stearns bill commanded wider Republican support in the Senate than any other health care legislation did in 1994.

Besides achieving neutrality in tax treatment among different sources of health insurance and types of health spending, these tax reforms also are designed to control costs. Many major approaches to health care reform control costs either by restraining medical prices through direct government controls on insurers and providers or by strengthening incentives on employers to curb their workers' utilization. But the tax reforms in the consumer-choice approach are designed to control health care costs by creating a set of market conditions more like those in other sectors of the economy, by establishing incentives for all consumers to "shop around" for the best value in plans.

Initial Steps on the Road to Reform

Even if sweeping tax reform implicit in the Nickles-Stearns legislation or elimination of the health care tax exclusion are not enacted immediately, several avenues are open to construct a consumer-choice health care system.

A New Health Care Deduction

Congress likely should not only continue the 25 percent tax deduction for purchases of health insurance by the self-employed, but also initiate a series of tax changes to reduce the general discrimination against health plans owned and chosen by families. The 25 percent deduction for the self-employed could be extended to purchases of insurance by any family lacking an employer-sponsored health plan and raised to a 100 percent deduction over time.

Introducing a new deduction for insurance purchases appears to be the most politically practical way of moving toward tax neutrality in the current climate and has strong bipartisan support. A proposal to extend that deduction to others without employer-based plans can be strongly defended on equity grounds and would probably garner strong popular support. Such a change would reduce revenues and could be accommodated in a general tax bill designed to reduce the income tax burden.

Critics may argue that a new deduction for workers without employer-sponsored plans would cause employers to drop existing plans in the knowledge that their employees could receive a tax break for buying their own plan. But moving away from employer-owned insurance is the aim of consumer-choice reform. Furthermore, employees would probably take the lead in demanding the elimination of existing plans, with the "cashing out" of existing benefits.

The only real concern would be if employers simply cut workers' total compensation package by the value of the health plan. But this practice is unlikely because employers still would be subject to labor market conditions regarding total compensation, and perhaps further constrained by bargaining agreements. The likelihood of a cut in the total compensation package also would be reduced if Congress required companies to indicate, as Uwe Reinhardt and others have suggested, workers' total compensation—including the value of health benefits—on each pay stub.[3] Further, Congress could attach temporary "maintenance-of-effort" rules for employers to the tax legislation. And the "cashing out" provisions in the Nickles-Stearns legislation, if added to a tax measure, would make it easier for a company's entire work force, if it so chose, to switch to an individual system without a loss of compensation.

Medical Savings Accounts

Medical savings accounts (MSAs) provide another way to reduce the current tax discrimination against direct payments for health care. Reducing the threshold for taking health care payments as an itemized deduction on household tax returns would promote the same goal. But support is stronger for establishing MSAs than for changing the itemized deduction. Such accounts could be established in a number of ways. One method, which has the disadvantage of being employment based, would be to change the tax rules governing cafeteria plans or flexible spending accounts to permit employees to roll over some amount of funds remaining in the account at the end of the year. Congress also could permit tax-free contributions to new MSAs, with families able to withdraw the funds tax free for medical purposes (making them, in effect, personal flexible spending accounts). Another approach would be to permit withdrawals from individual retirement accounts (IRAs) for medical purposes without penalty. This last option would have only a small revenue effect, by ending the penalty on younger Americans who withdraw IRA funds for medical emergencies.

These tax changes are not without their technical and political problems. One technical worry is that creating new tax deductions for medical care, while keeping the existing exclusion in place, makes health care spending more attractive at the margin than many other basic elements of a household's budget (such as paying for college). In isolation, this step would indeed raise health care costs, not lower them. This effect would be counteracted by the stronger cost control incentives felt by workers who were formerly enrolled in company-sponsored plans but now owned their own plans. Most economists favoring tax neutrality would prefer to see any new health care deduction balanced by a limitation on the exclusion or its outright elimination. But these steps face formidable political resistance.

The Heritage Foundation proposal and the Nickles-Stearns bill address the political problem by proposing to replace the exclusion with a sliding-scale tax credit. The credit percentage increases in steps according to a household's total health expenditures compared with its income (a structure similar to that of the child care credit).[4] According to an analysis of the Heritage proposal by Lewin-VHI, a budget-neutral "swap" of the credit for the exclusion means the vast majority of middle-class households would experience no net increase in taxes (box 10-1).[5] Yet because the credit applies to out-of-pocket expenses as well as to insurance, the marginal tax relief for middle- and upper-income families (typically 25 percent under the Nickles-Stearns legislation) is lower than under the current exclusion, encouraging greater cost-consciousness.

For the typical worker, the "deal" in the tax swap involves accepting

Box 10-1. Lewin-VHI, *The Individual Tax Credit Program: Estimated Cost and Impacts*

Under this plan individuals not covered by medicare or medicaid would be required to have insurance that paid for 80 percent of inpatient hospital services, outpatient hospital services, and extended or home health care and 75 percent of physician services, prenatal, well-baby, and well-child care, diagnostic tests, and inpatient prescription drugs, and 100 percent of the cost of emergency services, subject to deductibles of $1,000 per person ($2,000 per family) and a cost-sharing maximum of $5,000 on covered services. Mental health, dental, and vision care and outpatient prescription drugs would not be covered. Employers would not be required to continue sponsoring health insurance for their employees, but would be subject to a maintenance-of-effort requirement. The plan would also include a variety of insurance market reforms. State and local governments would be required to transfer to the public program any net savings in their health spending. The Lewin estimate assumes that all employers would drop their plans and (as required under the plan) raise wages by the amount they save. Currently insured employees in fair or poor health and people now covered by nongroup insurance are assumed to maintain their current level of coverage even if higher than the required package. Employees in good or excellent health and currently uninsured people are assumed to purchase only the required package. Administrative costs for workers in companies where employers arrange employee deductions are assumed to be unchanged, and administrative costs for individuals are assumed to fall to 16.5 percent from the current level of 40 percent for groups of one to four persons. Under these assumptions, the *average* change in net income changes negligibly after induced wage effects, changed health care spending, and tax credits. Despite negligible average changes within income brackets, individual families may experience significantly larger increases or decreases in net cost.

Final report prepared for the Heritage Foundation, November 10, 1993.

a lower marginal rate of tax relief in exchange for tax relief for out-of-pocket expenses and supplemental coverage of their own choice—and no net increase in taxes. This package is potentially attractive, especially because the credit would make it less expensive for an employee to "customize" a health plan with supplemental insurance or direct payments for medical care. In essence the politics of the exchange is a mirror image of the politics of tax simplification or the flat tax. In flat tax proposals, taxpayers give up tax relief for specific spending in return for lower marginal tax rates on all income. In the health care tax proposal, workers accept a lower rate of marginal tax relief on purchases of insurance (and hence a higher after-tax marginal cost) than under the exclusion, in return for tax relief for out-of-pocket spending and supplemental coverage, much greater control of spending, and the security of individual ownership.

An incremental version of the Nickles-Stearns bill might begin with a modest tax deduction or credit for out-of-pocket expenses or supplemental insurance available to taxpayers who do not itemize deductions financed by revenue from a cap on the tax exclusion. If carefully designed, this swap would leave the typical middle-class worker no worse off from a tax point of view (but with some tax relief for deductibles), upper-income workers somewhat worse off than today, and lower-income workers better off.

This incremental version would trigger a new political dynamic. Say a cap on the exclusion were used to finance tax relief for covering children not included in an employer-sponsored plan, or for the first $1,000 of out-of-pocket medical expenses. Pressure likely would grow for tax relief for adult dependents, or for additional out-of-pocket expenses to be tax-deductible. With a cap used to finance such tax relief, a constituency would emerge to lower the cap in the exclusion to finance this new tax relief. Thus the first, small step toward granting tax relief in this way would foster political pressure for the next step. This political dynamic is different, of course, from that associated with imposing a cap simply to foster cost-consciousness.

Assistance to Low-Income Families

General political support exists for some type of direct subsidy to lower-income working families for some insurance coverage. Unlike the current deduction, the tax credit in the Nickles-Stearns bill is refundable and so constitutes a net subsidy to lower-income families. In fact, if the wage-reducing effects of an employer mandate are taken into account, the Nickles-Stearns credit turns out to provide a larger net subsidy for these families than the Clinton plan would have provided.[6] Most major health reform proposals introduced in 1993 and 1994 also contain direct subsidies.

Therefore, a subsidy program might be one incremental reform that everyone can agree on. Despite this wide support, designing legislation to create such a subsidy is difficult, because a new subsidy on top of current income support programs that is also phased out as income grows, greatly reduces the incentive to work by raising the effective marginal tax rate. The Nickles-Stearns bill is much less prone to this problem than are other bills. The reason for this is that its refundable credit also restructures the whole tax treatment of health care expenditures. This restructuring allows the "tax expenditure" associated with the credit to be reduced very gradually over a large range of income—with only small work disincentive effects.

Any direct subsidy program enacted in the near future, assuming no radical change in federal means-tested income support programs, would have to be quite small if it is to limit the work disincentive effects. Of course, if Congress gives states wide discretion to reform means-tested income support programs, for example, by block-granting welfare and other programs to the states or granting generous waivers, designing a more generous federal subsidy program that minimizes additional work disincentive effects might be possible. But unless that happens, the apparent consensus on a subsidy program is unlikely to be translated into workable legislation.

Insurance Reform

Significant insurance reform is divisive because even small changes in the way the insurance system is structured would cause the health care system to evolve in sharply different ways. Thus the notion that many insurance reforms are items "everyone can agree on" is false, particularly if the long-term results of a reform are considered. Perhaps more than in any other area of health care reform, proponents of incremental steps must clearly state their ultimate objective.

STANDARDIZED BENEFITS. The Clinton plan and other Democratic reform strategies sought new federal rules to require insurance plans to contain a comprehensive standard benefit package. Opponents of these plans made blocking a comprehensive standard benefit package—especially one chosen by a federal commission—a top priority.

For those who believe that government should decide a comprehensive set of health care services to which a family has access, a federally mandated package should contain most of the services a family might need. Given the cost of such a comprehensive package, it would become a standard package for most Americans. By this view, a key objective of incremental insurance reform should be to take the first steps toward ensuring such a package, perhaps by introducing some general rules for insurance plans or by requiring comprehensive services for plans covering particular categories of the population. Most supporters of a consumer-choice health care system strongly oppose steps that would tend to lead to standardization. They argue instead for a relatively inexpensive core package, with more scope to add on selected services. Tax relief for health insurance under this view should require that families purchase only a minimal policy to cover catastrophic expenses.

Some supporters of standardization, such as Alain Enthoven, maintain that if families are free to choose the health benefits they want, that will lead to a "death spiral" of adverse selection in which the risk-spreading function of insurance will be undermined.[7] In other words, people would tend to buy coverage mainly for treatments they know they will need, meaning they are paying for a certainty, not insuring against a risk. The other side of the coin, they argue, is that insurance companies will be able to add or subtract benefits, to "cherry-pick" good risks and avoid bad risks, leaving sicker families unable to afford coverage.

Although adverse selection is inescapable if persons choose the benefits they want, it is far from clear that enough of a problem exists to justify standardization. The Federal Employees Health Benefits Program (FEHBP) has existed for more than thirty years. It covers more than nine million Americans, offers a wide range of benefits in the competing plans, and permits enrollees to switch plans without penalty every year. Because the program is also community rated, it creates strong incentives for adverse selection, with the sick seeking out high-benefit programs when they need them and healthier workers picking less expensive, leaner plans. Nonetheless, the program is quite stable.

The experience of the FEHBP suggests that the fear that choice of benefits makes insurance unstable is unfounded. Reform can further mitigate this fear in three ways. First, reasonable waiting periods and "entry fees" could be permitted for new coverage to discourage people from delaying certain types of coverage until they know they need the service. Such devices force consumers to make longer-term commitments to a particular plan. Second, the after-tax cost of direct payment for services could be reduced; this result would encourage families to use insurance more frequently to cover major, unforeseen costs than to cover routine services. The third way to protect against adverse selection is through underwriting reforms.

Congress may consider blocking measures to prohibit state insurance mandates. Concerns about federalism aside, state mandates directly conflict with what many conservatives believe to be basic economic freedoms. The Nickles-Stearns bill includes a provision to prohibit states from requiring anything more than catastrophic coverage in a plan that qualifies the policyholder for the bill's new tax credit.

PREMIUM RESTRICTIONS. Concern over adverse selection and cherry picking also leads to calls for some limit on the range of premiums insurers can charge. It also prompts the claim that a mandate on people to buy insurance is necessary to keep healthy Americans from staying outside of the insurance pool and driving up premiums for insured households.

Congress is extremely unlikely in the near future to pass any mandate, employer or individual, to purchase insurance. Congress is also unlikely to require community rating, as many younger Americans would forgo coverage if their premiums were raised to the community average. The intergenerational transfer of income implicit in community rating also makes it objectionable to most conservatives, who can accept income transfers based on individual need but resist transfers based merely on age. In addition, they worry that community rating distorts—and may undermine—the insurance system. Nevertheless, even conservative circles support some limitation on the freedom of insurance companies to vary premiums or cancel coverage. If consumer choice and vigorous competition in quality and price are to become a reality in health insurance, consumers must be able to count on long-term contracts with their insurers. Moreover, for consumer choice to be an effective check on quality and value in health insurance, consumers must in practice be able to switch policies even if their health deteriorates.

These considerations lead many conservatives to support guaranteed renewal of coverage and changes in how coverage is underwritten. A number of Republican bills introduced in 1994 contained limits on underwriting. Such limits could probably be enacted in an incremental package, especially if the new requirements allowed insurers to impose a reasonable waiting period for coverage, in order to discourage persons from seeking coverage or switching plans only when their health deteriorates. These underwriting restrictions also would protect against adverse selection. If health insurance premiums did not vary according to health status, purchasers of insurance would have little reason to form special pools consisting disproportionately of low-risk people in order to get good rates, thereby undermining other insurance pools.

The other alternative for Congress is to urge states to experiment with insurance regulation, as they can today, outside of plans covered by the

Employee Retirement Income Security Act (ERISA). Experimentation would permit alternative rate systems to be tested without requiring plans throughout the country to conform to federal underwriting requirements. Removal of ERISA protection for self-insured plans may be the only way to foster effective experimentation. The concern about this approach for supporters of consumer choice is that it may lead to standardization of all plans in a state, reducing the opportunity for employees to choose benefits by bargaining with their employer. From a conservative perspective a self-insured employer-sponsored system is certainly inferior to a system in which families are free to choose their benefits and own their plan, but it is better than having a state government choosing those benefits. In any case, if the tax system were more neutral and Americans less inclined to want employment-based coverage, ERISA-protected self-insurance would be less attractive.

CREATING NEW INSURANCE POOLS. Objections to the current employer-based system do not imply a rejection of group insurance. Insurance pools are necessary to spread risk and economize on administrative costs. A consumer-choice system allows people to establish their own contracts with insurers or providers. More important, it allows people to join a group other than one formed at work.

The place of employment typically is not the best setting for an insurance pool. Employment-based pools can make sense in large companies with a very stable work force. A consumer-choice system would not preclude them. But for persons who work for small companies or who change jobs frequently, an insurance pool could be based on another group such as a union, a church, or the local farm bureau—organizations with which the worker might have a more permanent affiliation. Such organizations offer insurance plans today. The problem is that the tax code discriminates against these alternative pools. When lawmakers discuss "small-group market reform" or other proposals to create insurance pools, however, they invariably consider only workplace pools. They should recognize that other groups, many of them already sponsoring insurance, could become an alternative to employer-sponsored groups if tax barriers were reduced.

Congress could also give Americans access to a wide range of additional group plans by opening up its own health program, the FEHBP. Recognizing the political potency of this strategy, several Democratic bills in 1994 would have allowed some people to join the FEHBP, albeit after standardizing the FEHBP benefit package. And Senator William V.

Roth, Jr., would allow small firms to join the program. Permitting individuals to join would be popular and would widen the insurance choices available to families. Once again, granting at least some tax relief to private-sector enrollees is essential to make the opportunity attractive for most Americans. To avoid any perceived threat to the stability of the existing FEHBP, new enrollees could be grouped in a separate pool and premiums established under limited underwriting requirements, not community rated.

REFORMING MEDICARE. While the consumer-choice approach to reform focuses on the problems of the private, employment-based system, it is possible to take compatible steps in some of the public programs, particularly medicare. Medicare today is the antithesis of a consumer-based system. To be sure, beneficiaries may choose among hospitals and physicians willing to accept the terms of the program. But the range of available services, the net prices charged to patients, and the payment schedule for providers is determined by the federal government. Cost control, such as it is, is achieved through price controls.

Given the political sensitivity of the program, even incremental reforms are difficult. One option would gradually transform the program into a consumer-choice health plan without disturbing current beneficiaries. Under this option, a new retiree would accept a medicare voucher equal in value to, say, 95 percent of the value of the anticipated medicare spending for a person of his or her age. The voucher could be used to purchase any plan that provided at least basic catastrophic coverage and was priced in line with the limited underwriting principles discussed earlier. If the voucher amount exceeded the cost of the chosen plan, the balance could be spent on out-of-pocket medical expenses.

In this way, a growing number of medicare beneficiaries would gain the right to coverage of their own choosing. Under the voucher proposal, especially if tax reforms had been instituted to encourage personal ownership of insurance by working-age Americans, many persons retiring at age sixty-five could continue coverage under the plan they found satisfactory at age sixty-four. And in any case, retirees opting for the voucher wold have a strong incentive to seek plans offering the best value for the money.

Still, it would be wise for Congress to introduce such a voucher system in a limited way, perhaps as a demonstration program, to assess the degree of adverse selection. This procedure would resemble that used to introduce managed care into medicare. A poorly designed voucher program could cause healthier retirees to take the voucher, buying the minimum required health plan, and to use the voucher to pay for services they would have to pay for out-of-pocket under the current medicare system. Meanwhile, sicker retirees might opt for the existing system, and total outlays would rise. On the other hand, limited underwriting requirements might offset those potential problems. It would be sensible to test different voucher designs before taking a needless gamble.

Conclusion

Good policymaking can be undertaken a step at a time. But if this process is to lead to a good outcome, in line with the wishes of the American people, each step must be consistent with a clearly stated objective. A consumer-choice system is one possible objective. So is a single-payer system, and so are other systems. Whatever the system, incremental reforms must be framed within the context of an ultimate reform. If instead "incremental reform" becomes an end in itself, Americans may discover too late that a "reformed" health care system is worse than the one they have now.

Notes

1. Lewin-VHI, "The Individual Tax Credit Program: Estimated Cost and Impacts," prepared for the Heritage Foundation, Washington, November 10, 1993.

2. Stuart M. Butler and Edmund F. Haislmaier, *The Consumer Choice Health Security Act* (Washington: Heritage Foundation, December 1993).

3. Uwe E. Reinhardt, "Reorganizing the Financial Flows in American Health Care," *Health Affairs*, vol. 12 (Supplement 1993), p. 183.

4. For a fuller description of the refundable credit in the Nickles-Stearns bill, see Butler and Haislmaier, *The Consumer Choice Health Security Act*. See box 10-1 for a summary of the Lewin-VHI study and the assumptions used.

5. The Nickles-Stearns legislation provided a refundable tax credit worth more in total cost to the Treasury than the value of the exclusion it eliminated, meaning that upper-income families typically experienced no net change in taxes, while middle-income and, to an even greater degree, lower-income households enjoyed a reduction in total taxes. The extra revenue loss in the bill was offset by various net spending reductions, chiefly in the medicare program.

6. See Stuart M. Butler, *How the Clinton and Nickles-Stearns Health Bills Would Affect American Workers* (Washington: Heritage Foundation, 1994), p. 11.

7. See Alain C. Enthoven, testimony before the U.S. Senate Committee on Finance, March 15, 1994, excerpted in Stuart M. Butler, *Reforming Health Insurance* (Washington: Heritage Foundation, 1994), p. 4.

CHAPTER ELEVEN

Cutting Costs and Improving Health

David M. Cutler

D ISCUSSIONS of large-scale health reform in the United States effectively ended in 1994. For the foreseeable future, policy debate must move away from systemwide health reform and focus on "incremental" reform. On the surface, increments seem easier than systemwide changes. After all, there is less that needs to be done. In reality, though, this simplicity is illusional. Consider the questions that incremental reform must address: Is partial reform better than no reform at all? What are the most urgent priorities? What can policymakers not afford to neglect?

In this chapter I offer two ideas for incremental reform. First, improving the efficiency of health care markets can reduce the level of health spending. Rising health care costs have contributed to fiscal imbalance in the public sector and to labor market and insurance market problems in the private sector. Addressing the cost problem is essential, even if nothing else is done. The proximate cause of rising health costs is technological change—new and better therapies, and the diffusion of existing therapies to new patients. Technological change is a symptom, however, not the underlying disease. The factor driving this technological change is an insurance market that overly rewards costly innovation and insufficiently rewards cost savings. To improve this market, I suggest four proposals: converting medicare into a choice-based system, opening the Federal Employees Health Benefits Program (FEHBP) to individuals and small companies, eliminating pre-existing condition restrictions for people who switch policies, and making individuals face the full cost of more expensive insurance.

The second area for reform begins with the fact that poor health outcomes largely result from adverse social behavior and not from medical factors. Although many see expanding insurance coverage as the key to improved health, the evidence to support this view is weak. I suggest instead that the United States put aside efforts at broad coverage expansions in favor of serious efforts to discourage poor social behavior, through increasing and indexing taxes on smoking, drinking, firearms, and bullets.

Health Care Costs

Slowing the growth rate of health care spending is the most pressing issue on the health reform agenda. Generally, economists do not care how much people spend on a particular good. In contrast to most goods, however, the rising costs of health care provokes several economic concerns. The most urgent issue is the large drain on the public budget from rapidly increasing health costs. Over the next several years virtually the only public spending item that is expected to increase significantly as a share of national product is health entitlements.[1] All other spending—infrastructure, environmental improvement, and transfer programs, to name a few—will likely decline. Is this really how Americans want to spend public money?

High health care costs also create a host of difficulties in the private sector.[2] Many workers, for example, feel "locked" into their current jobs because of pre-existing condition exclusions or other insurance restrictions that may come with a new job. As health costs rise, the problems of job lock increase. In the 1960s, for example, health costs were sufficiently low that time without insurance was not as worrisome as a similar time is today. Without reform, the problem of job lock will continue to increase along with health spending. If we slow the rate of health cost growth, we may correspondingly reduce the severity of job lock.

A second problem is growth in the number of contingent workers. Anecdotal evidence suggests that employers are increasingly switching from full-time employment to part-time workers, temporary workers, and contract service workers, in part because they need not provide contingent workers with health benefits. As health care costs rise, this problem too becomes more acute.

A third issue is risk selection in insurance markets. Much is made of the fact that insurance premiums vary with health status. Experience rating of insurance threatens people with loss of coverage or increased premiums if they become sick today. "Insurance market reforms" are generally designed to address this issue. It is worth noting, though, that the incentives for risk selection increase directly with health costs. When costs are low, the gains from finding the healthy and excluding the sick are small. When costs rise, the gains from risk selection increase. Thus reforms to slow the growth of health care costs will limit problems in insurance markets as well.

A final issue is the problem of free riders. In the United States, if an uninsured person becomes sick, he or she will be cared for, generally at low direct cost. When private insurance is cheap, this option is not that attractive. As private insurance costs increase, however, free care becomes ever more attractive. At least some of the recent reduction in private health insurance coverage reflects an increase in the number of free riders.

Failure to slow growth of health care spending will surely intensify all of these problems. Because prescriptions must be tailored to the diagnosis, I first present my view on why costs are so high and then suggest what to do about it.

The Cost Problem

Health care spending is arithmetically the sum of prices for each service times the quantity of those services provided. This identity suggests three sources for high health care costs. The first is high prices. Doctors' fees are up to three times higher in the United States than in Canada, and U.S. doctors earn up to 30 percent more than Canadian doctors do.[3] Since net income of physicians is about 10 percent of total health spending, this additional income is about 3 percent of health spending.

If physician prices were the whole story behind rising health costs, lowering fees would suffice as a reform. But prices are not the only issue. Furthermore, when provider fees fall, doctors increase the care they provide.[4] As a result, fee reductions alone cannot solve the cost problem.

The second source of high medical costs is excessive administrative expense, defined broadly to include all spending not devoted to patient care activities. Estimates of administrative expense range as high as 20 percent or more of total health spending.[5] Lack of coordination among insurers and money spent on risk selection waste society's resources. Promoting more coordination (for example, through universal claim forms) is therefore a generally accepted component of reform.

The third factor in explaining high costs, and the one I consider most important, is that people receive too much health care. The dominant fact about the use of health services is that for seriously ill persons with insurance, the marginal benefit of additional care is essentially zero. This conclusion shows up directly in studies estimating that up to one-quarter of many common procedures for the elderly are unnecessary or of equivocal value.[6]

Evidence of excessive health provision shows up indirectly in two ways. Several studies have found that persons who receive more intensive medical care do not experience better health outcomes than those who receive less intensive care. In the Rand Health Insurance Experiment, for example, persons with more generous benefits used more care than did persons with less generous benefits, but outcomes were no better. Similarly, a recent study of heart attack treatments found that persons living near high-tech hospitals are more likely to receive cardiac catheterization when they have a heart attack than are persons who live farther away from such hospitals, but these people do not have lower mortality rates.[7] In addition, recent evaluations of managed care suggest that it saves money without substantial effects on health outcomes.[8]

Other studies show that when providers are paid more for care, they perform more services and prolong the lives of their patients, but these health benefits are not very substantial. A comparison of patients who were treated by university-affiliated physicians versus community-affiliated physicians, for example, showed that the university-affiliated physicians used more resources than their community-based peers and had better survival rates in the first few months immediately following discharge but had no better survival rates nine months following discharge.[9] Related to this, evidence from changes in medicare reimbursement under PPS shows that hospitals that fared better under that system had more patients survive the first few months after discharge but did not have higher survival rates a year after discharge.[10] The implication of both of these facts is that "resources matter," but at the margin additional resources are not buying large health improvements.

Indeed, economic theory predicts just this finding. Patients who are well insured pay little for care. Often, providers are reimbursed for all care that is provided. As a result, there are substantial incentives to use any type of care that may improve health, regardless of the medical effectiveness or cost of the procedure. This is just what the accumulated evidence suggests.

Probably, little of the excessive care that is provided is truly unnecessary, in the sense that patients would be better off if they did not receive it. It is more likely that the care has value but is worth less than it costs. Some diagnostic procedures, for example, are performed to detect highly

Table 11-1. *Characteristics of Health Insurance, by Firm Size, 1991*

Employees	Firm size			
	<25	25–99	100–999	1,000+
Offered multiple plans (%)	6	17	30	63
Enrolled in managed care (%)	29	37	42	57

Source: Author's calculations and Health Insurance Association of America, "Employer-Sponsored Health Insurance in Private-Sector Firms in 1991" (Washington, 1992).

improbable conditions. Some medications relieve pain and suffering but do not cure the underlying injury. Some hospital days are spent "just to be sure" that the patient is all right. In each of these cases, society might not want to spend its money that way if it were given the choice.

Who, then, should eliminate this unnecessary care? Since patients typically pay little of the cost for their care, it is easy to see why they have few incentives to limit doctors' charges or refuse low-valued care. The real issue is why insurers do not do it for them, curbing low-value services and providers' fees so that they can in turn lower premiums and enroll more subscribers.

However, eliminating these costs is very difficult. Selling insurance policies with higher cost sharing, for example, lowers total spending but places more burden on patients. Monitoring the care delivered by providers and how much they earn for it requires constant battles with providers. Because intensive cost-saving measures are so difficult, an insurer undertakes them only if he stands to win many new subscribers in response.[11] If the demand response is low, insurers will not gain much from cost savings, and doctors will not need these insurers. If the demand response is high, providers will be forced to give in.

Solving the cost problem, therefore, boils down to two questions: do people have choices among enough different insurance policies to justify reductions in low-value care? And do people have financial incentives to choose appropriately? The answer to both questions, I believe, is no. People normally get health insurance in one of four ways: through employment in small companies; through employment in large companies; through individual purchase; or through the public sector. High fixed costs and restrictions by insurers make it hard for small companies to offer more than one health plan. As a result, as table 11-1 shows, fewer than 10 percent of small companies offer a choice of health care policies (compared with more than 60 percent of large companies), and the share of small-company employees in managed care is only half as large as the share of large-company employees.

In both small and large companies, tax subsidies for employer-provided health insurance lower the price of insurance. A dollar of compensation paid as wages is taxed by federal and state income taxes and by social security. A dollar of compensation paid as health insurance, in contrast, is not taxed. For a typical worker, the marginal tax rate from these three sources combined is about 30 percent. Thus if the employees of a company (or the companies' owners) collectively decide they want to spend less on health insurance and receive more in wages, their net income will rise by only $0.70 for each dollar of health benefits they forego. The result is a blunting of the incentives to seek out lower cost health plans.

Throughout the private sector, pre-existing condition restrictions limit the ability of insured people to change plans. Up to two-thirds of conventional insurance policies have restrictions on pre-existing conditions, as do most preferred provider organizations and point-of-service plans.

In public programs—particularly medicare—the situation is even worse. Medicare offers very few alternative plans, and beneficiaries receive none of the savings from choosing a lower-cost plan. As a result, fewer than 10 percent of medicare enrollees are in managed care, compared with more than half of persons with private insurance. The result of this antiquated system, evidenced in recent years in particular, is more rapid cost growth in the public sector than in the private sector (see figure 11-1).

The key to cost savings, therefore, is to use individual choice to make insurance markets more competitive. I propose four steps.

—Reform 1: Convert medicare into a choice-based system. To begin, I would establish regional pools for the medicare population, probably by state. Health plans would be encouraged to bid for medicare beneficiaries. Plans would have to take all beneficiaries who wanted to join (guaranteed issue) and would have to renew anyone who wanted to do so (guaranteed renewability). Initially, older elderly persons (age seventy and older) would be exempt from entering the pool. Over time, however, all medicare beneficiaries would be in the pool.

Premiums would vary by age, sex, and state. The government would contribute a fixed amount for each beneficiary. In the first year, the amount would be such that the individual contribution for the lowest-cost plan (the premium plus expected out-of-pocket payments) equals current average spending for medicare premiums and out-of-pocket expenses.

As an example, suppose that persons use $4,000 of services paid for by medicare and $800 of services that they pay for out of pocket. They also pay $500 for Part B premiums, for a total of $1,300 in individual

Figure 11-1. *Growth of Health Costs per Enrollee*

Percent real growth per enrollee per year

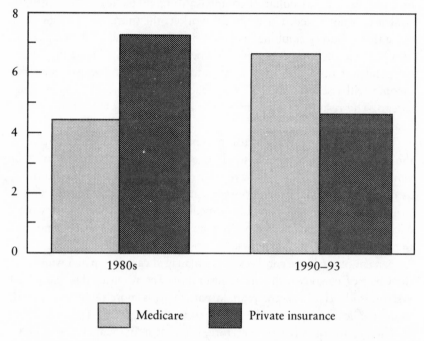

Medicare   Private insurance

Source: Author's calculations based on Katharine R. Levit and others, "National Health Spending Trends, 1961–1993," *Health Affairs*, vol. 13 (Winter 1994), pp. 14–31.

contributions. Now suppose that the low-cost plan is a health maintenance organization (HMO), with a premium of $3,900 (and thus $900 in total savings) and no cost sharing. The government contribution would be $2,600—the low-cost premium less current individual spending. If beneficiaries wanted to choose instead the plan they now belong to, they would need to pay the $1,400 additional premium, plus the expected out-of-pocket expenses of $800. Holding constant the beneficiary's spending for the lowest-cost plan automatically allocates any efficiency savings to the government.[12]

Over time, the government contribution would be indexed to the growth of average premiums, so that beneficiaries on average would pay the same share of total plan costs. Of course, if the government needs to cut medicare spending in the future, reducing the guaranteed payment would be one natural way to do so. I suspect that if indexation is the default, however, limiting the amount of indexation will only be done after considerable debate, as with social security cost-of-living increases.

This plan has several advantages. First, individual choice should promote efficiency, and these savings will directly reduce governmental savings. Second, this system offers medicare eligibles new benefits without substantial new spending. Because managed care plans generally cover prescription drugs, people who choose a managed care plan would receive additional covered services.

A choice-based system also seems more promising than other medicare reforms. In recent years medicare has cut costs by denying providers' increases in their fees. The fact that providers respond to these fee cuts by increasing the amount of services they perform reduces the efficiency of this form of cost containment. Indeed, the future of medicare with continued fee reductions is ever-lower prices, ever-higher utilization, and continuing budget problems. This is not a realistic option.

Increasing premiums for higher-income medicare beneficiaries is a second common proposal. Such fee increases may in fact be good social policy. Indeed, the choice-based system increases premiums for the average medicare beneficiary. Just increasing premiums, however, does nothing to reduce health spending. Rather, it just transfers to medicare beneficiaries costs that the government now bears. The choice-based system also encourages overall reductions in health costs.

Extending the diagnosis-related group (DRG) system by bundling outpatient and postacute care is the proposal most consistent with the choice-based idea. Indeed, the choice-based system extends bundling to the entire patient for the whole year. Because bundling at the hospital level creates numerous opportunities for care substitution—for example, movements into outpatient surgery and upcoding of DRGs—I prefer bundling at the patient level. Furthermore, by letting people keep the savings from choosing low-cost providers, the choice-based system creates additional mechanisms for reductions in health costs. Just extending DRGs, in contrast, does not allow patients to keep cost savings. For these reasons, I prefer the choice-based system.

Choice-based systems have traditionally raised three concerns.[13] The first is that quality will suffer. However, evidence suggests that this concern is baseless. Many studies in the private sector agree, as noted above, that managed care does not worsen outcomes. And the federal government could collect outcome data and monitor program quality. Finally, it is important to remember that the future of medicare without reform is ever-larger reductions in fees and less ability on the part of providers to shift losses to other payers. This development may have quality implications on its own.

The second concern is the possibility of risk selection by insurers. If insurers know that some medicare beneficiaries are healthy and others are sick, they will try to select the healthy and repel the sick. Risk selection may be more attractive to health plans than managing care more efficiently. I would attempt to limit risk selection by adjusting premiums according to age and sex and implementing more general risk adjustment methods.[14] Creating a risk pool for very high-cost cases, funded by a tax on all plans, would also help to limit risk selection. Although risk selection can be managed, it cannot be eliminated. Fundamentally, a choice-based system must have some selection. This selection is a necessary trade-off in achieving the cost savings resulting from individual choice.

Third, a choice-based system will cause some income redistribution. The most obvious source of this redistribution is between those with higher and lower incomes. If the government payment were the same for all medicare beneficiaries, those with low incomes would face a greater burden in purchasing the same level of care as those with higher incomes. Accordingly, some subsidies to low-income medicare beneficiaries should be provided to enable them to choose more expensive policies. These subsidies should be independent of the actual health plan chosen, however.[15]

—Reform 2: Open the FEHBP to small companies and individuals. My second reform proposal would allow small companies and individuals more opportunities to choose health plans. Small companies and individuals should be encouraged to join pools with other small groups and purchase jointly to achieve the economies of scale and choices that larger companies enjoy. Indeed, the pool for federal workers (FEHBP) is a natural pool that these groups could be allowed to join.

Expanding the FEHBP to include other groups would be relatively simple. Plans in each area that meet minimum conditions would be allowed to enter the pool. Guaranteed issue and renewability would be required. To reduce adverse selection, premiums would be based on age and sex. Further, separate rates would be established for government workers, workers in small companies, and individuals. In this way, each group would be shielded from adverse selection in the other two. There would be risk adjustment across plans.

Some analysts suggest going even further: encouraging employers to drop insurance coverage entirely and letting individuals join whatever pools they see fit.[16] In the current environment, however, risk selection and adverse selection dominate the individual market. As a result, dramatically expanded nongroup purchase might not lead to efficient outcomes. Establishing a framework in which individuals can buy adequate insurance seems a prerequisite to encouraging substantial nongroup purchase. My proposal should lead to a better-functioning nongroup market.

Others have suggested that just opening purchasing pools, without additional reforms, will not be enough.[17] Companies with healthy workers, for example, generally will be able to get lower rates outside of the FEHBP than in it. Furthermore, if someone becomes sick, the company may be able to join the pool at that point. Other insurance reforms—including more general rating restrictions—thus may be needed. It seems easier to start with the small steps, however, and evaluate how they work rather than to think that only implementing a major leap can be accomplished.

—Reform 3: Eliminate pre-existing condition restrictions for people who are changing policies. A third proposal is to reduce the barriers to plan mobility created by pre-existing condition restrictions. These restrictions limit the ability of workers to choose less expensive insurance and thus limit insurers' incentives to compete for these persons. Such restrictions do serve some purpose, however, in making it harder for people to delay purchasing coverage until they become sick. Accordingly, I would eliminate the exclusions only for people changing policies and would allow insurers to impose some exclusions on people who seek insurance after a period without it. Similar rules would be imposed on the FEHBP and other health purchasing groups or alliances.[18]

—Reform 4: Cap or eliminate the favorable tax treatment of health insurance. The final issue in cost reform is changing the tax treatment of health insurance. Employer payments for health insurance are not taxed as income to workers, nor are individual payments made through so-called cafeteria plans. As a result, a person who chooses less expensive health insurance will receive less as savings than they gave up in health insurance. Similarly, the workers in a company that chooses to provide less expensive health insurance but higher wages will not receive all of these savings as additional income. The result is less intensive cost containment, more generous insurance, and higher health spending.[19]

The solution to this problem is easy: limit the tax exclusion by capping the amount of employer payments that are tax preferred and eliminating employees' ability to pay for health insurance with pretax dollars. I would set the cap nationally: for example, $1,500 for an individual policy and $3,750 for a family policy. The cap would be indexed at the rate of general price inflation but would not rise with any additional health care cost increases.

Opposition to tax caps typically centers on two issues. The first is regional equity. Because health costs vary dramatically by region, equity would require regional variation in the exclusion amount. Regional caps are difficult to enforce, however. This point seems to me naive. The cost of living is higher in New York than in Mississippi, and yet taxes are the same for persons with the same income in the two states. Similarly, estimates of the poverty population do not take into account regional price disparities, and yet federal benefits for many programs depend on the size of the poverty population. Thus the argument for adjusting health exclusions by region does not seem compelling.

A more serious criticism is that this proposal may induce some employers to stop providing health insurance. The current tax subsidy undoubtedly encourages some employers to offer insurance who otherwise would not and some people to take insurance when they otherwise would not. There are several answers to this concern. One answer is to set a high exclusion amount to minimize the loss in coverage. The key issue for economic incentives is that marginal spending on insurance be subject to taxation, while the subsidy that encourages employers to offer insurance depends on the average amount of the exclusion. By setting the cap reasonably high, marginal incentives for cost-conscious purchase of insurance are preserved, with only small effects on the total value of the subsidy. A second answer is that if the reforms work as intended and costs are lower than they otherwise would have been, it will be easier for people to afford insurance after the tax cap is imposed. Thus total coverage may not fall by nearly as much as simple estimates suggest.

Addressing Cost Growth

Historically, real per capita health care costs have grown more than twice as fast as real per capita income. As long as cost growth is so high, financing problems in the public and private sectors are inescapable.

Many are skeptical that the reforms noted above will lower the growth rate of health costs.[20] Economic research strongly suggests that the growth of health costs is attributable to technological change in the practice of medicine—new and better devices and drugs, and the diffusion of existing treatments to new patients.[21] If technological change is a result of exogenous factors such as general scientific advance, it will not be amenable to changes in tax policy, insurance competition, or other market-based incentives.

On the other hand, technological change may respond to the economic environment. Weak competition in insurance markets, for example, may encourage doctors to adopt new procedures readily or pharmaceutical companies to develop expensive new treatments.[22] And, perhaps more important, even if the same technologies are ultimately made available, reform of insurance markets could help limit the application of these technologies to only cases where the benefits are greater than the costs.

Unfortunately, empirical evidence on how various reforms will impact the development and diffusion of new technologies is only anecdotal. My own sense is that the cost reforms outlined above will affect the growth rate of health costs. Although medical progress undoubtedly will bring new technologies at very high cost, better economic incentives could limit the diffusion of low-valued technologies or increase the diffusion of cost-reducing technologies throughout the health care system. Thus I would not deal separately with the issue of cost growth beyond enacting the reforms.

The issue of cost growth does reinforce the conclusion, however, that implementing incentives for cost containment is essential. If cost reform could reduce resource waste, both at any time and over time, the social cost of not enacting these reforms is enormous. Even if no other reform is possible, a more effective market in health care delivery could yield large benefits.

Improving Health Outcomes

The second structural reform is implementing measures to improve the health of Americans. Americans are rightly amazed and saddened by their health outcomes. On most measures of health, the United States ranks at or near the bottom of the other countries in the Organization for Economic Cooperation and Development.[23]

Coverage expansions are generally promoted as the best way to improve health outcomes. Indeed, empirical evidence suggests that the uninsured are less likely than the insured to receive care and are more likely to die in the hospital.[24]

Nevertheless, coverage expansions are not the best way to improve health, for several reasons. First, the cost of such expansions is extremely high. When the uninsured receive health insurance subsidies, the insured with the same income must receive subsidies as well. Among people with incomes between 100 percent and 200 percent of poverty, two people have insurance for each one that does not.[25] Thus the "target efficiency" of subsidies in this range is at best one-third, and the subsidy cost will be very high relative to the increase in coverage.

Second, since health care costs are rising faster than incomes, subsidy costs grow faster than income too. Ideally, a coverage expansion would be funded through revenues growing at the rate of cost growth (for example, the added revenues from a cap on the exclusion of employer-financed premiums). These sources are scarce, however.

Third, coverage expansions often fail to encourage appropriate preventive care. A study in Tennessee, for example, found that increasing the share of women who could receive medicaid coverage for prenatal care did not improve health outcomes. Instead, hospitals just signed women up for medicaid when they came in to give birth. As a result, spending increased without improving health.[26] This result is not universal; other evidence suggests that medicaid expansions have improved health outcomes.[27]

Finally, even if the goal is to provide more medical care to the uninsured, increased insurance coverage may not be the way to do it. Alternatives such as school-based health care and expanded outlays on such programs as Women, Infants, and Children and Head Start may be much more cost effective than expanded insurance coverage. Sufficient resources to pay for everything are unavailable. I suspect that among the available options, subsidies for insurance rank relatively low. In this light, the now-recurrent calls to cut back on these public health programs gives me great concern.

Rather than devote resources to expanded insurance coverage, I believe the best way to improve health is to change social policy rather than medical policy. More than two-thirds of higher infant mortality rates in the United States compared with rates in other countries, for example, is attributable to a greater prevalence of low-weight births rather than a higher mortality rate conditional on birthweight.[28] Low birthweight is largely a result of poor social conditions, not of a lack of medical care. Focusing on social factors influencing health outcomes may therefore be the most important health policy. Indeed, Victor Fuchs has argued that the cigarette tax in the Clinton plan would have accomplished more than universal coverage would have to promote health.[29]

—Reform 5: A rather simple proposal to improve the health of Americans would be to tax sins against good health. The best way is to tax the instruments of sin: cigarettes, alcohol, firearms, and bullets. More specifically, I would increase the tax on each of these items and index the rates.

Sin taxes improve health.[30] Doubling the price of cigarettes would cut smoking of adults about 30 percent and 50 percent among teenagers. Taxation of alcohol, beer in particular, cuts alcohol use and lowers motor vehicle fatalities. One estimate suggests that if alcohol taxes had remained at their 1951 value in real terms, there would be 5,000 fewer motor vehicle fatalities annually.[31] Although no estimates have been made of the health benefits of taxes on firearms or bullets, if these too respond to price, taxes would improve health outcomes.

In many cases, taxes can also be justified on efficiency grounds. If people do not know the true risks of smoking or drinking, for example, discouraging these activities through taxation will help to reduce unwanted consumption. In other cases, the costs that these users impose on others—through higher insurance premiums, auto fatalities, or second-hand smoke—may justify increased taxation.[32]

If we tax cigarettes, why not fat and cholesterol as well? And why not subsidize bran? I am not opposed to any of these measures. The medical case to be made against smoking, drinking, firearms and bullets, however, is far greater than for other products. It seems sensible to start with the most egregious items first and then worry about the rest. I have no illusions that sin taxes will dramatically improve the welfare of Americans. Then again, I have no illusions that coverage expansions will, either. If we want to improve health, however, it pays to start with that which we do to ourselves, rather than that which we would have to do for others.

Notes

1. *Economic Report of the President, February 1994.*

2. More discussion of these issues is in David M. Cutler, "The Cost and Financing of Health Care," *American Economic Review*, vol. 85 (May 1995), pp. 32–37.

3. Victor R. Fuchs and James S. Hahn, "How Does Canada Do It?: A Comparison of Expenditures for Physicians' Services in the United States and Canada," *New England Journal of Medicine*, vol. 323 (September 27, 1990), pp. 884–90. There are no estimates available of how much of this 30 percent differential is attributable to more highly trained physicians in the United States.

4. A summary of the evidence on this question is in Health Care Financing Administration, "Medicare Program: Fee Schedule for Physicians' Services, Proposed Rule," *Federal Register*, vol. 56 (June 1991), pp. 25792–978.

5. Not all administrative costs are wasteful. Some administrative costs (monitoring doctors' incomes and practices; checking for fraudulent bills) may lower total costs or improve the quality of care, some measures do both.

6. Mark Chassin and others, "Does Inappropriate Use Explain Geographic Variations in the Use of Health Care Services?" *Journal of the American Medical Association*, vol. 258 (November 1987), pp. 2533–37; Constance M. Winslow and others, "The Appropriateness of Carotid Endarterectomy," *New England Journal of Medicine*, vol. 318 (March 24, 1988), pp. 721–27; Constance M. Winslow and others, "The Appropriateness of Performing Coronary Artery Bypass Surgery," *Journal of the American Medical Association*, vol. 260 (July 22, 1988), pp. 505–09; and Allan M. Greenspan and others, "Incidence of Unwarranted Implantation of Permanent Cardiac Pacemakers in a Large Medical Population," *New England Journal of Medicine*, vol. 318 (January 21, 1988), pp. 158–63.

7. Mark McClellan, Barbara J. McNeil, and Joseph P. Newhouse, "Does More Intensive Treatment of Acute Myocardial Infarction in the Elderly Reduce Mortality?" *Journal of the American Medical Association*, vol. 272 (September 1994), pp. 859–66.

8. Robert H. Miller and Harold S. Luft, "Managed Care Plan Performance Since 1980," *Journal of the American Medical Association*, vol. 271 (May 18, 1994), pp. 1512–19.

9. Alan Garber, Victor Fuchs, and James Silverman, "Case Mix, Costs and Outcomes," *New England Journal of Medicine*, vol. 310 (May 1984), pp. 231–37.

10. David M. Cutler, "The Incidence of Adverse Medical Outcomes under Prospective Payment," *Econometrica*, vol. 63 (January 1995), pp. 29–50; and Douglas Staiger and Gary Gaumer, "The Impact of Financial Pressure on Quality of Care in Hospitals: Post-Admission Mortality under Medicare's Prospective Payment System," mimeo, 1990.

11. Alain C. Enthoven, "Why Managed Care Has Failed to Contain Health Costs," *Health Affairs*, vol. 12 (Fall 1993), pp. 27–43; and Jack Zwanziger and Glenn Melnick, "The Effects of Hospital Competition and the Medicare PPS Program on Hospital Cost Behavior in California," *Journal of Health Economics*, vol. 7 (December 1988), pp. 301–20.

12. Some of the $900 in total savings could be given to the beneficiary by increasing the government contribution.

13. Paul B. Ginsburg and Glenn M. Hackbarth, "A Private Health Plan Option Strategy for Medicare" (Santa Monica, Calif.: Rand, July 1987).

14. For more discussion, see Joseph P. Newhouse, "Patients at Risk: Health Reform and Risk Adjustment," *Health Affairs*, vol. 13 (Spring I 1994), pp. 132–46.

15. Ideally, subsidies would be given on the basis of lifetime income (as with social security benefits) rather than annual income.

16. See, for example, Stuart Butler's contribution to this volume.

17. See, for example, Paul Starr, "Design of Health Insurance Purchasing Cooperatives," *Health Affairs*, vol. 12 (Supplement 1993), pp. 58–64.

18. Potentially, limitations of pre-existing condition restrictions could be waived only for those moving between similar policies, so that individuals could not buy a very limited policy just to qualify for more comprehensive coverage without restrictions. One way to accomplish this would be to have a minimum that guaranteed the right to unrestricted changes.

19. Mark V. Pauly, "Taxation, Health Insurance, and Market Failure in the Medical Economy," *Journal of Economic Literature,* vol. 24 (June 1986), pp. 629–75.

20. William B. Schwartz, "In the Pipeline: A Wave of Valuable Medical Technology," *Health Affairs,* vol. 13 (Summer 1994), pp. 70–79.

21. Joseph P. Newhouse, "Medical Care Costs: How Much Welfare Loss?" *Journal of Economic Perspectives,* vol. 6 (Summer 1992), pp. 3–21; and Henry Aaron, *Serious and Unstable Condition* (Brookings, 1991).

22. Burton Weisbrod, "The Health Care Quadrilemma," *Journal of Economic Literature,* vol. 29 (June 1991), pp. 523–52.

23. George J. Schieber, Jean-Pierre Poullier, and Leslie M. Greenwald, "Health Spending, Delivery, and Outcomes in OECD Countries," *Health Affairs,* vol. 12 (Summer 1993), pp. 120–29.

24. Mark B. Wenneker, Joel S. Weissman, and Arnold M. Epstein, "The Association of Payer with Utilization of Cardiac Procedures in Massachusetts," *Journal of the American Medical Association,* vol. 264 (September 12, 1990), pp. 1255–60; and Jack Hadley, Earl P. Steinberg, and Judith Feder, "Comparison of Uninsured and Privately Insured Hospital Patients," *Journal of the American Medical Association,* vol. 265 (January 16, 1991), pp. 374–79.

25. Employee Benefit Research Institute, *Sources of Health Insurance and Characteristics of the Uninsured* (Washington: EBRI, January 1994).

26. Joyce M. Piper, Wayne A. Ray, and Marie R. Griffin, "Effects of Medicaid Eligibility Expansion on Prenatal Care and Pregnancy Outcomes in Tennessee," *Journal of the American Medical Association,* vol. 264 (November 7, 1990), pp. 2219–23.

27. Janet Currie and Jonathan Gruber, "Saving Babies: The Efficacy and Cost of Recent Expansions of Medicaid Eligibility for Pregnant Women," Working Paper 4644 (Cambridge, Mass.: National Bureau of Economic Research, 1994).

28. Korbin Liu and others, "International Infant Mortality Rankings: A Look behind the Numbers," *Health Care Financing Review,* vol. 13 (Summer 1992), pp. 105–18; and Allen Wilcox and others, "Birth Weight and Perinatal Mortality: A Comparison of the United States and Norway," *Journal of the American Medical Association,* vol. 273 (March 1, 1995), pp. 709–11.

29. Victor R. Fuchs, "The Clinton Plan: A Researcher Examines Reform," *Health Affairs,* vol. 13 (Spring I 1994), pp. 102–14.

30. Frank J. Chaloupka, "Public Policies and Private Anti-Health Behaviors," *American Economic Review,* vol. 85 (May 1995), pp. 45–49; and Michael Grossman and others, "Policy Watch: Alcohol and Cigarette Taxes," *Journal of Economic Perspectives,* vol. 7 (Fall 1993), pp. 211–22.

31. Frank J. Chaloupka, Henry Saffer, and Michael Grossman, "Alcohol Control Policies and Motor Vehicle Fatalities," *Journal of Legal Studies,* vol. 22 (January 1993), pp. 161–86.

32. There is some debate about this in the case of cigarettes. For alcohol taxes, the externality benefits alone suggest higher taxes. See Willard G. Manning and others, *The Costs of Poor Health Habits: A Rand Study* (Harvard University Press, 1991).

CHAPTER TWELVE

Bite-Sized Chunks of Health Care Reform—Where Medicare Fits In

Gail R. Wilensky

AFTER spending two years discussing the "big bang" of health care reform—reform that simultaneously would have changed the rules governing insurance for the private sector, the conditions under which employers contribute to health insurance for their employees, the way employees purchase health insurance for themselves and their families, how governments support low-income families, medical education, public hospitals, and other "essential" providers, plus a myriad of other changes—the nation seems clearly, though reluctantly, to have recognized that health care reform will occur the way most other legislative changes happen in this country, piecemeal and incrementally. It may seem ironic that formally legislated reforms almost always occur in a slow deliberative manner, while the private sector brings change tumultuously. Nonetheless, incremental changes to the medicare program are inescapable because of the financial problems that program faces. These changes should be done in a way that supports and augments the changes occurring in private insurance for other Americans.

Medicare: Large, Popular, and Growing

Medicare is the world's largest insurance company and has been one of this country's most popular programs. Congress enacted it in 1965 to provide coverage for the aged and later expanded it to cover the disabled and patients with end-stage renal disease. In 1994, 32 million beneficiaries are aged, 3.5 million are disabled, and about 75,000 are on the ESRD program.[1]

Medicare is popular for several reasons. First and foremost, medicare has fulfilled its original mission well. Medicare was enacted to increase and extend access to care for the elderly. Before 1965, the elderly experienced great difficulties purchasing insurance and receiving adequate and appropriate health care. This problem was most serious for the elderly poor, but even those elderly with adequate income found it hard to buy insurance.

Congress designed medicare to mimic the prevailing structure of health care financing in 1965, typified by the reimbursement arrangements used by the Blue Cross and Blue Shield plans. Medicare is generally regarded as having accomplished this fundamental objective exceedingly well, some might even say too well.

Medicare is popular not only because it fulfilled its mission, but also because it places few restraints on the elderly as consumers of health care. With few exceptions, mostly concerning coinsurance payments for hospital care after ninety days of care, medicare payments are open-ended and come with few restraints on the elderly. They enjoy substantially free choice about which physicians to use, which hospitals to enter, and which home care providers to employ. Medicare beneficiaries have little reason to care about what their care costs and face little or no pressure to seek cost-effective providers or cost-efficient health care plans. The more than 85 percent of the elderly with either private insurance or medicaid eligibility escape most of the remaining financial pressure from medicare's deductibles or coinsurance. Although some concerns have been raised about potential future problems of access to physicians as a result of medicare payment levels, no evidence to date suggests that beneficiaries are yet having any systematic problems securing access to care under medicare.

The Need for Reform

Medicare has some major weaknesses and is in serious need of reform. The most important concern is financing. In the short term, medicare spending acts as a major drain on the budget and therefore exacerbates the deficit. In the longer term, medicare hospital insurance is not financially viable, and its future fiscal insolvency raises serious questions about the nature and design of a program that will be sustainable for the twenty-first century.

Hospital Insurance (HI) is funded through the HI trust fund. According to the Congressional Budget Office (CBO) March 1995 baseline estimates, spending on benefits financed through the HI trust fund will grow at an annual average of 8.8 percent between 1995 and 2000. Hospital spending is projected to grow at 5.8 percent, but the other services are projected to grow much faster. Spending on home health services is projected to grow 26 percent from 1994 to 1995, slowing to a comparatively lower 9 percent annual growth by the end of the decade. Spending on skilled nursing facilities, also projected to grow 26 percent from 1994 to 1995, is projected to moderate to 8 percent annual growth by the end of the decade.[2]

The HI trust fund is running out of money. Using intermediate actuarial assumptions, which some consider optimistic, the latest HI board of trustees report projects that the trust fund will be bankrupt in the year 2002 and that the imbalance between revenues and cost will grow rapidly thereafter. Under current projections, for example, by the year 2020 HI trust fund spending is projected to be more than double the income. General revenues pay for about three-quarters of the cost of part B, the portion of medicare that pays for physicians' benefits and other outpatient services. Premium payments from the elderly cover the remaining one-quarter. Part B poses a different set of problems from those facing part A. Part B is draining the federal budget. According to CBO estimates, part B spending will grow 10.9 percent in 1995 and 12 percent or slightly more annually over the remainder of the decade. Even growth of spending for the physician component, which is projected to run at slightly less than 6 percent in 1995, is projected to run between 9 percent and 12 percent a year throughout the rest of the decade. Growth rates for durable medical equipment, laboratories, outpatient hospital spending, and other part B spending are projected to be even higher.

At a time when hints are appearing that spending in the private sector may be slowing, medicare spending continues to grow at more than 10 percent annually. Between 1983 and 1991, medicare spending grew more slowly than spending did in the private sector. But since 1991, spending in medicare has grown substantially faster than that in the private sector, 6.5 percent versus 4.7 percent growth in real spending, per capita. The difference appears to be even larger for 1993–94, although most of the data for this period remains preliminary. According to the latest CBO estimates, private expenditures grew about 5 percent in 1994, while those of medicare outlays grew more than 10 percent. Some evidence suggests that private spending, or at least some segments of it, may have slowed down even more than the CBO projections suggest.[3] A recent Foster-Higgins National Survey of Employers study indicated, for example, that for all companies, health care premiums declined 1.1 percent, with the decline being largest for large companies, −1.9 percent.[4] Another indication comes from the changes in the consumer price index. In 1994 the medical component of the consumer price index rose 4.9 percent as opposed to 2.7 percent for the entire CPI. What this means is that for the first time in a long while the MCPI is less than twice the overall CPI, and a substantial proportion of the upward pressure is coming from medicare and medicaid. Whether these indications of even greater differentials in spending rates between medicare and the private sector are true and continue is something that only the future will determine, but that total medicare spending has been growing at least 50 percent faster than private sector spending since 1990 is fact.

This outcome should not be surprising. Medicare is primarily *á la carte* fee-for-service medicine with government-administered pricing and a volume control on physicians. The payment system encourages hospitals to game the way inpatient admissions are coded and to encourage increased hospital admissions. It rewards physicians for doing more even when less care may be better care. It offers few incentives to beneficiaries to seek cost-effective providers or to their physicians or medical suppliers to limit the spending. Increased spending on hospital outpatient services, clinical lab procedures, home health care, and skilled nursing facilities has been a particular problem, but moderating spending on physician services has also been difficult. An individual physician's behavior has little bearing on the change in fees for that individual physician. Rather, the fees are determined by the aggregate behavior of all physicians. Rates of growth are differentiated only according to whether doctors are in primary care, a nonsurgical specialty, or surgery. As a result, the system provides no rewards for physicians who practice cost-efficient and prudent medicine.

In this third-party-financed, fee-for-service world, policy can slow growth of spending in only four ways: by reducing prices (and guarding against volume increases); by tying price changes to spending targets; by increasing deductibles and co-pays; and by controlling access to providers and technology.

Medicare has relied primarily on the first three, and this country has shown little interest in using the fourth. No one should be surprised that direct controls can moderate spending for a few years (particularly when compared with a passive private sector), or that this moderating force dissipates after a short time.

Present Structure of Medicare

Despite all of the changes occurring in the private sector, medicare continues to remain a fee-for-service program, with limited availability of and participation in managed care. Projections indicate that 2.5 million medicare beneficiaries, or 6.6 percent of all enrollees, will enroll in health maintenance organizations in 1995. Medicare HMO enrollment has grown rapidly over the last few years relative to that of the nonmedicare population, but that is because the base was so small.

Several reasons explain why so few medicare beneficiaries choose managed care. First, medicare subsidizes the main competitors to HMOs. Fee-for-service medigap plans receive no direct subsidy but are implicitly subsidized because they eliminate medicare's cost-sharing. Employer-provided supplemental insurance is subsidized this way and also because it is provided tax free to the beneficiary. In addition, medicare's method of paying HMOs has been flawed. Inadequate adjustment for risk appears to have produced overpayments to some HMOs and probably underpayments to others. This flaw explains why the Health Care Financing Administration (HCFA) appears to have saved little and may have experienced increased costs because of HMO growth, although that finding has been subject to some dispute. Of greater relevance is the substantial variation in payment levels between counties and the substantial year-to-year variation in payments. Questions have been raised about the accuracy of HMO payments in terms of component measurements and about the effects of a potential "spillover" on medicare from having a large HMO enrollment in the nonmedicare population.

The most significant deterrent to growth of managed care, however, is the paucity of non-HMO managed care options currently available to the medicare population, the very population that most needs and probably most desires flexibility. Medicare Select, a Preferred Provider Organization (PPO) offering, was limited to offerings to fifteen states, with a three-year sunset provision. That authority is in the process of being renegotiated, but its need for reauthorization reflects the difficulty that managed care plans have had within the medicare framework. Point-of-service plans, which allow patients to opt out of their network and choose other physicians or facilities, are not currently allowed. Risk-based "carve-outs," like the package price heart bypass demonstration, are also not allowed except on a demonstration basis. And HMO group-only contracts that would permit employers to establish an HMO/Complete

Medical Plan, which enrolls only their own retirees who are medicare beneficiaries, are also not allowed.

If the medicare program is to increase managed care enrollment significantly, the first requirement must be to make available the more varied and flexible options that are available in the private sector. But availability will probably not suffice. To see substantial growth in managed care, it will also be necessary to change the incentives facing the elderly.

Goals and Strategies for a Reformed Medicare Program

Changing a popular program is always difficult, and changing a popular program involving the elderly is especially difficult because the income of the elderly and disabled is generally set and because they can not easily respond to new incentives or rules. This means that political support for medicare reform must be strong, and the goals and strategies for accomplishing the goals must be clear. I believe that these goals should include at least the following: increasing consumer choice for beneficiaries; providing incentives for accessible, high-quality, patient-oriented care; encouraging cost-conscious decisionmaking; incorporating the innovative, cost-reducing delivery system reforms from the private sector into the medicare program; and restoring fiscal solvency of the medicare program.

To achieve these goals it will be necessary to change medicare's incentives, to expand the options available to beneficiaries, and to provide them with the information needed to make informed choices. Ultimately, beneficiaries should reap tangible benefits from choosing more cost-effective health care. Physicians and hospitals should gain from providing cost-effective medicine. And federal payment formulas should share the savings that an aggressive reorganization of health care can produce.

I believe that the use of a better-designed adjusted average per capita cost (AAPCC) payment, the payment currently used for reimbursing HMOs, could become the basis of a voucher or medicare certificate that would encourage cost-effective choices. To make this transformation, several steps are necessary. One is to redesign the determinants of the AAPCC to make it more stable and to take better account of the risk selection that appears to occur. A second is to open up more choices toward which that payment can be made. Varying the amount of the payment with the income or wealth of the beneficiary may prove appropriate or desirable, thus transforming medicare into an income-related

voucher or payment. I recommend several specific changes. First, medicare select, the preferred provider payment system, should be available
in all fifty states. Second, this program should include point-of-service
plans and allow partial capitation or risk-based "carve-out" plans. Third,
the capitation rate should be refined and revised by breaking the link to
fee-for-service spending by experimenting with basing medicare's contribution on competitively bid premiums, which amount would define medicare's contribution for fee-for-service plans as well, and finally by experimenting with alternative calculations of the capitation payment for areas
that can't support competitive bids. Fourth, medicare should institute
annual open enrollment periods for all changes in medicare-related policies; this policy would end the thirty-day disenrollment policy for
HMOs. Fifth, medicare should discontinue the 50/50 rule for HMOs
serving medicare beneficiaries. As part of this change HMOs should be
required to provide outcome-based reports plus consumer satisfaction
measures and make this information available to all potential enrollees.
Finally, HMOs should be permitted to price underneath the medicare
payment and rebate savings to beneficiaries (and share savings with the
government).

These changes would substantially increase the availability of managed care to medicare beneficiaries, remove provisions that inhibit managed care growth, and, provide some incentives to choose the more cost-
effective health care plans. To the extent that medicare payments are set
at the price of the "lowest cost plan" in an area or determined by the
difference between the lowest- and the average-cost plan, medicare would
encourage beneficiaries to choose cost-effective health care plans that
meet their needs and demands, which may or may not turn out to be
managed care plans.

In the short term, budget pressures will influence medicare policy. Some budget-cutting policies are consistent with the move to an
incentive-based system, some are neutral, and some would move medicare in the wrong direction. Which changes are made will have important
ramifications for the long run. For example, adding a 10 percent coinsurance for home health, or a fixed copayment for rehab hospital admissions, would raise some additional revenues, lower utilization of these
services, and make managed care options more attractive. So would
"bundling" payments for hospitalization and postacute care services.
Capitating the areas of part A that have been growing very rapidly and
will continue to grow more rapidly than the remainder of part A will
also increase the attractiveness of managed care plans that cover these

components and discourage their use in the fee-for-service world. Reducing payments to indirect medical education or direct medical education would be neutral with respect to its effect on the choice of the elderly regarding cost-effective health care plans, although it will obviously affect academic health centers and teaching hospitals. But large reductions in overall physician fees could cause physicians to increase volume, offsetting the savings and exacerbating the divisions between fee-for-service and at-risk medical practice.

I believe it is possible to accommodate the need for short-term budget policy while setting the stage for the more fundamental change in the incentives, information, and options that are needed to reform medicare. Since it will take some time to realize the gains from restructuring and reforming medicare, it is important that these reforms be started as soon as possible.

Notes

1. *1995 Annual Report of the Board of Trustees of the Federal Hospital Insurance Fund.*
2. Congressional Budget Office, fact sheet, Washington, March 1995 baseline.
3. Ibid.
4. *1994 National Survey of Employer-Sponsored Health Plans* (New York: Foster Higgins and Co., April 1995).

CHAPTER THIRTEEN

Using Tax Credits for Health Insurance and Medical Savings Accounts

Mark V. Pauly and John C. Goodman

W ITH the demise of efforts for large-scale health care reform, policymakers have turned their attention to incremental reforms. A reform of particular interest is the use of the tax system to encourage the purchase of insurance coverage and the creation of medical savings accounts (MSAs). We outline a proposal to combine these devices in a way that strengthens the acceptability and desirability of catastrophic insurance coverage, structures MSAs so that they do not distort incentives, and avoids individual or employer mandates.

The generic objectives of our proposal are efficiency and equity. Efficiency does not necessarily mean less medical spending; it means that each dollar citizens spend on medical services generates benefits that exceed costs. One way to promote efficiency is to make sure that individuals' incentives are not distorted. Thus beyond encouraging access to a basic level of medical care, public policy should be neutral, neither encouraging nor discouraging medical insurance or out-of-pocket medical spending relative to the consumption of other goods, or savings. Equity is more difficult to define. We assume that people with the same income should be treated the same. Many people also believe in helping low-income people more than higher-income people. But this objective usually reduces efficiency because redistribution almost always distorts incentives.[1] We propose alternatives that limit this distortion.

Problems with the Current System of Financing Private Insurance

The current tax system in the United States offers tax advantages to people who obtain their insurance in connection with employment, by excluding compensation that employers pay as fringe benefits from federal income and payroll taxation. This exclusion creates two kinds of distortions. First, the system favors the financing of medical services via insurance and offers a larger tax break the more costly the employer-provided insurance is. This incentive encourages people to devote more of their total compensation to insured medical services, rather than to uninsured services, other consumption, or savings. Second, this subsidy is available only to people whose employers arrange such coverage. It is not available to the nonemployed or people who work for firms that do not provide health insurance.[2] Thus it distorts decisions people make on whether to work, which firm to work for, and whether to work as an employee or as a self-employed person.

The subsidy also violates the principle of horizontal equity, since it offers tax breaks to some people but denies them to others earning the same incomes. Moreover, the value of the exclusion, which rises with a person's marginal tax rate, is greater for higher-income workers than for lower-income workers.

Current tax policy makes it possible for people to reduce their income and payroll taxes if they elect more generous insurance policies. Defenders of the current system sometimes argue that it encourages the purchase of health insurance. However, it is poorly designed for this purpose. It creates no incentive for those who pay no taxes and only very weak incentives for those with low incomes and low marginal tax rates. Thus it is no surprise that such lower-wage families make up a large fraction of the working uninsured. In short, the current tax treatment of insurance biases choices toward insured medical care and away from other consumption or saving and does so unfairly.[3] These problems could be eliminated by repealing the exclusion, taxing employer premium payments as part of employee wages, and using any revenue increase to lower everyone's taxes. However, this tax advantage has substantial political durability.

Analysts therefore have been searching for an alternative policy that does not tackle the tax exclusion head on but instead eliminates some of its most harmful effects without running into a political firestorm. Such a policy would not be as efficient as complete elimination of the exclusion but could still do much good.

In this chapter we propose income-related tax credits for the purchase of combinations of catastrophic coverage and MSAs.[4] Instead of abolishing the current tax advantages, we propose to make a new system that individuals and groups could voluntarily substitute for the existing tax treatment of health insurance. We believe that this plan eliminates many of the distortions caused by a tax subsidy for third-party payment of medical bills and yet prevents the use of MSAs to shelter out-of-pocket spending on medical care. Our plan reduces the likelihood that people will purchase catastrophic coverage with unaffordable deductibles.

Three Policy Goals

We propose to change incentives so that citizens will choose the appropriate level of medical care. To achieve this objective, public policy should encourage people to buy adequate insurance coverage to accumulate sufficient resources to pay for out-of-pocket expenses and provide for fair and efficient financing. These three broad goals are achieved by tax credits fixed in amount for each household based on income to reward those who voluntarily purchase insurance; basic catastrophic insurance coverage to cover the large medical bills that families cannot afford; and MSAs to pay small medical bills and to offer rewards for prudent purchasing decisions.

These three characteristics complement one another. Catastrophic coverage protects against the risk of large medical bills above a deductible. The ability to choose higher deductibles without tax penalty gives families proper incentives to hold down the cost of insurance. Paying small medical bills from one's own resources encourages wise purchases. A way to fund medical expenses below the deductible is to have an earmarked savings account. We propose a tax credit to help people pay for insurance and finance their MSAs. It offers a specific dollar reduction in taxes (or a refund or voucher, if the family owes no taxes) for those families who obtain at least the catastrophic coverage. The tax credit would not increase if people purchased additional insurance coverage or added to their MSAs.

The result would be a decent insurance policy, a spending account to permit rational decisions on out-of-pocket amounts not covered by the policy, and a tax credit to help finance medical care in a nondistortive and fair way. In what follows we explain why these three pieces make possible major gains in extending insurance coverage and slowing the growth of health care spending, offer some examples of how they might work in practice, and predict the impacts of these changes.

Health Insurance: Protecting Resources or Distorting Incentives?

In redesigning tax policy toward medical care, two approaches are open. One is to use tax policy to direct citizens toward types of care or insurance determined by experts or by politicians to be socially appropriate. We specifically reject this approach, because the current knowledge does not permit determination of what medical services or insurance are best for everyone and because a choice as personal as medical care ought to be left up to citizens, not tailored by government. The other approach is to provide citizens with the financial means and the information to make good choices, without distorting their incentives. This approach is more suitable in a democracy that treats voters as adults able to make rational and responsible choices in their personal lives just as they do in the political process.

A premise of this approach is that political decisionmakers must resist the temptation to engineer choices for other citizens even if people sometimes choose unwisely or make choices the decisionmakers would not make. Government policy should ensure that people face prices for insurance and for medical care that reflect true costs.

All third-party insurance contains an inherent distortion that cannot be entirely avoided, but can be contained. Risk-averse consumers demand insurance against the unpredictable cost of medical care, but insured patients need not consider the cost of the services, even though any costs they incur will eventually raise premiums.

To minimize this distortion, one good idea is for people to buy insurance that covers only large medical expenses and permits them to pay-out-of pocket for smaller ones. (The other alternative is managed care, which encourages providers to refuse or discourage low-value services.) People should be able to make their own choices about how much risk they will accept and how much they will transfer to insurance, as long as that exposure does not create unreasonable financial burdens for others or cause moral burdens that might stem from seeing some people go without needed care. The primary social objective here, in our view, is not to discourage people from accepting risk they find tolerable, but instead to help them handle that risk in a way that makes them take costs into account and benefit from efforts to limit those costs. The best way to achieve this objective is to permit people to take catastrophic coverage with relatively high deductibles, but to make it possible for them to finance those payments as efficiently as possible.

MSAs and Catastrophic Insurance

A number of companies and their employees already use individual MSAs to pay medical bills.[5] Under these plans, employees buy catastrophic insurance instead of full-coverage policies and create a special account with after-tax dollars, earmarked to cover expenses below the plan's deductibles. This account means that the family will not have to risk incurring bad debts and defaulting on its obligation to pay for the care received.

With an MSA, even a family of moderate income could tolerate insurance with a substantial deductible, thus holding down the insurance premium they have to pay and the administrative expense associated with small claims. Deductibles that might be judged unacceptable become tolerable cost containment devices when joined to an MSA. Families should be free to decide that they wish to pay for coverage with lower deductibles, for more protection against risk, if that is how they prefer to spend their money. But the combination of an MSA and catastrophic coverage will, we expect, appeal to many. Tax incentives surely should not inhibit them as is now the case.

MSAs have a further administrative and social advantage. No one wishes to encourage the current situation in which an important minority of middle-class families now forgo insurance and must count on the charity of providers and their fellow citizens if they need costly care. Such bad debtors impose a burden on others, either providers or other consumers. Companies that sometimes sell on credit often give discounts to buyers they are sure will pay. Integrating an MSA with a catastrophic policy should also permit insurers administering catastrophic policies to get better prices from providers and transfer this advantage to consumers. A discount for fiscal responsibility should benefit everyone.

People obviously can and should use the funds in their MSAs for their deductibles. We believe they should be able to withdraw unused funds for other purposes at the end of each insurance year. Because this account (like any savings account) can eventually be used for purposes other than medical services, strong and proper incentives would exist to avoid medical services that are not worth their cost. People would be able to finance highly valuable care, but in contrast to the current system they would be deterred from seeking care of low benefit relative to its cost.

The ideal MSA does not distort incentives. The taxes a family pays should be neither higher nor lower if the family chooses an MSA accompanied by catastrophic coverage or a low-deductible managed care plan or low-deductible conventional insurance. Some MSA proposals extend the tax exclusion now limited to employer premium payments to uninsured medical spending made out of MSAs. This removes the distorted incentive to overinsure, but at the risk of offering incentives to overconsume medical services paid out of the MSA.[6] The MSA proposal described below avoids both of these distortions by making a person's taxes (after the MSA is set up) independent of how much he or she deposits in or spends out of an MSA. This is accomplished by designing the program so that MSA deposits come from after-tax dollars, just as do expenditures on health insurance, other current consumption, or other mechanisms for saving and investing.

Tax Incentives and Tax Credits

As noted earlier, the current tax subsidy does not offer well-designed incentives to purchase health insurance. A better subsidy should take the form of a fixed-dollar tax credit, contingent on the purchase of at least basic catastrophic insurance coverage that does not increase when more costly insurance or medical care is purchased.

The tax credit is intended not to encourage any particular form of insurance but an adequate package of savings accounts and insurance coverage. People who purchase benefits above the basic minimum will be paying entirely with their own after-tax income, not shifting the cost of such purchases to others via the Treasury.

The credit is intended to help families set up and maintain an MSA and purchase insurance but is not itself intended to fully fund the insurance and care for families above the poverty line. Rather families must use some of their own after-tax income to pay for the insurance they choose, a requirement we regard both as fair and conducive of economic efficiency.

The tax credit approach can be made available to all citizens, regardless of their employment status, thus removing the distortion and inequity associated with subsidizing only those who are labeled "employees." Indeed, the most sensible first step might be to make tax credits available to the self-employed as a substitute for the temporary 25 percent insurance deduction that expired in 1994 and was restored in 1995. Making the same tax break available whether an insured person worked as an employee or decided to become self-employed would reduce tax-related "job lock."[7]

Closing the Exclusion Loophole Voluntarily

If we were devising tax policy toward health insurance from the start, we would propose tax credits for catastrophic coverage and MSAs as the only (minimal) government intervention in citizens' choices about medical care and medical insurance. However, the U.S. tax system provides a subsidy of nearly $100 billion a year to people who buy private health insurance through their employment. Removing the tax subsidy by wholesale revisions of the tax code seems politically improbable and likely to harm people who made their employment choices based in part on expectations about the tax advantages of the fringe benefit packages some firms offer. Though we do not, therefore, want to snatch away the tax exclusion, we do want to persuade people, voluntarily, to trade it for a tax system with better incentives. Creating the option for groups and individuals to give up the old system of exclusions and take a refundable tax credit instead would achieve this goal. If a fixed-dollar tax credit really is better for people than the old distortive subsidies, many people should be willing to switch.

A simple example illustrates why people would wish to switch to our plan.[8] Imagine a medium-sized company with employees who all earn close to the median annual wage. This firm now pays part of its compensation in the form of a fully paid health insurance policy that covers the employee only, with a $500 deductible. The tax subsidy to this policy is assumed to be about $750 a year.[9] Expected or average expenses under this plan are assumed to be approximately $2,900. We propose to offer an alternative to the firm's employees: pay income and payroll tax on the $2,500 employer premium and receive instead a personal income tax credit of $750 a person. The requirement to qualify for the credits is that employees obtain at least a catastrophic policy with a specified maximum deductible and protect the deductible by establishing or maintaining an MSA for after-tax dollars.[10]

For example, assume that a catastrophic policy with a $2,000 deductible, rather than the $500 deductible, reduces the premium by $1,100. By depositing this $1,100 in an MSA, each employee would have funds immediately available for the first $1,100 of medical expenses. The next $900 would be paid out-of-pocket, as shown in table 13-1.[11]

The expected or average value of all health expenditures is assumed to drop by $800, from $2,900 to $2,100, when the deductible is increased from $500 to $2,000. So, although the maximum exposure to uninsured

Table 13-1. *Detailed Calculations of Cost Implications of Medical Savings Accounts (MSAs)*

	Old policy	New policy	Difference
1. Premium	$2,500	$1,400	−$1,100
2. Deductible (maximum)	500	2,000	1,500
3. MSA deposit	0	1,100	1,100
4. Expected values of expenses beneath deductible	400	700	300
Total expected expenses (line 1 + line 4)	2,900	2,100	−800
Net maximum exposure (line 2 − line 3)	500	900	400

Source: Authors' calculations.

expenses is increased by $400 (from $500 to $900), in return the average saving in total health care spending is twice as great, at $800.[12]

If the employees agree to give up the tax exclusion (and therefore pay taxes on the part of their compensation that formerly went to employer-paid health insurance premiums), they will pay $750 more in income and payroll taxes (on an additional $2,500 in money income) but will receive an exactly offsetting $750 personal income tax credit. They could remain with their old policy and be no better or worse off than before. But by electing the catastrophic coverage-MSA combination, they would save, on average, $800 on medical care and medical insurance.

To be sure, employees could have chosen to set up an MSA and purchase catastrophic coverage under current tax laws. But if they did so, and reduced their premium by $1,100, they would have to pay additional taxes on the higher money wages. The additional taxes ($300 at a 30 percent marginal rate) would wipe out 41 percent of the $800 savings on medical expenses. So under current law they would be deterred from making this choice, because they would have to share their savings with the government. Under the tax credit, in strong contrast, they would keep all of the savings, since they would receive the same $750 credit regardless of whether they chose the catastrophic or the low-deductible policy.

Additional Policy Choices

So far we have presented the broad outlines of an MSA-minimum catastrophic insurance proposal. We now describe some additional policy decisions needed to implement that proposal.

Individual versus Group Choice

Should individual employees be allowed to exercise the tax credit option, or should the entire group be required to do so? The latter strategy probably would induce the largest number of people to join the new, efficient tax system. Allowing individual employees to declare "employer contributions" as taxable income and receive a credit in return would not lead directly to a change in the types of coverage offered if only some took advantage of it. (However, permitting individual employees to "defect" might be less cumbersome than requiring a group decision and would eventually put pressure on the group.)

This change in tax treatment in no sense gives individual employees the "right" to opt out of a group and demand a full premium refund. Employers or unions may still choose to require all employees to participate in the group plan (by the financial device of making premium payments for each employee before the money wage paycheck is written). Such group purchases can hold down the administrative cost of insurance, provide a form of risk spreading that is not possible with individual insurance purchases, and can inhibit adverse selection.

Putting Limits on Deductibles not Covered by MSAs

As the numerical example suggests, the MSA balance may be smaller than the insurance deductible. This gap represents an out-of-pocket risk for the individual. Since one purpose of public subsidies for medical insurance is to encourage people to limit their exposure to risk, some upper limit on out-of-pocket exposure that people are allowed to have and still qualify for a tax credit is necessary. There is also an argument for capping out-of-pocket payments by lower-income families, as out-of-pocket payments may deter them from obtaining the most beneficial care.

Putting Limits on the Catastrophic Deductible

There are also good reasons to restrict the size of the deductible. Someone who chooses a $100,000 deductible and deposits $100,000 in an MSA is obviously using the MSA to shelter interest earnings rather than achieving an optimal exposure to risk. (The premium savings become quite small as the deductible grows beyond $3,000.) In addition, it probably would not be desirable to permit a lower-income family to select a policy with a very high deductible and put their entire life savings

Table 13-2. *Examples of Maximum Deductible and Out-of-Pocket Limits under a Medical Savings Account (MSA) Proposal*

	Option A	Option B
Maximum deductible	$3,000	$2,000
Maximum out-of-pocket payment	1,000	500
Minimum MSA balance	2,000	1,500

Source: Authors' calculations.

into an MSA, since fear of wiping out their assets may deter them from seeking beneficial care.

The precise deductible-MSA combination a family at a given income level should be required to have in order to qualify for a tax credit is a policy decision. The lower the maximum deductible, the less likely the chance of underuse of beneficial care, but the greater the chance of overuse of less valuable care. Moreover, the higher the required MSA deposit, the more likely lower-income families would forgo insurance (even with a credit), unless they received a very generous credit.

Putting the Pieces Together

A simple version of the plan would entitle people to a $750 tax credit if they are not receiving a tax-shielded employer contribution and if they buy insurance with a deductible no greater than some amount protected by an MSA with no more than some (smaller) amount to be paid out of pocket. Table 13-2 gives examples of two such specifications. Such an easy-to-understand message sets a floor to the coverage people must have to receive a tax credit, permits (but does not require) them to purchase more coverage if they wish, and helps via a tax credit. The fixed-dollar tax credit has the desirable incentive property that if people are not forbidden from buying more generous coverage than the minimum, but they receive no additional tax reduction if they do, they will be paying with their own money.

Tax Treatment of Rollovers

The only tax break in this plan so far is the tax credit. If people deposit $2,000 in their MSA in the first period and use no medical care, they will have available $2,000 plus interest at the end of the period. Since the MSA would be created with after-tax dollars, they could use these funds for any purpose. To offer an incentive to retain the funds in the MSA, the plan would offer the same $750 credit for the next period if the same

MSA-catastrophic insurance combination was maintained. (A person would not need to add another $2,000 to an MSA if he or she carried over the previous period's protection.) In addition, it may be desirable, as an optional design feature, to permit the interest to be rolled over or withdrawn without tax penalty. If it is desired to limit the Treasury's revenue loss on tax-free interest, there would be a maximum amount that an MSA could earn tax free.

Varying the Tax Credits by Income

How to relate the credit to income poses a design challenge. The value of the current tax exclusion rises moderately with income. To get maximum participation of persons who now enjoy the tax exclusion, the credit would also have to increase with income (as marginal tax rates increase). But such a policy would offer little incentive for participation by lower-income families—since they benefit little from the current exclusion. To get them to participate in greater numbers, the credit should be large for lower-income families, especially if the goal is for them to obtain more generous coverage, and decline with income to limit aggregate cost.

Offering lower- and middle-income families credits larger than the $750 target has a cost to other taxpayers. There is also a cost in that work effort is deterred, since high effective marginal tax rates are created if the value of the credit is scaled down as income rises. However, if such income-related refundable tax credits replace current medicaid, they offer the possibility of reducing deterrent effects of the medicaid phase-out.

Tax Credits, MSAs, and Managed Care

The argument for MSAs and tax credits is not limited to their encouragement of catastrophic coverage as a cost containment device. They also would help to encourage the use of appropriate forms of managed care and would discourage the use of inappropriate care. Just as catastrophic coverage contains costs by putting patients at risk for paying for care, managed care contains costs by putting providers at risk, encouraging them to limit care that is judged by the insurance plan to be worth less than its cost. Under the principle of incentive-neutrality, we do not want tax policy to favor either type of cost containment device. Different people, with different preferences, will appropriately choose one or the other.

Current tax policy governing the choices between managed care and catastrophic coverage in the employment setting is not neutral, and the choices among managed care plans are distorted as well. If an employee group chooses a managed care plan with low out-of-pocket payments under current tax treatment, virtually all medical expenses are tax subsidized. If the group chooses catastrophic coverage, less compensation is excluded from federal taxes—thus penalizing the catastrophic plan, even if it is more efficient. If the group is choosing between two managed care plans—one more costly and more lavish than another that is somewhat more inconvenient or constraining—it will find that it will raise its members' taxes if it chooses the less costly plan. This loss of the tax subsidy will bias it away from lower-cost managed care plans.

The arrangement we have proposed avoids both of these biases because the tax credit is independent of the insurance chosen. In the choice between managed care and catastrophic coverage, the tax credit is not increased if the managed care plan is chosen; the tax credit "covers" both the insurance premium and the out-of-pocket expenditures from an MSA. In the choice between more and less expensive managed care plans, the tax credit does not fall for those who choose a less attractive but less costly plan or rise for those who purchase a more costly plan. Under our proposal, we expect that many people would voluntarily choose managed care plans. Since people do not have to share their savings with the government, they would face proper incentives.

Our proposal is consistent with the recent trend in managed care to increase out-of-pocket payments, either as user charges or as extra payments for people who exercise a point-of-service option and pay out-of-pocket to use nonnetwork providers. Under our proposal, MSA funds can cover the "risk" that individuals will decide, once they are sick, to see a doctor or enter a hospital not in the managed care plan's network.

The Problem of Adverse Selection

Some critics fear that increased use of catastrophic insurance coverage protected by MSAs will worsen risk segmentation and adverse selection in the private health insurance market. A similar argument has been made over the years against all innovative forms of private insurance, most especially against health maintenance organizations (HMOs)—which do seem, in some circumstances, to be attractive to low risks. The natural tendency in competitive insurance markets is for premiums to reflect risks. To the degree that this process creates unreasonable burdens for some people, government intervention in the form of tax-financed risk pools or risk-related tax credits for unusually high risks are the correct solutions. The alternative strategy, of using regulation to forbid insurers from pricing risk, will itself have undesirable consequences—it either will induce insurers to avoid bad risks and to attract good risks (thereby causing even worse adverse selection) or will offer incentives to good risks to purchase too much insurance. A full treatment of this exceedingly complex and confusing issue is beyond the scope of this chapter.[13]

There is little reason to believe that the specific form of tax credits we have proposed will alter the situation appreciably, however. Our proposal is limited to solving what we believe to be the more serious problem of tax-distorted insurance, and it need not worsen current risk segmentation. Under our proposal, we expect that most people will continue to obtain health insurance through employment-based groups.[14] Our proposal would permit employers or unions to continue to require payment for group health insurance as part of the compensation package. If the group switched to a higher-deductible plan, and all employees were switched, higher-risk employees would continue to be members of the same group as lower-risk employees. And all would have access to an MSA to meet expenses below the deductible. Moreover, our proposal offers those who most typically drop out of the current insurance system—young, healthy, but low-wage workers—a larger subsidy to stay in and obtain catastrophic coverage. Our plan also offers people at all risk levels, including the small minority at high risk, the option of a credit toward a decent minimum insurance policy.

If the group decides to allow individual employee choice between a high-deductible and a low-deductible (or managed care) option, it would be expected to adjust the premium differential between options to limit adverse selection or excessive risk segmentation, since such behavior is not in the interest of the employer, the union, the employee group, or whoever is arranging the terms of coverage. Therefore, even if better risks would choose catastrophic coverage, and other risks would stick with more generous but more expensive coverage, negative consequences of this choice need not occur.

To be sure, the employer or union may decide that the advantages of risk pooling are not as great as the advantages of individual choice in the individual insurance market, which can better tailor coverage to individual demands. In that case, they might no longer require universal participation, or they might no longer discourage dropouts by returning only a fraction of premiums to those who forgo coverage. The tax incentives we have designed are neutral in this regard. We do not wish to encourage or discourage employers or unions from being in the health insurance business. But this trade-off is one of many that the group would have to make, and should be trusted to make, under proper incentives.

Finally, in the individual market, people are already free to select high-deductible options and often do so. The availability of MSAs therefore is unlikely to further affect the risk segmentation in this market.

Impact on the Budget and the Economy

A required exercise in Washington for any health care reform proposal is the "scoring" of its impact on the budget. We believe that the desirability of the qualitative characteristics of the plan we have outlined does not in any way depend on how it scores. If a plan with these characteristics appears to the taxpayers to cost too much, some less costly plan with a smaller tax credit—but one that still represents an improvement over the current state of affairs—can be substituted.

However, a voluntary plan with a tax credit close to the current average tax subsidy need not increase the federal deficit. Such a credit should appeal to workers for whom the value of the current tax exclusion is close to the tax credit. For those people, the impact on the Treasury is roughly neutral, since the tax credit is just offset by tax collections on what were formerly tax-excluded employer contributions. The real benefit, to citizens and to the economy, comes from lower spending on medical care, which will occur when people have the opportunity to choose between medical care and other goods and services on a level playing field.

People at higher income levels, who will pay more taxes than they receive in credits, may still make the trade. They might do so because the savings on their medical spending will more than offset any extra taxes they would have to pay. In the numerical example presented earlier, a person subject to a high marginal income tax rate would have to pay about $400 more in taxes as a result of trading in the tax exclusion. Yet the reduction in average or expected medical expenses from switching from a convention insurance policy to a catastrophic/MSA combination would be on the order of $800.[15] If such people switch the exclusion for a tax credit, they will pay more to the Treasury.

The Treasury will lose money on lower-wage workers who trade in a tax exclusion for a more generous tax credit. Some of these workers will be insured for the first time, however—a social gain. Moreover, the drain on the Treasury only represents a more equitable and more efficient way of treating lower-wage workers. Delivering a tax cut to low-income households through health insurance credit reduces taxes for people who cannot afford high taxes and also helps them afford protection against medical care costs.

Will trading in a tax exclusion for a tax credit and a lower-cost insurance policy really appeal to many people at moderate income levels? The answer to this question depends critically on the answer to another question: How serious is the distortion in insurance choices now produced by the tax exclusion? Economic analyses suggest that the distortion is substantial. If this analysis is correct, an opportunity to save money by seeking the tax credit and changing their health insurance will appeal to reasonable consumers. If economics is wrong, and people tend to buy the same insurance plan no matter what the tax advantages, then removing the exclusion will not cut medical costs (although it will quiet the chorus of economists), but it will cause no harm.

Conclusion

One lesson from the debate on health care reform is that no magic bullets exist to solve the health care problem. In this chapter we have outlined a plan for a careful combination of some of the good ingredients. MSAs, tax credits, and catastrophic coverage all have to carry the freight, and no one component is more important than any other. Given the maturing of the debate that has occurred, we believe that the electorate will see these policies as a good step in the right direction.

Notes

1. For further discussion of these objectives, see Mark V. Pauly and others, "A Plan for 'Responsible National Health Insurance'" *Health Affairs*, vol. 10 (Spring 1991), pp. 5–25.

2. In early 1995 Congress restored the exclusion of 25 percent of premium payments by the self-employed.

3. See Martin S. Feldstein and Bernard Freidman, "Tax Subsidies, the Rational Demand for Insurance, and the Health Care Crisis," *Journal of Public Economics*, vol. 7 (April 1977), pp. 155–78; Mark V. Pauly, "Taxation, Health

Insurance, and Market Failure in the Medical Economy," *Journal of Economic Literature*, vol. 24 (June 1986), pp. 629–75; Congressional Budget Office, *The Tax Treatment of Employer Based Health Insurance* (Washington, March 1994); and Sherry Glied, *Revising the Tax Treatment of Employer-Provided Health Insurance* (Washington: American Enterprise Institute for Public Policy Research, 1994).

4. For a description of the MSA concept, see John C. Goodman and Gerald L. Musgrave, *Patient Power: The Free Enterprise Alternative to Clinton's Health Plan* (Washington: Cato Institute, 1994).

5. See National Center for Policy Analysis, "Medical Savings Accounts: The Private Sector Already Has Them," NCPA Brief Analysis 105 (Washington: NCPA, 1994). For a discussion of the problems of eliminating distortions through the design of MSAs, see John C. Goodman and Gerald L. Musgrave, "The Economic Case for Medical Savings Accounts," paper presented to the American Enterprise Institute for Public Policy Research, April 1994.

6. For an analysis and critique of these tax-subsidized MSAs, see Mark V. Pauly, *An Analysis of Medical Savings Accounts: Do Two Wrongs Make a Right?* (Washington: American Enterprise Institute Press, 1994).

7. If employees could remain members of the same plan regardless of employment status, this combination of features would end job lock.

8. The numbers are purely illustrative, but they are chosen to be reasonable; the examples are constructed only for employees who buy insurance for themselves but could be modified to illustrate family coverage.

9. This is approximately the value of the tax exclusion if the employees' marginal income tax rate is 15 percent (combined with the 15 percent payroll tax rate), and the employer contribution toward an individual insurance is $2,500.

10. The method by which the account to protect the deductible would be created would be determined by the insurer: insurers might require an initial deposit of $2,000 (less any permitted out-of-pocket amount) or might collect the deposit in monthly or quarterly installments, along with the insurance premium. The key requirement is that the minimum MSA balance be available to cover any large expense incurred in the first month of coverage.

11. As indicated in the first column of table 13-1, the original policy has a $500 deductible, a $2,500 premium, and the average or expected expense of $2,900. As indicated in the second column, moving to a policy with a $2,000 deductible would lead to a premium savings of $1,100—a sum that may be deposited in an MSA. The third column shows that at the higher deductible (partly protected by the MSA), the maximum individual expense for out-of-pocket spending has increased by $400. However, total expected spending on medical care will be reduced by $800.

12. This implies that the new lower premium, $1,400, covers 67 percent of all expenses and that expected expenses under the deductible rise from $400 to $700.

13. See Mark V. Pauly, "Killing with Kindness: Why Some Forms of Managed Competition Might Needlessly Stifle Competitive Managed Care," in Robert

B. Helms, ed., *Health Policy Reform: Competition and Controls* (Washington: American Enterprise Institute Press, 1993), pp. 149–75.

14. After all, for most people the substantially lower administrative cost for group insurance (compared with individual insurance) is at least as large an advantage as is the tax subsidy.

15. The value of the tax exclusion of $2,500 in premium at a marginal income tax rate of 31 percent (plus the 15 percent payroll tax) is $1,150, $400 more than the $750 for the 15 percent income tax rate in our example.

Contributors*

HENRY J. AARON
The Brookings Institution

DREW E. ALTMAN
*Henry J. Kaiser Family
Foundation*

LINDA BILHEIMER
Congressional Budget Office

KARLYN H. BOWMAN
*American Enterprise Institute for
Public Policy Research*

STUART M. BUTLER
The Heritage Foundation

DAVID M. CUTLER
Harvard University

HELEN DARLING
Xerox Corporation

ALAIN C. ENTHOVEN
Stanford University

JUDITH FEDER
*Department of Health and
Human Services*

JOHN C. GOODMAN
*National Center for Policy
Analysis*

FRED GRANDY
Former Representative, Iowa

HUGH HECLO
George Mason University

JULIE KOSTERLITZ
National Journal *and The
Brookings Institution*

*Affiliation at the time of the conference.

291

LARRY LEVITT
Department of Health and
 Human Services

JAMES J. MONGAN
Truman Medical Center

LEN M. NICHOLS
The Urban Institute

MARK V. PAULY
University of Pennsylvania

UWE REINHARDT
Princeton University

ROBERT REISCHAUER
Congressional Budget Office

WILLIAM L. ROPER
Prudential Center for Health
 Care Research

JOHN F. SHIELS
Lewin-VHI, Inc.

SARA J. SINGER
Stanford University

THEDA SKOCPOL
Harvard University

STEVEN C. SUNSHINE
Department of Justice

KENNETH THORPE
Department of Health and
 Human Services

MARGARET WEIR
The Brookings Institution

GAIL R. WILENSKY
Project HOPE

GRAHAM K. WILSON
University of Wisconsin

DANIEL YANKELOVICH
The Public Agenda

Index

Adverse selection, 194, 227, 244, 247, 285–87
Affirmative action, 36
Agricultural Adjustment Act, 24
Alliances. *See* Health alliances
American Association of Retired Persons (AARP), 42, 51, 68, 52, 123, 126–27
American Farm Bureau Federation, 113
American Federation of Labor–Congress of Industrial Organizations (AFL–CIO), 112, 119, 121
American Medical Association (AMA): Clinton health plan and, 116, 124, 125, 129–30; Clinton task force neglects, 121; employer mandates, 119; federal financing of medical care, 113; labor union dispute, 112; medicare opposition, 115–16; social security and, 47; universal health insurance plan, 36
Antigovernment campaign, 44–49, 58, 80
Antitrust policy, 207–22
Archer, Bill, 140
Archey, William T., 117
Armey, Dick: "flow chart" on health care bureaucracy, 45; on health care for the poor, 101–02
Association of American Physicians and Surgeons (AAPS), 120, 130

Association of Private Pension and Welfare Plans, 131

Behavioral responses, to health care reform, 152, 175, 178–79
Benefit packages: lacking for contingent workers, 251; standardized, 152–53, 201, 243–45
Bipartisanship: health care commission, 37, 51; policy reform and, 15, 51
Blendon, Robert, 36
Blue Cross/Blue Shield, 19, 119
Bonner and Associates, 124
Bromberg, Michael, 121
Buber, Martin, 83
Budget (U.S.): balancing the, 5, 147–48; deficit reduction, 38, 52
Bush administration: health insurance reform, 29, 36; on play-or-pay proposals, 38; tax reform issues, 37
Business interest groups, 116–18, 122
Business Roundtable, 117, 119, 122, 125, 129

California Public Employees Retirement System (CalPERS), 43, 156–57, 192
Canadian-style health plan. *See* Single-payer insurance plans
Cantor, Joel, 117
Capitation, 190
Carter administration: health insurance

reform, 19, 22, 26; political resources, 28; universal coverage proposals, 2
Catastrophic health insurance. *See* Medical savings accounts
Center for Public Integrity, 45
Chamber of Commerce, 117–18, 119, 122, 124, 125, 129–30
Choice in health care. *See* Free choice in health care
Christian Coalition groups, 46
Civilian Health and Medical Program of the Uniformed Services (CHAMPUS), 189
Civil rights movement, 19–20, 22, 32, 10
Clean Air Act of 1990, 18
Clinton administration:
   health reform proposal: causes of failure, 70–71; failure of, 25–31, 34–69, 70–109; gestation period, 28–31, 57; nature of the objective, 25–27; political resources, 27–28, 54–57; security theme, 25
   health reform task force, 39; health security plan, analysis of, 34–69
Clinton, Bill: Health Security speech (1993), 34, 40, 75, 126, 131; presidential election campaign, 1–2, 36
Clinton, Hillary Rodham, health reform and, 30, 110, 111, 112, 117, 120–21, 122, 132–33
Colvinaux, Paul, 16
Committee for Economic Security (1934), 2, 24
Communication. *See* Public communication model; Public deliberation
Community-rated pool, 153–56, 186, 192–93, 200–201, 228, 245
Comparison of health plans, 196–97
Concord Coalition, 53
Congressional Black Caucus, 122
Congressional Budget Office (CBO):
   health spending estimates, 4–5, 41, 133, 147–81; Hospital Insurance trust fund estimates, 268; medicaid and medicare reductions and, 38
Congress (U.S.): health care reform, 57, 121, 132–35; rules governing congressional campaigns, 2

Consolidated Omnibus Budget Reconciliation Act (COBRA), 204, 218
Consumer-based health system, 236, 246–47
Contract with America, 34
Cooperatives. *See* Health plan purchasing cooperatives
Cooper-Grandy bill, 137, 139
Cooper, Jim, 50, 132
Costs of health care. *See* Health care costs; Health care spending
County Business Patterns (CBP), 150, 167
Coverage: estimating, 158–59; expansion of, 230–31. *See also* Universal health insurance
Crosby, John B., 116
Current Population Survey (CPS), 149, 154, 179

Democratic Action Network, 27
Democratic Leadership Council, 38
Democratic National Committee (DNC), 27, 42, 110
Democratic party: election of 1994, 34; Health security bill and, 39–44; political strategy, 55. *See also* Clinton administration
Diagnosis-related group (DRG) system, 257
Dingell, John, 133, 138
Dole, Robert J., 126, 153, 156, 238
Donelan, Karen, 36

Employee Retirement Income Security Act (ERISA), 192–93, 200, 214, 221–22, 230, 246
Employer contribution policies, 197–99
Employer-mandates, 59, 116–17, 137, 153
Employment-based systems, 35–36, 37, 203, 236, 237, 246
Evans, Roland, 117
Experience-rated pool, 154, 186, 229

Faris, Jack, 118
Federal Employees Health Benefits Program (FEHBP), 244, 246–47, 250, 258–59
Fee-for-service model, 188–89

Fenno, Richard F., Jr., 129
Foster-Higgins National Survey of Employers, 268–69
Free choice in health care, 97–98, 103, 188–89
Free riding, 187, 191, 193, 252
Future of health care, 201–04

Gallup polls, 75, 76, 81, 97
Garamendi, John, 38
Gaylin, Will, 86
Geertz, Clifford, 82
Gephardt bill, 134–35, 153, 158
Gephardt, Richard, 136
Gibbons, Sam, 137
Gingrich, Newt, 45, 116, 119
Gore, Al, on government waste, 204
Gradison, Bill, 134
Great Society. *See* War on Poverty
Guaranteed issue, 187, 191, 228, 245

Harris polls, 75, 76, 79
Harry and Louise commercials, 93–94, 118, 120, 124, 132–33, 136
Health alliances, 40, 43–44, 51, 52, 67
Health care, as a right, 75–76
Health care costs: administrative expenses, 252; containment policies, 156–58; cost sharing proposals, 254; cutting costs, 250–65; doctors' fees, 252; estimating reform costs, 147–81; excessive health provisions, 252–54; existing data, 172; growth of, 256, 260–61; responsibility for, 76–77; vs. benefits, 87–88. *See also* Medical technologies
Health Care Financing Administration (HCFA), 150, 151, 270
Health Care Leadership Council, 123, 124
Health Care Reform Project, 42
Health care spending: annual estimates, 150; demand-side problems, 191–200; federal role, 5, 10; growth rate, 511; projections, 151; supply-side problems, 186–90
"Health Care That's Always There" (Clinton security theme), 25
Health Insurance Association of America

(HIAA), 44–45, 118–28, 130, 136, 139, 167. *See also* Harry and Louise commercials
Health maintenance organizations (HMOs), 8, 103, 116, 118, 185, 210, 270–72
Health outcomes. *See* Quality of health care
Health Plan and Employer Data Set (HEDIS 2.0), 218
Health plan purchasing cooperatives (HPPCs), 43, 52, 164–65, 193, 202–04
Heritage Foundation, 238, 240–41
Herman, Alexis M., 121–22
HMOs. *See* Health maintenance organizations
Hospital Insurance trust fund, 267–68
Hospitals: antitrust issues, 207–22; consolidations, 150, 210–13; excess capacity, 187–88

Independent practice associations, 8
Individual retirement accounts (IRAs), 240
Insurance industry, health care reform and, 118–19, 120, 123
Interest groups: advertising dollars, 123, 138; antihealth reform lobbying efforts, 45, 93, 171; Clinton administration strategy toward, 119–23; growth of, 111; health care debate and, 110–43, 171; impact of, 125–27; insider and outsider campaigns, 124; performance evaluation, 127–30; policy issues, 113–14; strategies of, 123–24. *See also* Lobbyists

Jamieson, Kathleen, 42
Jefferson, Thomas, 21
Job-lock: in employment-based systems, 251, 279. *See also* Employment-based systems
Johnson, Lyndon Baines, 31

Kaiser Family Foundation, 35, 91
Kennedy, Edward, 29
Kennedy, John F., social reforms, 18, 21, 23, 24
Kennelly, Barbara B., 170

Kerr-Mills package of *1960*, 24
Kerry, Robert, 37, 38
Kettering Foundation, health care reform plan agenda, 87–88
Kids First Insurance, 95
Koop, C. Everett, 140
Kristol, William, 45–46, 136

Labor unions, health care insurance supporters, 116, 119, 125, 126
Lawrence, David, 221
Leadership, health care reform and, 82–83, 99–100, 100–101, 106–07
Lesher, Richard, 117
Lewin-VHI: health reform modeling, 165–69, 170, 173; tax credit program, 241
Lobbyists: for health sector, 123; number of registered, 111. *See also* Interest groups
Long-term care, 5, 232–33

McDermott, Jim, 136
McInturff, William, 126
Magaziner, Ira, 30, 39, 113, 120, 122
Managed care: bargaining for services, 6; chiropractors' response to, 134–35; cost containment and, 9–10; definition of, 7–8; medicaid beneficiaries and, 150; medicare beneficiaries and, 270; provider protection legislation and, 189–91; public worries concerning, 49, 68*n*., 56
Managed competition: 38, 52, 55, 65, 118, 119; effectiveness ratings, 157
Managed Competition Act of *1993*, 132, 153, 157–58, 204
Market-based reforms, 37, 50, 185–206
Marmor, Theodore, 112, 113
Martin, Cathie Jo, 117, 122
Media: disinformation, 104–05; education role, 94, 100; newspaper coverage, 42, 104; news-talk radio shows, 41, 46, 131; radio ads, 124; slogans vs. explanatory messages, 41; television coverage, 41–42, 103–04, 131; Whitewater scandal, 66, 30. *See also* Harry and Louise commercials
Medicaid: costs of beneficiaries, 155–56; coverage, 7; enactment of, 2; long-

term care costs, 5; managed care and, 150; spending cuts and, 5, 233
Medical savings accounts (MSAs), 239–40, 274–90
Medical technologies: access to, 9, 221; cost controls, 87–88; costs of, 5, 7, 87–88, 250; future of, 150; public opinion about, 80; standardization of coverage, 195
Medicare: acute care costs, 5; adjusted average per capita cost (AAPCC), 271; AMA opposition to, 115–16; annual open season proposal, 185; choice-based system reform, 250, 255–58; coverage, 7; enactment of legislation, 2, 53; fee-for-service program, 189; health care reform and, 24, 266–73; present structure of, 270–71; reimbursement policies, 150; social security analogy and, 43–44; spending cuts and, 5, 233; voucher proposal, 247–48
Mentally ill, health care for, 220
Mergers. *See* Antitrust policy
Michel, Robert H., 117, 119
Minnesota State Employee Insurance Program (SEIP), 157
Mitchell, George, 136, 153, 158, 159, 229
Mondale, Walter, 37
Moynihan, Daniel Patrick, 49, 159

National Center for Health Statistics, 173
National Committee for Quality Assurance (NCQA), 216, 218
National Federation of Independent Businesses (NFIB), 46, 114–28, 138
"National Health Care Campaign," 42
National health insurance. *See* Universal health insurance
National Health Interview Survey (NHIS), 149, 166
National Leadership Coalition for Health Care, 37
National Medical Expenditure Survey (NMES), 149, 156, 166, 173
Natural monopolies: in health care markets, 9, 190. *See also* Antitrust policy

Nichols, Sara, 120
Nickles, Don, 238
Nickles-Stearns bill, 238–42, 245, 248
Nixon administration: social reforms, 22; universal coverage proposals, 2
North American Free Trade Agreement (NAFTA), 40–41
Novak, Robert, 117

Old Age Assistance program of 1956, 24
Old age insurance, 2, 18–19
O'Neill, Tip, 140

Pepper Commission. *See* U.S. Bipartisan Commission on Comprehensive Health Care
Pharmaceutical Manufacturers' Association, 111, 112
Play-or-pay insurance plans, 37, 38, 52
Point-of-service plans, 8, 270
Policy reform. *See* Social policy reform
Political action committees (PACs), 111, 123
Political parties, elections (1994), 34–35
Porter Novelli (firm), 111
Pre-existing medical conditions, 187, 200, 228, 250, 259–60, 264
Preferred-provider organizations, 6, 185, 214–15, 270
Premiums: compressing costs, 227; estimating, 152–58; payment of, 160–64; restrictions, 245–46; sources of payment, 160–64; subsidies, 161–63
Private insurance coverage: market developments, 7–10; population, 7
Professional review organizations (PROs), 215
Prohibition, as social reform effort, 16–17, 20–21
Project for the Republican Future, 45–46
Provider protection legislation, 189–91
Prudential Health Care System, 214, 216
Public Agenda Foundation, 99
Public Citizen, 120
Public communication model, 83, 88–90
Public deliberation on health care, 71–74, 80–91
Public Judgment Model (PJM), 89–90
Public opinion: costs of medical care,

76–77; crisis in health care system, 76; favorable-unfavorable ratio, 75; grass-roots movements, 27; health care as a right, 75–76; health care costs, 76–78; knowledge of Clinton plan, 78–79; leadership attitudes and, 82–83; on universal health insurance coverage, 35, 64; polling and, 94; quality of health care, 81; raw opinion stage, 81; satisfaction with health care, 76
Public power, policy reform and, 16
Purchasing cooperatives. *See* Health plan purchasing cooperatives

Quality of health care, 197, 216, 218, 261–63

Radio. *See* Media
Rand Health Insurance Experiment (HIE), 163–64, 177, 253
Rauch, Jonathan, 134–35
Reagan administration, supply-side economics, 106
Reconstruction Finance Corporation, 24
Reed, Ralph, 46
Reform. *See* Social policy reform
Regulation of health care industry, 9–10, 200–01, 230, 236
Republican party: antigovernment campaign, 45–46, 58; election results (1994), 3–4, 34–85; interest groups and, 126
Ridley Group, 124
Risk selection, 186, 199–200, 251–52
Rockefeller, Jay, 42
Roosevelt, Franklin Delano: health insurance plans, 19, 47; New Deal reforms, 24; social security and, 47
Roosevelt, Theodore, national health insurance and, 28–29
Roper surveys, 76
Rostenkowski, Dan, 137
Rother, John, 42
Roth, William V., Jr., 246–47

School-based health system, 262
Schultze, Charles, 3, 185
Single-payer insurance plans, 37, 50, 119, 126, 135

Slattery, Jim, 132
Social policy reform: estimating effects
    of, 147–81; gestation periods, 23–
    25; historical perspective, 15–33;
    major reform efforts, 17–19, 21–22,
    31–32; morality and, 19; nature of
    reform objectives, 17–20; political
    environment resources, 20–22, 48;
    presidential role, 24; public power
    and, 16
Social security: antigovernment cam-
    paigns and, 47; opposition, 53; pay-
    roll taxes and, 47–48; political envi-
    ronment, 47–48; as universal social
    insurance program model, 53
Social Security Act of 1935, 2, 48
Specialists, excess supply, 188
Sponsored-group model, 202–03
Stark, Pete, 121, 137
Starr, Paul, 38, 121
Stearns, Cliff, 238
Steurle, Eugene, 159
Stillwell, Lee J., 116
Subsidies: for access, 200, 236; for cost
    sharing, 163–64; for low-income
    families, 242–43; for premiums,
    161–63; work disincentive effects
    and, 243

Tax reform: act of 1986, 106; health
    care deductions, 30, 237–38, 239,
    255–56, 259–60; raising taxes, 37;
    sin taxes, 78, 251, 262–63; social
    security and, 47–48; tax credits,
    198–99. See also Medical savings
    accounts
Technology. See Medical technologies
Television. See Media
Truman, Harry S, national health insur-
    ance proposal, 2, 21, 24, 53
Tsongas, Paul, 38

Uninsured: composition of, 156; number
    of, 6–7, 25, 149; plans for coverage
    of children, 95; rationing of health
    care, 102–03
Unions. See Labor unions
U.S. Bipartisan Commission on Compre-
    hensive Health Care, 37
Universal health insurance: compromises
    to coverage, 60–62; conservative
    agenda, 236–49; historical perspec-
    tive, 53; incremental steps toward,
    225–35; percent coverage, 4; presi-
    dential plans for, 4; public opinion
    polls, 64; public support, 79–80;
    Truman proposals, 2. See also Clin-
    ton administration
The Urban Institute, 159

Vogel, David, 113, 129

Wagner-Murray-Dingell health insurance
    bill of 1943, 24
War on Poverty, 17–18, 24, 31, 53, 115
Wellstone, Paul, 131, 136
White House, Office of Public Liaison,
    120, 122
Whitewater scandal, 30, 66
Will, George, 104–05
Wilson, James Q., 113
Wofford, Harris, Senate election (1991),
    27, 29, 35
Wolfe, Sidney, 120

Xerox, managed care plan, 217–22

Yankelovich Partners, surveys, 76

Zelman, Walter, 38